Evidence-Based Chiropractic Practice

Michael T. Haneline, DC, MPH
Associate Professor
Palmer College of Chiropractic West
San Jose, California

JONES AND BARTLETT PUBLISHERS
Sudbury, Massachusetts
BOSTON   TORONTO   LONDON   SINGAPORE

World Headquarters
Jones and Bartlett Publishers
40 Tall Pine Drive
Sudbury, MA 01776
978-443-5000
info@jbpub.com
www.jbpub.com

Jones and Bartlett Publishers
Canada
6339 Ormindale Way
Mississauga, ON L5V 1J2
CANADA

Jones and Bartlett Publishers
International
Barb House, Barb Mews
London W6 7PA
UK

Jones and Bartlett's books and products are available through most bookstores and online booksellers. To contact Jones and Bartlett Publishers directly, call 800-832-0034, fax 978-443-8000, or visit our website at www.jbpub.com.

Substantial discounts on bulk quantities of Jones and Bartlett's publications are available to corporations, professional associations, and other qualified organizations. For details and specific discount information, contact the special sales department at Jones and Bartlett via the above contact information or send an email to specialsales@jbpub.com.

Copyright © 2007 by Jones and Bartlett Publishers, Inc.
Cover Images: © Andrzej Windak/ShutterStock, Inc. and Konrad Lewandowski/ShutterStock, Inc.

All rights reserved. No part of the material protected by this copyright notice may be reproduced or utilized in any form, electronic or mechanical, including photocopying, recording, or any information storage or retrieval system, without written permission from the copyright owner.

Library of Congress Cataloging-in-Publication Data
Haneline, Michael T.
  Evidence-based chiropractic practice / Michael T. Haneline.
    p. ; cm.
  Includes bibliographical references and index.
  ISBN-13: 978-0-7637-3571-5
  ISBN-10: 0-7637-3571-X
  1. Chiropractic. 2. Evidence-based medicine.   I. Title. [DNLM: 1. Chiropractic—methods. 2. Manipulation, Chiropractic—methods. 3. Evidence-Based Medicine—methods. 4. Patient-Centered Care—methods. 5. Physician-Patient Relations. WB 905.9 H237e   2007]
  RZ244.H36   2007
  615.5'34—dc22   2006022677
6048

Production Credits
Executive Editor: David Cella
Production Director: Amy Rose
Editorial Assistant: Lisa Gordon
Production Editor: Renée Sekerak
Associate Marketing Manager: Laura Kavigian
Manufacturing Buyer: Amy Bacus
Composition: Pageworks
Cover Design: Timothy Dziewit
Printing and Binding: Malloy, Inc.
Cover Printing: Malloy, Inc.

Printed in the United States of America
10 09 08 07 06   10 9 8 7 6 5 4 3 2 1

Dedicated to my wife, Melanie, who has always supported me in my professional endeavors, and my son, Mick, who encouraged me to write this book.

CONTENTS

Foreword xi
Preface xiii

PART I
Fundamentals of Evidence-Based Practice

CHAPTER ONE
Introduction 3
What Is Evidence-Based Chiropractic? 3
Why Evidence-Based Chiropractic? 11
When to Use Evidence-Based Chiropractic 16
Steps Involved in the Practice of Evidence-Based Chiropractic 18
Relationship of Chiropractic Philosophy to Evidence-Based Chiropractic 32

CHAPTER TWO
Types of Evidence 39
Peer Review 40
Indexing 42
Sources of Evidence 43
Journals 44
Newsletters 45
Websites 48
Anatomy of a Scholarly Article 55
Red Flags for Untrustworthy Information 58
Appraising Evidence 59

CHAPTER THREE
Literature Searching   65

The Databases   66
Searching Essentials   70
Advanced Strategies   76
Summary   86

CHAPTER FOUR
Biostatistics Basics   89

Populations and Samples   90
Descriptive Statistics   91
Inferential Statistics   109
Statistical Tests Commonly Encountered in Research   119

PART II
Research Designs Commonly Encountered in the Chiropractic Literature

CHAPTER FIVE
Experimental Designs   145

Research Methods   145
Group Clinical Trial Designs   151
Design Options   162
Chiropractic Interventions and Experimental Methods   167
Ethics in Biomedical Research   169
Appraisal Tactics   172

CHAPTER SIX
Literature Review Designs   179

Narrative Reviews   181
Systematic Reviews   182
Meta-analyses   187
Comparison of Literature Review Designs   195

Structure of a Review Article 198
Appraisal Tactics 202

CHAPTER SEVEN
Case Designs 211

Case Reports 211
Case Series 220
Single-Subject Time Series Designs 223
Appraisal Tactics 236

CHAPTER EIGHT
Epidemiology 243

Measurement of Disease Frequency and Occurrence 244
Causation in Epidemiology 246
Cross-Sectional Studies 252
Case-Control Studies 254
Cohort Studies 260
Appraisal Tactics 265

CHAPTER NINE
Reliability and Validity Designs 275

Estimating Reliability 278
Validity 285
Clinical Disagreement 300
Appraisal Tactics 301

PART III
Practical Applications of Evidence-Based Chiropractic

CHAPTER TEN
Evidence-Based Chiropractic and Documentation 311

Supporting Diagnostic and Treatment Protocols
   Through Good Documentation 311

Guidelines 313
Outcome Measures Commonly Used in Chiropractic 317
Measures of Pain 319
Measures of Function 327

CHAPTER ELEVEN
Putting It All Together 349

Practical Clinical Scenarios 349
What If Evidence Is Lacking for Your Topic? 360
Improving the EBC Process 364

Appendix 1	Health Information Website Evaluation Checklist	373
Appendix 2	General Checklist for the Appraisal of Journal Articles	375
Appendix 3	Checklist for the Appraisal of Therapy Articles	377
Appendix 4	Checklist for the Appraisal of Literature Review Articles	379
Appendix 5	Checklist for the Appraisal of Case Reports	381
Appendix 6	Checklist for the Appraisal of Epidemiologic Articles	383
Appendix 7	Checklist for the Appraisal of Diagnostic Accuracy Articles	385
Appendix 8	Characteristic Pain Intensity (CPI)	389
Appendix 9	Short-Form McGill Pain Questionnaire and Pain Diagram	391
Appendix 10	Revised Oswestry Low Back Disability Index	393
Appendix 11	The Roland-Morris Low Back Pain and Disability Questionnaire	397

Appendix 12	Neck Disability Index	399
Appendix 13	Whiplash Disability Questionnaire	403
Appendix 14	Headache Disability Inventory	407
Appendix 15	Migraine Disability Assessment Score (MIDAS)	411
Appendix 16	RAND 36-Item Health Survey Instrument (Version 1.0)	413

Glossary **419**
Index **441**

FOREWORD

Just as houses are made of stones, so is science made of facts. But a pile of stones is not a house and a collection of facts is not necessarily science.
                                              (Jules Henri Poincare, 1851–1912)

Without systematic evaluation and the ability to critically appraise information that one uses in practice, it is easy to fool oneself. The purpose of science is to provide tools that limit the likelihood of a doctor being misled. In the last quarter of the 20th century, the emphasis in health care shifted from the purely experiential practice base to that of integrating experience and science. Clinical practice is seductive. The process of helping patients sculpts self-image and can delude the practitioner into believing his or her role is the central feature of health delivery or maintenance rather than the inherent recuperative power of the body.

The doctor's role is that of an advisor and teacher. He or she can guide the patient to better health by listening and integrating information specific to the patient with knowledge, prior experience, and when necessary, personal intervention.

Thirty years ago, few chiropractors were cross-trained sufficiently to comprehend and implement the tools of science to critically appraise and interpret evidence, in order to improve the quality of healthcare delivery. One who worked diligently to extend beyond training of the typical doctor of chiropractic for the age was Michael Haneline, the author of this work. Here he provides the basic knowledge for the doctor of the future to understand the confounders of practice. The gamut of misunderstandings include

- how patients honestly lie (termed acquiescence) as they inform their doctor on how much better they are feeling from treatment—even when they aren't.
- how placebo effects of all treatments confuse understanding the true benefit of care.

- how placebo effects, unabashedly, are a treatment that can be used to facilitate care.
- how research methodology and analysis can serve to drive clinical decision making for the betterment of patient care and outcomes.

The future of Chiropractic depends on the ability to articulate its effective role in guiding and managing patients. The toolbox provided in this work is essential to accurate interaction with patients, payers, and policy makers responding to critics and working to keep the system honest for the future. These tools are as valuable as learning the next adjusting technique or examination procedure for casting the success of practice in defensible terms. Each of us now carries that charge.

John J. Triano, DC, PhD, FCCS(C)

PREFACE

The primary recommendation of the Institute for Alternative Futures (IAF) regarding the most important activity the chiropractic field should pursue is to accelerate research.[1] The IAF identified the need for more research that would demonstrate the efficacy and cost-effectiveness of chiropractic for both neuromusculoskeletal and somatovisceral conditions. Considering the magnitude of this recommendation, one would think that doctors of chiropractic (DCs) would be proficient in the utilization of research-related resources, such as scientific journals and conferences. However, a cross-sectional study by Feise[2] revealed that most DCs do not comprehend the most basic research principles. It would then appear that a large portion of the profession is in need of some form of training to be brought up to date on this topic. Fortunately, research methods are now emphasized in chiropractic education, so future practitioners will be much better prepared than their predecessors.

Early in my chiropractic career, I was caring for a patient who had injured his lower back at work, and, based on follow-up examination findings and feedback from the patient, I thought he was improving satisfactorily after three weeks of care. Nevertheless, the insurance company sent him to an independent medical examiner for a second opinion. The examiner called me following the evaluation to tell me that the patient reported that he had experienced virtually no improvement while under my care; as a result, he was referring the patient to another provider. At the time, I did not believe the report to be true and was incensed about the examiner challenging my opinion. Later in my career, however, when I too began to evaluate the patients of other doctors, I regularly observed similar situations in which patients reported to their treating doctors that they were improving, when in reality they were not. This phenomenon is known as patient acquiescence and has the potential to completely misrepresent the patient's true condition.

The moral of this story is that practitioners cannot simply rely on patient reports as the sole validation of the procedures they utilize in practice. In addition to evaluating patient progress using valid and reliable clinical outcome measures, research is necessary to establish whether these procedures are actually effective compared with another type of treatment or a placebo. Because of the problem with patient acquiescence, as well as many other confounding issues, it is not possible for practitioners to adequately evaluate the effectiveness of a given treatment in the course of routine practice.

Another example of why research is needed to verify the effectiveness of treatments comes from outside the chiropractic profession. A surgical procedure known as internal mammary ligation was in common use prior to the 1960s as a treatment for angina. The surgery involved a small incision in the chest and then knots being tied in two small arteries in an attempt to increase blood flow to the heart. The procedure was popular among doctors as well as patients and was reported to be effective in 90% of cases. However, a cardiologist named Leonard Cobb[3] carried out a unique trial that compared internal mammary ligation with a placebo surgery in which incisions were made but the arteries were not tied off. Amazingly, the sham operations were just as successful as the real ones; as a result, the procedure was soon abandoned.[4] This example emphasizes the necessity of research for all health care professions and demonstrates how useless therapies can persist in its absence.

Practitioners who want to utilize the best available clinical methods are obliged to stay current by consistently reading (and comprehending) relevant journal articles. Once the validity of a particular procedure has been verified through scientific methods, practitioners should be capable of interpreting the results of the studies that are subsequently published. However, journal articles are often very difficult to understand; consequently, they are not read by the majority of the profession. When they are read, they may easily be misinterpreted. Accordingly, much of the material presented in this book is designed to help practitioners read, understand, and interpret the content of research articles.

The primary purpose of this book is to enable healthcare practitioners and students (particularly those in the chiropractic profession) to care for their patients as effectively and efficiently as possible. Patients who receive evidence-based health care have the potential to reach a maximum level of recovery as quickly and economically as possible. To practice this way, however, practitioners must become familiar with the best and most current information on the specific health issue that confronts them. Textbooks and prior education are not the best sources for this kind of information because they become outdated rather quickly. For this reason, the most useful information for patient care must be derived from current research (e.g., journal articles and conferences). There is no way of getting around the necessity for healthcare providers to be proficient at locating, evaluating, and applying the findings of research to patient care.

Some members of the various healthcare professions have been resistant to the evidence-based practice model because they think their independence will be lost to the dictates of scientists, who really don't understand or relate to the complexities of patient care. This is not true, since the ultimate decision to utilize research evidence and apply its findings to a given patient rests with the practitioner. Practitioner know-how, which results from past education and practice experience, continues to be a big part of the evidence-based practice model.

As an instructor of evidence-based chiropractic (EBC) at Palmer College of Chiropractic West, I am acutely aware of the need for a textbook on this subject. The influence of evidence-based health care on the chiropractic profession is increasing; as a result, DCs will in due course be required to become familiar with its concepts in order to remain competitive. It is wonderful that today's chiropractic students are being taught evidence-based methods, but, as was previously mentioned, many in the profession are without this knowledge. Given that some readers may have limited research-related backgrounds, the material in this book is presented in as simple terms as possible. It can be used by students as well as practitioners for instructional purposes or as a reference.

Many of the examples presented are from actual journal articles, but at times they are hypothetical in order to introduce difficult concepts in an uncomplicated way. This book covers EBC widely, but because of the expansiveness of the subject, some points may be absent or covered only in part. If the reader desires additional information, refer to the list of references for each chapter.

References

1. Institute for Alternative Futures. *The Future of Chiropractic Revisited: 2005–2015.* 2005. http://www.altfutures.com.
2. Feise, R. *The Evidence-Based Approach. J Amer Chiropr Assoc.* 2002. **39**(8):30–3.
3. Cobb, L.A., et al. *An evaluation of internal-mammary-artery ligation by a double-blind technic. N Engl J Med.* 1959. **260**(22):1115–8.
4. Talbot, M. *The Placebo Prescription. New York Times Magazine.* 9 Jan. 2000, 34–9.

The author(s) has made every effort to ensure the accuracy of the information herein. However, appropriate information sources should be consulted, especially for new or unfamiliar procedures. It is the responsibility of every practitioner to evaluate the appropriateness of a particular opinion in the context of actual clinical situations and with due considerations to new developments. The author(s) and publisher disclaim all responsibility for any liability, loss, injury, or damage incurred as a consequence, directly or indirectly, of the use and application of any of the contents in this volume.

PART I

Fundamentals of Evidence-Based Practice

ONE

Introduction

What Is Evidence-Based Chiropractic?

Evidence-based chiropractic (EBC) is an offshoot from a movement that was started by a group of medical educators at McMaster's University in Ontario, Canada, during the 1980s.[1] These physicians observed that a certain gap had developed between what occurred in the clinical practice of medicine and the vast amount of information from clinical research that was being produced. Essentially, the authors noted that clinicians could not stay abreast of all of the new research because it was being produced so fast; consequently, they were not putting into practice the most current information. In response, the McMaster's group began in earnest to educate physicians about the importance of integrating research evidence into their clinical practices, and also how to combine this newfound knowledge with their expertise as clinicians and the desires and preferences of the patients they cared for. This method of practice eventually became known as evidence-based medicine (EBM). Many in the chiropractic profession have embraced these concepts in recent years and, as a result, EBC has evolved.[2,3]

David Sackett, who was one of the key originators of evidence-based practice (EBP), provided the following often-cited definition of EBM: "Evidence-based medicine is the conscientious, explicit, and judicious use of current best evidence in making decisions about the care of individual patients. The practice of evidence-based medicine means integrating individual clinical expertise with the best available external clinical evidence from systematic research."[4]

It should be emphasized that *individual clinical expertise* is a very important part of EBM, and likewise of EBC. Clinical expertise can be thought of as the skills and knowledge that clinicians acquire through clinical experience and practice. Accordingly, the practice of EBC relies heavily upon past experience as a practitioner and does not propose blind acceptance of information that might not apply to the given clinical circumstances. EBC involves more than simply reading the right scientific article at the right time and then changing your clinical behavior in response to this new information. Because of this supposed fault, some have criticized EBP as being a "cookbook" way to practice.[5] However, since it is actually a continuing process of integrating the best evidence (that which is the most current and as strong as possible) with the past training and expertise of the clinician, it results in better care for patients. The addition of evidence to patient care serves to supplant outdated information, which also leads to better practices.

Rosenberg and Donald defined EBM as "a process of turning clinical problems into questions and then systematically locating, appraising, and using contemporaneous research findings as the basis for clinical decisions."[6] However, EBC is much more than simply finding an article in the literature to either guide or support the treatment of a particular patient. At best, evidence from research only answers questions that have to do with the averages of groups of patients, whereas patient care involves an individual. Thus, decision making that entails a specific patient is based on clinical expertise and awareness of the patient's preferences, coupled with evidence from research. Patient input therefore becomes an essential part of the EBC process, and individual outcomes will vary accordingly. For instance, a patient with low back pain may refuse to participate in home care advice that is supported by research evidence because of time constraints. Bolton[3] provided a definition of EBP as follows: "clinical decision-making based on 1) sound external research evidence combined with individual clinical expertise and 2) the needs of the individual patient."

You may not have previously thought that patient preferences would be an element of EBC, but taking them into consideration is actually a crucial step in the process. Patient preferences are related to the *personal values, concerns*, and *expectations* that patients have as they receive care or contemplate receiving care.[7] Regardless of what you as a practitioner determine to be an appropriate course of treatment, it is the patient who has the final say in accepting, rejecting, or modifying care. *Personal values* have to do with the beliefs patients have concerning the care that is being offered to them and may be related to philosophical or even religious issues. For example, if a Doctor of Chiropractic (DC) recommends increased meat consumption to an undernourished patient and the patient happens to be a vegetarian because of his or her religious beliefs, the advice will have to be modified or noncompliance will likely be the end result. *Patient concerns* may include such things as financial issues, time constraints, and even the geographical location of your office. *Patient expectations* have to do with their degree of acceptance of your recommendations for the management of their condition. A patient with chronic neck pain, for example, may expect relief after one or two adjustments and may balk when confronted with your suggestion that he or she will require prolonged care involving multiple modalities. Kravitz[8] indicated that medical patients' expectations are wide-ranging and can have a significant impact on clinical results.

Considering the earlier mentioned definitions of EBP and EBM, I will now provide one for EBC that is admittedly derived from previous works. For the purposes of this book, a definition of EBC is as follows: *actively seeking support for and improvement of chiropractic clinical practices through the integration of the best available research evidence, combined with clinical expertise and patient values* (Figure 1.1). EBC becomes essential when, in the course of providing chiropractic patient care, clinical situations arise for which practitioners do not have adequate answers. Essentially, the practitioners' clinical expertise is incomplete. Rather than evading these clinical questions by simply referring involved patients to other providers or providing substandard care, EBC advocates that the best evidence on the topic be searched for, evaluated for its validity and relevance to the clinical problem at issue, and then applied to the management of involved patients.

Various types of practitioners on an international level have accepted EBP, but it does have its critics. As mentioned previously, it has been maligned for being too robotic. In addition, Hunink[9] pointed out that although the process of EBP can be considered helpful in the critical appraisal of scientific articles, one needs to be critical of the EBP approach itself. The author pointed out that the hierarchy of evidence that is utilized in EBP, which considers systematic reviews and randomized controlled trials (RCTs) to be the highest level of evidence, can sometimes be misleading. Indeed, many of the conditions that are currently being

FIGURE 1.1 **Evidence-based chiropractice combines the best research evidence with clinical expertise and patient values.**

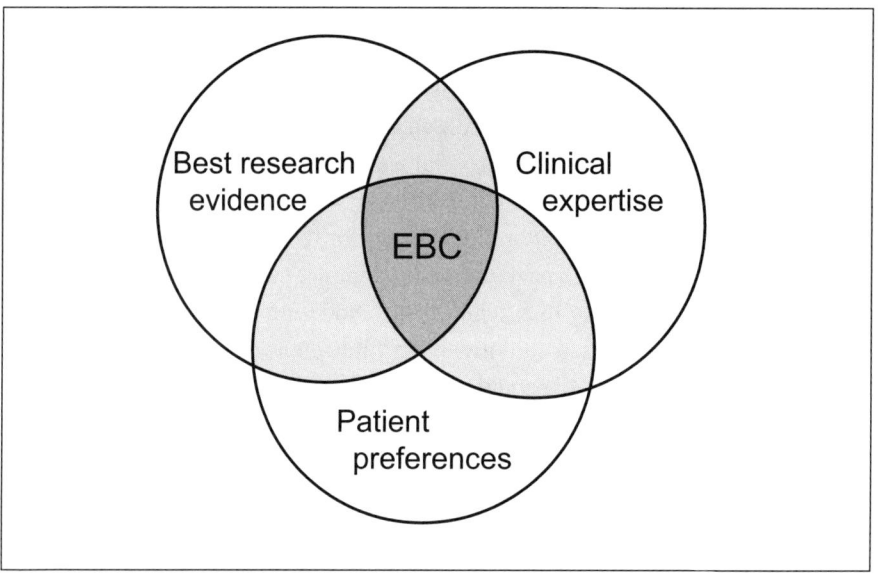

managed by chiropractic methods have not been investigated in this manner. Table 1.1 provides a hierarchy of research evidence taken from the Agency for Health Care Policy and Research, with the study types listed in order of strength of evidence. Stronger evidence is higher in order, with systematic reviews of RCTs being the strongest and expert opinion the weakest. EBP has also been criticized because empirical evidence cannot be directly applied to individual patients. This is because clinical research deals with groups of individuals who had a variety of outcomes and did not include the patient in question. Consequently, the knowledge gained from clinical research does not specifically establish what is best for particular patients.[10]

Because one of the fundamental steps of EBP is to locate the highest quality of evidence that is available and then apply its findings to individual clinical circumstances, a conundrum occurs when no high-quality evidence is available. In these cases, lower levels of evidence must be utilized, although this type of evidence will accordingly generate less confidence for making clinical decisions. For conditions in which there is little or no evidence supporting management by

TABLE 1.1 A hierarchy of research evidence

1. Systematic reviews and meta-analyses of randomized controlled trials
2. Randomized controlled trials
3. Nonrandomized intervention studies
4. Observational studies
5. Nonexperimental studies
6. Expert opinion

Source: Agency for Healthcare Research and Quality (formerly Agency for Healthcare Policy and Research). http://www.ahrq.gov

chiropractic methods, practitioners will have to decide whether to render treatment (perhaps on a time- and improvement-dependent trial basis) or refer to an appropriate specialist for autonomous or co-management of the case or just to obtain a second opinion.

It should be noted that the process of EBP itself has not been rigorously tested, so we do not know for sure if it actually results in improved health.[5] No RCTs that have compared EBP with standard methods of practice have been carried out in any of the health care professions because of the methodological difficulties and exorbitantly high costs that would be associated with attempting to execute such studies.[9] A case-control study was carried out concerning lower back pain, which indicated that evidence-based care was more helpful over the long term than good-quality usual care, with fewer patients requiring continuing care and remaining in pain.[11] The problem with this type of study, as you will in due course discover, is that it is not a design capable of determining whether one event caused another. Thus, in this case, one could not say that the evidence-based care actually caused better outcomes than usual care based on a case-control study. It takes a study design that is a higher level of evidence to establish causation. On the other hand, it should be readily apparent that clinical decisions based on up-to-date evidence would be preferable to the alternative. In reality EBP is simply a method that facilitates the process of practitioners finding solutions to their patients' individual clinical problems.

Evidence-Based Practice and Evidence-Based Chiropractic

As mentioned earlier, the roots of EBC can be traced to evidence-based medicine, a phrase that was first mentioned in print in an article by Gordon Guyatt that appeared in the *ACP Journal Club* in 1991.[12] Around this time, the previously mentioned medical educators from McMaster's University, which included such renowned personalities as David Sackett, Andrew Oxman, and Gordon Guyatt, produced a series of 25 articles titled "Users' Guides to the Medical Literature." The series provided training in EBM methods and was published in the *Journal of the American Medical Association* between 1992 and 2000. It was a natural progression for EBC to develop from this initial work because of the similarities between the practice of medicine and chiropractic. Moreover, the practice of EBC involves the same steps as EBM, but is preceded by questions that are pertinent to chiropractic patients. EBC is just one of the many varieties of EBP, a model that has been applied to virtually all of the health care disciplines (e.g., evidence-based dentistry, nursing). EBC has been well received by a sizeable portion of the chiropractic profession and is taught in some form at all chiropractic colleges.

Despite its similarities with EBM and EBP, EBC is unique in several ways. First, chiropractic interventions (primarily manipulation) are more difficult to investigate by experimental methods than are drugs, homeopathic preparations, herbs, and even surgery. Drug trials, for example, can be designed without much difficulty to represent a proper experiment, which involves the comparison of a group of patients receiving an active medication with another group that receives a counterfeit (placebo) medication. If the drug group has a significantly better outcome at the end of the trial, then the researchers involved can say that the drug was effective. To reduce the influence of circumstances that might confound the study's results, such as placebo effects or patient acquiescence, it is very important that neither the doctors nor the patients involved know which intervention they were giving or receiving. This method of keeping investigators and subjects in experiments unaware about which treatment is involved is known as *blinding*, and it is not easy to achieve when manipulation is under study. The reason it is so difficult to blind DCs during manipulation trials is they will almost always know whether they are delivering a real versus a counterfeit manipulation. Likewise, patients are not easily fooled about whether they are receiving real or a placebo manipulation.[13] To solve this problem, placebo manipulation is often designed so that it is very similar to real manipulation—so similar that patients in the placebo group may actually receive a treatment effect.[14,15] Conversely, if the placebo is too dissimilar to real manipulation, patients will realize they are not actually being treated and are likely to respond poorly. Because blinding and the use of placebos are difficult to accomplish in chiropractic trials, there are fewer articles available that meet these criteria than there are for medical trials. Consequently, EBC practitioners will at times have to be content relying on less rigorous evidence.

In the course of treating patients, DCs commonly utilize multiple modalities that include a variety of different manipulations, rehabilitative procedures, ergonomic advice, physiotherapy, and so on. On the other hand, clinical trials usually prohibit the use of procedures other than the specific intervention under investigation. The reason for this limitation is to isolate the manipulative procedure so that it can be compared with a placebo or some type of alternative therapy. If other procedures are utilized in addition to manipulation, one really wouldn't know whether it was the manipulation or one of the other procedures allowed in the study that influenced its outcome. *Pragmatic* (real-world) studies, which permit the treating DCs to practice as usual, exist, but their results are not as convincing as studies that are more tightly controlled. All health care interventions that are investigated face this same dilemma: Tighter control of the intervention yields a study that is capable of showing a cause-and-effect relationship, but often does not represent what clinicians actually do in practice; on the other hand, pragmatic studies, while being more relevant to clinical practice, have limited ability to offer conclusive results. This state of affairs represents another reason that the evidence we find in EBC may not be entirely comparable to other types of EBP.

EBC may also be considered unique because finances have historically been very limited for conducting chiropractic research. Because high-quality research is very expensive to carry out, progress has been hampered in this area. This inadequate financial situation has been changing, however, and there have been quite a few elegant chiropractic-related studies conducted in recent years. Additionally, federal funds are increasingly becoming available for chiropractic research, especially since the formation of the National Center for Complementary and Alternative Medicine[16] (formerly the Office of Alternative Medicine) in 1992. As a result, EBC practitioners can look forward to an increasing supply of high-quality evidence to support their clinical practices in the future.

The particular research needs of the chiropractic profession give rise to a correspondingly unique evidence base for DCs to rely on. The pharmaceutical industry is well suited to using strict experimental methods: these methods are almost exclusively used for drug trials. Conversely, chiropractic methods are not well suited for this model of research,[17] with some of the reasons outlined previously.

Additional reasons will be explained when experimental research designs are covered more thoroughly in later chapters. At this point, the main thing to consider is that chiropractic evidence will more frequently be derived from studies that are comparatively less stringently controlled than many other interventions. DCs should not be too concerned about this situation, however, since other types of studies are available to support and help direct chiropractic patient care. On the other hand, critics from outside the profession may not understand the unique constraints of chiropractic research and point out that evidence is lacking in certain areas.

One final issue to mention concerning the distinction between EBC and EBP involves the recognized prejudice of medical authors against the practice of chiropractic that is present in the biomedical literature.[18] There have been instances in which adverse effects associated with manipulation have been attributed to chiropractors, when in fact the practitioners involved were actually from other professions or even lay manipulators.[19,20] In addition, after looking at the accumulated evidence on a specified topic, medical authors may come to a more pessimistic conclusion about the aggregate findings as compared with chiropractic authors. This problem becomes apparent when medical and chiropractic authors are contrasted regarding their conclusions about the treatment of low back pain using manipulation. As an example, Bronfort and associates,[21] chiropractic authors, reported, "Our data synthesis suggests that recommendations can be made with some confidence regarding the use of SMT (manipulation) . . . as a viable option for the treatment of . . . low-back pain." On the other hand, Assendelft and colleagues,[22] medical authors, reporting on the same topic, concluded, "While some patients with low back pain may prefer spinal manipulation to traditional therapies, there is no evidence that it achieves better outcomes than standard treatments."

Irresponsible reports in the literature about the safety and effectiveness of chiropractic negatively affect the opinions of readers about the practice of chiropractic and may influence their decisions regarding patient referrals to DCs as well as their opinions on public health policy matters. EBC practitioners should be cognizant of this prejudice and look for it as related evidence is being appraised. Unfortunately, there is a subjective aspect to interpreting the results of research, which often results in conflicting opinions that you will have to sort out for yourself; the knowledge of EBC methods is the best way I know of to deal with this problem.

Why Evidence-Based Chiropractic?

Not infrequently DCs are confronted with clinical problems that they are not familiar with and for which they lack the necessary skills.[23] In the past, clinicians were taught to seek answers to these problems based on information gleaned from textbooks, field experts, or respected colleagues. However, these strategies are often inadequate and are not likely to generate the best information possible. There are several reasons why sources such as these frequently do not lead to optimal solutions for clinical problems. Textbooks that were acquired during chiropractic schooling may be of little or no help because they rapidly become obsolete as new information becomes available.[7] In fact, many are already outdated by the time they are published and continue to depreciate the longer they sit on a bookshelf. Experts may convey somewhat more current information, but it will only be as current as the latest reference that they have cited. In addition, experts are not typically readily accessible. Colleagues are apt to rely on the same outdated information sources as you would, although they might be more current on a given topic and therefore may have something useful to offer. Knowledge that was received during primary chiropractic training also becomes outdated very quickly, in addition to being forgotten.

Another resource that may be utilized in making chiropractic clinical decisions is past clinical experiences. Although experiential problem-solving strategies such as these may provide useful information, the information will likely be incomplete and out of date. A practitioner relying on past clinical experience alone may reason: "I used this method successfully in the past with patients having similar conditions; therefore, I will now use it with this patient." This is not to say that clinical experience is worthless; quite the opposite, it is extremely valuable. Indeed, it is one of the major steps involved in the practice of EBC, which integrates evidence from research with clinical expertise (see Table 1.2, later in this chapter). Furthermore, combining clinical expertise with the best available research evidence is complementary to and has a synergistic effect on patient care.

I don't want to leave you with the impression that some of the previously mentioned problem-solving strategies are useless. Indeed, they work together to form the foundation of clinical problem-solving skills. EBC builds on this foundation by using supplementary problem-solving strategies to help you locate research articles that are relevant to the clinical problem under investigation, critically appraise these articles, and then apply the results of the best studies to help solve the clinical problem under consideration.

One of the most essential components of EBC is, of course, evidence in the form of research findings. Hence, DCs should be competent at interpreting the articles that report this research in order to integrate EBC into their practices. Yet a survey of 165 randomly selected DCs from across the United States found that the majority of DCs do not understand even basic research methods. Moreover, the survey found that 80% of the respondents did not know the difference between a retrospective and a prospective research design.[24] This is a very elementary research concept that should be familiar to all doctoral-level health care practitioners. Much of this lack of knowledge can be attributed to the fact that research was essentially ignored for many years by the chiropractic profession. During the early years of the profession, chiropractic schools were struggling financially and did not have the resources needed to carry out research.[25] Unfortunately, the priorities of the schools were almost exclusively focused on improving education; consequently, there was very little emphasis on research. This situation has radically changed in recent years; as a result, a sizeable amount of quality chiropractic research is being produced from within the profession. In addition, chiropractic students are now being taught to interpret scientific evidence, which will eventually improve the research-related awareness level of DCs. The majority of the profession who lack knowledge in this area can improve themselves through a variety of available methods, such as self-study, taking classes in research methods, regularly reading journal articles, and attending scientific conferences.

The Information Explosion

An information explosion has occurred as a consequence of widespread access to the Internet. As a result, patients are more frequently asking difficult questions about the effectiveness of chiropractic care, the safety of manipulation, the existence of alternative treatments, and so forth. Yet some of the information sources that patients utilize to formulate their questions are not trustworthy and may be extremely biased for or against chiropractic methods. Biased information sources are in general based on a degree of truth, often quoting respected references. They do so selectively, however, and do not present a balanced account of the topic. Patients may ask probing questions based on this misinformation. To deal with their questions effectively, clinicians should be proficient at finding and appraising applicable evidence. To facilitate the evaluation of Internet health information resources, a checklist for evaluating health information websites is presented in Appendix 1.

A great deal of new information emanates from the vast supply of new research articles published in the biomedical literature, with which DCs are expected to keep reasonably current. This represents another reason to consider becoming familiar with and making use of EBC. Much of this information is either not valid or not applicable to chiropractic practice, and careful assessment is needed to discern which of it should be accepted and which should be rejected. Accordingly, one of the major objectives of EBC is to enable practicing DCs to distinguish quality evidence from that which is flawed. Because numerous types of studies are utilized in research, another objective is to recognize which articles are relevant to the given clinical circumstances.

Best Practices

Reliance on anatomical and pathophysiological principles has historically played a large role in the development of chiropractic theories. This process is fundamental to the advancement of any science, but may prove to be insufficient as a basis for clinical practice. Eventually these theories need to be tested to discover whether they are valid and can be reliably employed in practice. Yet many such theories operational in the practice of chiropractic, as well as in all other health care disciplines, have not been rigorously tested. Moreover, some have only been described in case reports and case series, study designs that are not capable of showing cause-and-effect relationships. When diagnoses and treatments stem from information derived in this manner, there is a possibility that they may be erroneous. Therefore, one should strive to locate the highest-quality evidence that is available, although at times you will be forced to rely on weaker evidence.

Knowledge about, and subsequent use of, the most valid diagnostic and treatment protocols leads to better patient care, which should be the ultimate goal of anyone involved in the field of health care. Often termed *best practices*, the most valid clinical tools available can be established by interpreting the research that has addressed these issues. Some studies are capable of determining whether a particular treatment is effective or if there is harm associated with it, whereas others explore diagnostic methods to establish the level of reliability or validity, or both, of tests.

Certainly you would want to know about an investigation that had previously shown that a condition you were considering treating had been nonresponsive to chiropractic manipulation, or if a diagnostic procedure you were using was shown to be unreliable (it was not reproducible) or was not valid (it did not really measure what it was supposed to). With this knowledge you could alter your practices accordingly. One needs to keep in mind, however, that the evidence needed to make these decisions is often not definitive, especially when there are disparate findings among the studies that were used to make them. The evidence may be very weak at times (e.g., the unmethodical observations of a lone clinician or generalizations from animal studies), but there is almost always something available.[26]

The treatment of childhood asthma with manipulation is a prime example. Studies using manipulation have not shown an effect on changes in objective lung function measures, yet subjective measures, such as quality of life, symptoms, and bronchodilator use, are improved.[27] Motion palpation, a diagnostic method commonly used by DCs, has been the subject of numerous investigations. Most of these studies have concluded that it is not a reliable method for evaluating the spine, and, as a result, some authors have questioned its continued use.[28] However, there is a small amount of evidence pointing to its reliability,[29] and it has been the analytical procedure of choice in many trials dealing with manipulation.

What, then, is a practitioner to do when confronted with similar circumstances? There are no easy answers to this conundrum, and this is one of the main points at which biomedical science falters. It is a problem that practitioners from all disciplines occasionally face, since good evidence does not exist to support every form of treatment that is available. One thing is very important to bear in mind regarding studies that fail to produce significant findings, however: *No evidence of effect* is not the same as *evidence of no effect*.[30] It is tempting to conclude that because a certain treatment method was not supported in a clinical trial it is therefore not effective. This assumption would be a mistake, although some authors do in fact make such statements. It is entirely possible in these cases that the treatment actually did work, but the study design was simply not able to demonstrate the effect. Stated another way, it is wrong to cite a "failed study" as evidence that the treatment under investigation is not clinically useful.

Practitioners from all health care professions have expressed fears about EBP in that the resulting evidence could potentially contradict their current practices. This evolution of health care is inevitable as new research findings bring about professional advances that call for changes of practice. This is a process that should be welcomed by all and not feared. What is best for the patient in any given clinical situation should always take priority over the traditions and beliefs of practitioners. Moreover, EBP believes that the patient takes precedence over specific professions as well as the individual practitioners.[31]

Reimbursement Issues

Insurance companies often look to practice guidelines and experts in the field as they determine for which diagnostic and treatment methods they will pay. However, this scheme may be problematical when these sources of information do not correctly evaluate the evidence, a scenario that is not uncommon and can lead to either incorrectly portrayed or improperly extrapolated research findings. These players will frequently change their minds and pay for the services that were provided when given an explanation that is grounded in credible evidence and justifies the clinical procedures at issue. This approach is not as difficult as one might think, but knowledge of how to locate and evaluate scientific articles is necessary to carry it off, topics that will be discussed in later chapters of this book.

Practice guidelines too are not infallible.[32] Even though they are typically prepared by experts in the field and involve an extensive and methodical process of evaluating the available evidence on a given topic, mistakes can occur. Not only that, but guidelines become outdated very quickly as new evidence is published. Indeed, the well-known *Mercy guidelines*[33] caution users that their legitimacy will diminish as time progresses and that they should be updated regularly, an undertaking that has never been carried out. A recent revision to some practice guidelines that were produced by the American College of Occupational and Environmental Medicine (ACOEM) was shown to be biased against manipulation and chiropractic,[34] yet the guidelines were adopted by several insurance companies as well as by government agencies because they were considered the best evidence at the time. Payers may not be aware of the limitations of the guidelines that they rely on, but when presented with the appropriate data, they will often change their opinions.

The point of presenting this material on reimbursement is that it is possible to influence decision makers if you can provide a rational explanation for your clinical procedures that is based on sound evidence—evidence that must first be located, next appraised for validity, and then applied to the clinical circumstances. Fortunately, a major portion of this book involves instruction that deals with these topics.

When to Use Evidence-Based Chiropractic

Patient-Specific Issues

Patients regularly present to chiropractic offices with conditions that are unusual or possibly even unknown to the practitioner. Is this patient a likely candidate for chiropractic care? What are the best options for managing this patient's condition? Are there any contraindications to manipulation? Questions such as these should stimulate interest in EBC methods for those who have thus far been reluctant to become involved. Moreover, finding answers that are derived from the best evidence available is nearly impossible unless EBC is utilized.

As was previously mentioned, patients ask questions that may at times be quite sophisticated due to the widespread availability of health-related information in recent years. Frequently they look to you for answers to questions that may not specifically deal with chiropractic issues, especially when seeking alternatives to drugs and surgery. It is common for patients who do not receive help from allopathic health care to seek alternative therapies[35] and growing numbers who do not trust the medical system seek alternative practitioners in the first place.[36] Accordingly, such patients may seek your opinion regarding out-of-the-ordinary conditions that compel investigation on your part or referral to another provider.

Condition-Specific Issues

It is advantageous for DCs to acquire knowledge about unfamiliar conditions, hopefully before patients with these types of complaints present for treatment. However, these patients will undoubtedly turn up at chiropractic offices, and implicated DCs will somehow have to make sure they are provided with the optimal treatment. Preferably the decisions involved in this process will be based on the best available evidence. This form of learning is reactive; nonetheless, it is often successful and leads to knowledge that will facilitate care of similar patients in the future. A more proactive approach that involves consistently exploring professional journals and educating oneself about unfamiliar topics is a superior strategy. Rather than having to rush around to find answers when patients with unusual conditions appear, these DCs will already be prepared and will be able to focus entirely on the problem at hand.

Very few, if any, DCs are experts in all areas of chiropractic practice. In fact, many are not authoritative in any specific area, instead taking a broad view of the field. However, it is prudent to have one or two conditions that you are very familiar with—enough that you could consider yourself to be an expert. DCs have made a name for themselves by becoming well informed about a variety of conditions, such as carpal tunnel syndrome, whiplash, and temporomandibular joint syndrome, to name a few. Basic instruction can be obtained at various seminars covering these and other conditions, although further study using the techniques of EBC is needed in order to advance to the higher levels of practice and to remain current on the subject.

Self-Education

Self-education is an extension of the scenario just described and is an excellent way of learning. Many practitioners attend seminars to be educated about a variety of clinical topics, and this method certainly has its place in the didactic process. Then again, one must speculate about how informed the speaker is and how accurate and current the material being presented is. A preferred method would be to gather the best available evidence on the topic yourself and then assimilate this information into your practice. Although this type of self-teaching may not always be practical and instructors are often indispensable, knowledge acquired through application of EBC is very gratifying. The development of lifelong learning skills is a fringe benefit, so to speak, of utilizing EBC.

Regular use of EBC methods is one of the best ways to stay current on the subject of innovative chiropractic care and is also an excellent means of learning the intricacies of research. Journal articles represent the most authoritative source available with regard to treatment, diagnosis, and other health issues that are related to chiropractic practice. As a result, the education acquired from them will be more accurate, credible, and applicable to practice than that gained from other resources. The knowledge gained from reading and understanding these articles can be especially gratifying, which then stimulates confidence as a practitioner.

Regardless of what situation prompts the use of EBC, it is important to immediately write a note to yourself in sufficient detail so that you will be able to recall what was involved and look for appropriate evidence at a more convenient time.

Learning Curve Involved

It takes time and practice to learn EBC methods. In fact, EBC has some elements that are fairly difficult to master, particularly research methods and biostatistics. It is definitely worth learning EBC, however, since this information is what supports and justifies what you do in practice. Additionally, once learned, EBC requires continued practice in order for you to become an expert.

You should not expect to make progress as an EBC practitioner unless you regularly implement the procedures outlined in this book. Hunting down relevant information, reviewing and critiquing it, and then applying this new information to the clinical situations you encounter gets easier when repeated over time. It is very helpful to read an assortment of journal articles on a regular basis, and you should make time in your busy schedule to do this; perhaps setting aside 30 minutes to one hour per day specifically for reading research-related material. Subscribe to a few peer-reviewed chiropractic journals and read them regularly. Don't feel compelled to read every article in every issue, but peruse the abstracts and then read the entire articles of those that are of interest to you. That way, you will sharpen your EBC skills and, at the same time, be on the cutting edge of knowledge within the profession. As stated so accurately by Keating,[37] "Chiropractors who cannot (or do not) follow the chiropractic literature can never be more than second class citizens." In addition to having access to journal articles, Internet access is essential in order to effectively practice EBC, since relevant resources can best be found with its use. Set aside some time each day to search for answers to clinical questions as they arise in your practice. If more than a few unanswered, questions accumulate, the time required to research them can become overwhelming and they could go unanswered to the detriment of the patients.

Although some may find it easier to become proficient in EBC and some may have better availability of the necessary tools (e.g., computers and library access), learning the basic procedures involved in EBC is achievable for all DCs who are willing to put in the necessary time. It does, however, require a fairly large commitment in order to fully master the skill, and once learned, like just about anything else, it must be used regularly in order to retain the knowledge and skills involved. When considering the teaching of EBP, there is little evidence to support the notion that it actually changes learners' practice behaviors, either in the near or distant future.[38] Therefore, it appears that follow-through in this area is essential and is ultimately the responsibility of the individual practitioner.

Steps Involved in the Practice of Evidence-Based Chiropractic

There are five steps involved in the practice of EBC (Table 1.2), which are adapted from the work of Sackett and associates:[1]

Steps Involved in the Practice of Evidence-Based Chiropractic

1. Ask a clinically relevant question.
2. Search the literature to find the best available evidence to answer your question.
3. Appraise the evidence for validity and applicability to the clinical circumstances.
4. Apply the relevant evidence to the clinical situation.
5. Evaluate your effectiveness in carrying out steps 1 through 4 and revise if necessary.

These steps constitute the substance of this book, especially the third step (appraising the evidence), which requires about half of the book to explain. Even though EBC is a systematic process with specific elements involved, it cannot be considered "cookbook" practice.[4,39] As a matter of fact, the practitioner's clinical expertise is of paramount importance in the application of external clinical evidence to patient circumstances. Although external evidence often provides valuable information, it is ultimately up to the clinician to decide how and if it should be utilized.

Asking an Appropriate Clinical Quesion

An appropriate question is clinically relevant—something that will help you with the management of a particular patient or patients that you encounter with a certain type of health problem. Before leaping headlong into the various sources of evidence looking for answers to clinical problems, it is important to generate a relevant question that will help guide your search. Otherwise, a great deal of time

TABLE 1.2   Evidence-based chiropractic

Definition
Actively seeking support for and improvement of chiropractic clinical practices through the integration of the best available research evidence, combined with clinical expertise and patient values.

Steps of EBC
1. Ask a clinically relevant question.
2. Search the literature to find the best available evidence to answer your question.
3. Appraise the evidence for validity and applicability to the clinical circumstances.
4. Apply the relevant evidence to the clinical situation.
5. Evaluate your effectiveness in carrying out steps 1 through 4 and revise if necessary.

may be wasted aimlessly reading irrelevant material. Questions of this type contain certain elements of the clinical problem that enable purposeful searching strategies;[40] however, there are some crucial steps involved that must be followed so as to ensure that the final product will indeed help you solve the clinical problem. Of course, without an appropriate question, it is difficult to know where to even start looking for information, and, as you will soon discover, there are many possible choices.

Background Versus Foreground Questions
There are two general types of questions: those that are based on *background information*—broad knowledge about the condition at issue regarding its anatomical and pathophysiological basis—and those based on *foreground information*—focused knowledge that will lead to the best diagnostic and treatment strategies for the involved patient. Background questions are simple two-part questions that address the basic facts about a patient's health problem. Background questions are limited because the information that is obtained does not fully address issues about the best diagnostic or treatment options. On the other hand, this knowledge is essential to a practitioner who is not well-read on a given topic, and it facilitates the construction of a more complex question. Familiarity with background information on a given topic is needed prior to dealing with matters in the foreground and for progressing to the point of asking a useful foreground question. For instance, if a patient presents with suspected multiple sclerosis, a general definition of the condition and information about its common characteristics would be helpful. This type of information can best be acquired from sources such as current textbooks and electronic publications that are thoroughly referenced and regularly peer-reviewed (e.g., *Harrison's Online*[41] and *UpToDate*[42]). Journal articles, in contrast, are typically not efficient sources of background information.

Foreground questions deal with issues that are more involved than background questions and apply to decisions practitioners must make about establishing the most favorable treatment or diagnostic strategies. Answers for these types of questions are derived from sources that provide primary and secondary information. Primary (also called *unfiltered*) sources are original journal articles; secondary (also called *prefiltered*) sources include expert reviews of all available original articles on a given topic. Essentially, prefiltered information sources have teams of experts from the various specialties who perform a topic-specific literature search, methodically evaluate each of the articles discovered, and then provide a synopsis and overall conclusion from this evidence. Because much of the work has been done for you, prefiltered information sources are often a preferable first step in obtaining evidence. The biggest disadvantage for DCs with regard to this type of information is that the reviewers are almost always medically trained. As a result of their background, they may provide potentially biased reports and may not cover topics germane to chiropractic and other forms of natural health care.

Foreground questions, being more complex than background questions, are more difficult to compose and require targeted conceptualization. Better clinical questions are made up of several components, being divided into three or four sections. The general idea is to produce a question that considers whether a relationship between the involved patient and some type of treatment, diagnostic test, or risk is associated with some specific outcome.

The mnemonic *PICO* is frequently used to help remember the components of a correctly formatted clinical question (Table 1.3). The letter *P* represents the patient or problem that is under consideration and can involve a single patient or group of patients with a particular condition. When composing this part of a question, consider characteristics such as age, ethnicity, and risk factors that may be clinically relevant. An example is an elderly man with lower back pain. Letter *I* concerns the intervention or exposure that is being considered. An example is: treatment with manipulation. Letter *C* may not apply to all questions; hence, it is optional. It has to do with treatments that you might want to compare with the primary intervention. An example is comparison of manipulation with exercise. Letter *O* represents the outcome of interest, which preferably will be patient-relevant. By *patient-relevant*, I mean outcomes that are of interest to patients, such as less pain or disability. Although you as a practitioner may be interested in watching a patient's straight leg raise test go from 30 to 60 degrees or his or her surface electromyographic findings normalize, patients simply want to feel and

TABLE 1.3 **Components of PICO questions**

Patient or problem
Intervention
Comparison intervention
Outcome(s) of interest

function better. Joining these elements into a single question would result in something like this: In an elderly man with lower back pain, would manipulation be preferable to exercise in reducing pain and disability?

The previous example was straightforward, involving a type of patient that is commonly seen in chiropractic offices. Consider now another example involving a not so common condition that may or may not call for chiropractic management. A middle-aged female patient enters your practice complaining of lower back pain with radiation to both legs involving the posterior thighs. She also notices numbness of both feet affecting the S1 nerve distribution after prolonged sitting or standing. The radiology report, based on plain films and CT, points to mild to moderate spinal stenosis, but there are no objective neurological signs present. You consider accepting this patient for a trial of manipulation and wonder if there is evidence that supports this type of management and if there are alternative therapies that might be superior. The PICO-formatted question: Is manipulation effective at reducing back and leg pain in a middle-aged female patient with lumbar spinal stenosis and concomitant radicular pain, or are any alternative methods more favorable? A dissection of this question into its elements is as follows:

P A middle-aged female patient with lumbar spinal stenosis and concomitant radicular pain
I Manipulation
C Any alternative method that might be superior to manipulation
O A reduction of lower back and leg pain

One more example will be presented that should help make this very important subject more understandable. A 50-year-old female patient with a family history of breast cancer is told by another physician that she should consider hormone replacement therapy as a preventive strategy for Alzheimer's disease since both of her parents with progressive dementia were recently diagnosed with Alzheimer's. She asks you for your opinion and wants to know what risks are involved with the intervention and if indeed it does prevent Alzheimer's. The PICO-formatted question: Would hormone replacement therapy in a 50-year-old female with a family history of breast cancer and Alzheimer's disease actually prevent the occurrence of Alzheimer's, and would it offset the added risk of breast cancer?

P A 50-year-old female patient with a family history of breast cancer
I Hormone replacement therapy
C None
O Prevention of Alzheimer's disease

Asking good clinical questions is not as difficult as it may seem and can be mastered quickly with a little practice. Making use of appropriate clinical questions in your practice can be very helpful in sorting out your thoughts, finding solutions to problems, and directing patient management. It is not an exercise in futility that will ultimately just waste your time, as some think. Remember that there is a goal involved in asking these questions, and, once achieved, the end result will facilitate better-quality patient care.

As was mentioned earlier, outcomes that are patient-relevant and of significance to patients as well as to practitioners are preferred. In response, Shaughnessy and colleagues developed the concept of patient-oriented evidence that matters (POEMs).[43] The POEMs concept can be used in selecting evidence and involves finding valid research that meets three criteria:[44]

1. The outcome investigated in the study should be something that patients are expected to care about, such as morbidity or quality of life.
2. The problem that was studied should be widespread, and the intervention involved should be feasible.
3. The information should have the potential to change the practice of many practitioners.

In contrast, disease-oriented evidence (DOE) deals with outcomes that may be of interest to researchers and practitioners but are of little interest to patients. DOEs involve what are often termed *surrogate end points* (outcome measures that are used as a substitute for a clinically meaningful POEM), such as changes in x-ray or examination findings. These surrogate outcome measures are not actually capable of determining whether a given treatment works, but may provide evidence as to how it works. It is not that uncommon for an intervention to have a positive effect on a surrogate outcome but not on clinically relevant outcomes.[45]

What Is Evidence and Where to Find It?

Evidence that is needed to support the use of manipulation, modalities, and diagnostic tests utilized in chiropractic practice can primarily be found in biomedical journals. A number of these journals specifically deal with chiropractic-related issues, and there are many others that deal with the various medical specialties, health issues, epidemiology, basic sciences, and so forth. Articles that are of interest to EBC practitioners in these journals deal with subjects such as the effectiveness and safety of treatments, the validity and reliability of diagnostic tests, and the incidence and prevalence of diseases in populations. Chapter 2 identifies many of the publications that are helpful to EBC practitioners and discusses how to determine which ones are trustworthy. In addition to biomedical journals, evidence can also be derived from books.

The first step in finding evidence is to conduct a search of one or more of the databases that are designed to help locate relevant articles. This pursuit, termed *literature searching*, is the fundamental way to find articles of interest. It is a subject matter that requires more than just a few paragraphs to cover; it is thoroughly dealt with in Chapter 3. At this point, just realize that there are thousands of journals to choose relevant articles from that are referenced in one or more of the available biomedical databases, and that this is where one goes to find evidence.

When searching the literature for evidence, one's efforts should be directed toward locating the types of studies that are capable of answering questions about the particular clinical circumstances being considered. For instance, when looking for answers to questions about the effectiveness of various treatments, one should search for RCTs. On the other hand, if clinical questions have to do with risk, prospective cohort studies usually offer the best evidence.[46]

It would be wonderful if we could simply trust all of the biomedical journals and every article that they contain as being valid, but that is not the case. Unfortunately, it is common for scientific articles to contain errors, making it a necessity for practitioners to learn how to discriminate good-quality from poor-quality evidence before applying research findings to their practices.[47] In addition to being concerned about the quality of these articles, a topic to be covered later on, the hierarchy of evidence must also be assessed.

The Hierarchy of Research Evidence

The hierarchy of evidence that was previously mentioned, with RCTs and systematic reviews of RCTs being at the pinnacle, is considered by most to be the gold standard for determining whether a given treatment is effective. However, many therapies have not yet been studied in this manner and no RCTs or reviews have been carried out. This is true concerning the use of manipulation for some conditions that are commonly managed by DCs (e.g., acute neck pain). When you as a practitioner are presented with a clinical problem for which appropriate evidence is lacking, you cannot wait for the necessary trials to be conducted before moving forward with the care of that particular patient or similar patients. In situations such as this, you will have to utilize external evidence that is lower in the hierarchy of research and work from there. Examples of lower-level evidence include cohort studies, case series, case reports, and expert opinion. Figure 1.2

FIGURE 1.2 **Hierarchy of evidence pyramid.**

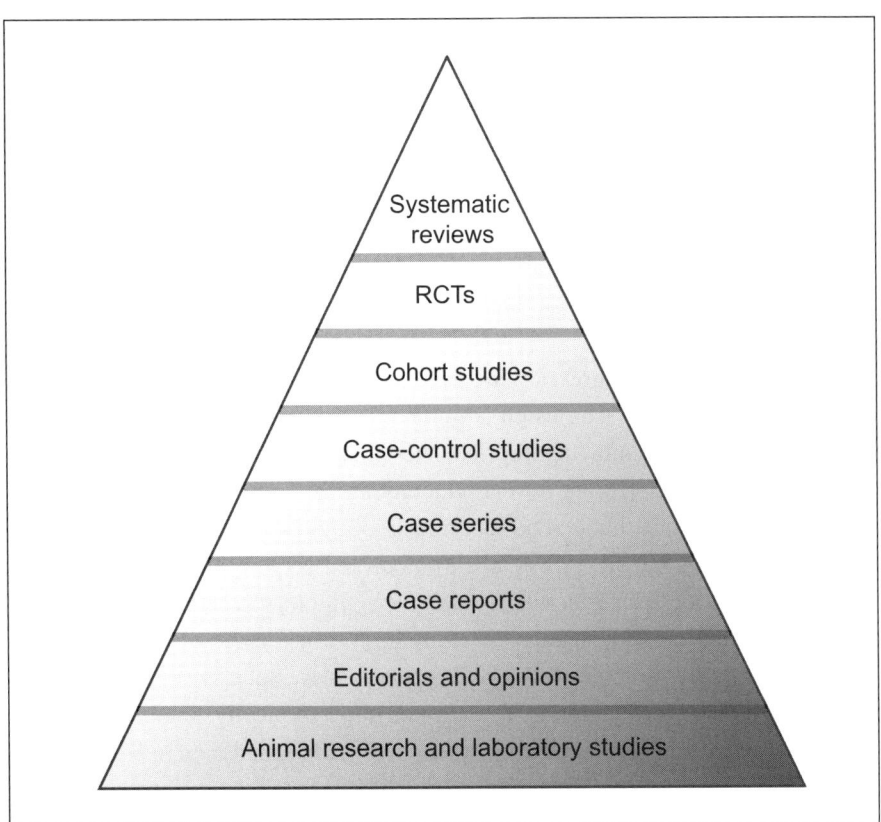

represents the hierarchy of the levels of evidence as a pyramid, with the highest-level evidence on top and the lowest on the bottom. The reason for the pyramidal shape is that there are progressively fewer studies available as one advances from the lowest to the highest levels. In cases where no evidence exists, you should be cautious in making clinical decisions, and in cases where there is evidence of no positive effect (or possibly even a negative effect), you may opt to avoid utilizing that diagnostic or treatment modality. On the other hand, it does not make sense to withhold treatment from a patient just because there are no RCTs or systematic reviews available. In these cases, the best evidence that can be obtained should be utilized to make the best clinical decision possible.

You may be asking why systematic reviews (meta-analyses are included in this category) have been placed in the highest position of evidence, even above RCTs. The main reason, which will be further clarified in Chapters 5 and 6, is that systematic reviews take into account all of the RCTs on a specified topic and then draw a conclusion based on the collective information derived from all of these studies. Note, however, that Sackett[48] points out that in evidence-based clinical practice, "use of the current best evidence in making decisions about the care of individual patients . . . is not restricted to randomized trials and meta-analyses. It involves tracking down the best external evidence with which to answer our clinical questions." In other words, when there are no high-level studies available, use the best evidence that you are able to find. Locating systematic reviews or evidence-based clinical practice guidelines is an efficient approach to finding the best evidence.[49]

There is a normal progression involved in the investigation of clinical topics, wherein a specific research design is more appropriate at one point in the progression and others are more appropriate later on. For example, it would not make much sense to dive headlong into conducting an RCT intended to study a new chiropractic technique that had not previously been described in the literature in any form. Carrying out an RCT is an enormous and very expensive undertaking. Consequently, prior to an undertaking of this magnitude, researchers want to have a good idea that the subject of their study has a fair chance of demonstrating effectiveness based on lower-level (and typically less expensive) designs. Thus, the progression of investigation for a given topic typically begins with case reports or series, then advances to observational studies, and then to RCTs. After a few RCTs are reported in the literature, the final step is to conduct a systematic review (Figure 1.3).

Steps Involved in the Practice of Evidence-Based Chiropractic

FIGURE 1.3 **Progression of investigations for a clinical topic. Note how they correspond to the hierarchy of evidence shown in Figure 1.2.**

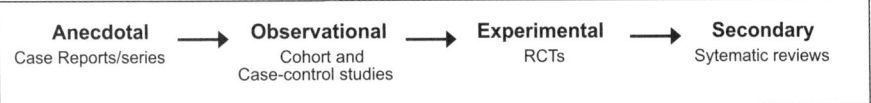

Just because a study ranks higher on the hierarchy of evidence does not necessarily mean that it can automatically be considered at a higher level of evidence than a lower-level study. For example, the results from a single RCT involving a small number of subjects are not necessarily more credible than reliable results from several high-quality trails that did not involve randomization. Systematic reviews are often helpful at sorting out this type of problem, although the position assigned in the evidentiary scheme is somewhat subjective and one ultimately has to trust the acumen of the review's authors.

Evidence Rating Systems

A number of different systems have been developed and subsequently described in the literature to facilitate rating the quality and class structure of biomedical evidence. Rating systems are used by authors of review articles, by experts involved in guidelines development,[46] and others. You too can utilize them as you consider incorporating evidence from the findings of various studies that you encounter into your EBC practice.

The position a given study has in the hierarchy of evidence plays a big part in the final determination produced by rating systems. The hierarchy schemes used to determine levels of evidence that are utilized by a few of these systems are presented in Table 1.4, which provides a sampling of the different methods that may be employed. All three methods shown in the table are quite similar, although my favorite is the one developed by the Scottish Intercollegiate Guidelines Network (SIGN).[50] As one might surmise from the title of the SIGN group, this evidence rating system was designed to be utilized to evaluate evidence in the process of developing guidelines. Also included are the systems from the Agency for Healthcare Research and Quality (AHRQ)[51] and the Oxford Centre for Evidence-based Medicine (CEBM).[52] The latter group's *Levels of Evidence* guide is designed to evaluate articles that deal with therapy/ prevention or etiology/harm.

TABLE 1.4 Comparison of the levels of evidence utilized by several sources

Scottish Intercollegiate Guidelines Network (SIGN) [50]		Agency for Healthcare Research and Quality (AHRQ) [51]		Oxford Centre for Evidence-based Medicine (CEBM) [52]
1++	High-quality meta-analyses, systematic reviews of randomized controlled trials (RCTs), or RCTs with a very low risk of bias	1	Randomized controlled trials	1a Systematic reviews (SR) with homogeneity* of randomized controlled trials
1+	Well-conducted meta-analyses, systematic reviews of RCTs, or RCTs with a low risk of bias	2	Controlled before–after (CBA): Contemporaneous observation periods for control and intervention groups before and after an intervention	1b Individual RCT with a narrow confidence interval
				1c All or none†
1−	Meta-analyses, systematic reviews of RCTs, or RCTs with a high risk of bias		Interrupted time series (ITS): Well-defined time period for intervention implementation and at least three time points both before and after intervention	2a SR with homogeneity of cohort studies
2++	High-quality systematic reviews of case-control or cohort studies, or high-quality case-control or cohort studies with a very low risk of confounding, bias, or chance and a high probability that the relationship is causal		Quasi-randomized trials: Contained at least two cohorts of patients assembled prospectively based on an allocation procedure that was nonrandom, but arbitrary, in the sense of bearing no apparent	2b Individual cohort study (including low-quality RCT; e.g., <80% follow-up)
				2c "Outcomes" research; ecological studies
				3a SR with homogeneity of case-control studies

Steps Involved in the Practice of Evidence-Based Chiropractic

2+ Well-conducted case-control or cohort studies with a low risk of confounding, bias, or chance and a moderate probability that the relationship is causal

2− Case-control or cohort studies with a high risk of confounding, bias, or chance and a significant risk that the relationship is not causal

3 Nonanalytic studies (e.g., case reports, case series)

4 Expert opinion

connection to patient or provider factors that might affect intervention outcome (e.g., alternation, date of birth, even/odd character of provider or patient identification)

3 Observational studies with controls: Includes before–after and time series not meeting strict definitions of CBA and ITS (see above), case-control studies, cohort studies with controls

4 Observational studies without controls (e.g., cohort studies without controls and case series)

3b Individual case-control study

4 Case series (and poor-quality cohort and case-control studies‡)

5 Expert opinion without explicit critical appraisal, or based on physiology, bench research, or "first principles"

---

* Systematic reviews that are free of worrisome variations in the directions and degrees of results between individual studies.
† Has to do with all patients dying before a treatment became available, but some now surviving once it is available.
‡ A poor-quality cohort or case-control study is one that fails to clearly define comparison groups, fails to measure exposures and outcomes in the same (preferably blinded) objective way in both exposed and nonexposed individuals, fails to identify or appropriately control known confounders, or fails to carry out a sufficiently long and complete follow-up of patients.

The levels of evidence used in these rating systems are presented side by side in Table 1.4, with corresponding levels of evidence aligned horizontally, although they do not match up precisely because of differences between the systems. Although there are subtle differences between the systems, essentially they all follow the pattern presented in the hierarchy of evidence pyramid in Figure 1.2.

Grading systems are an attempt to depict the relative strength of the evidence that is provided by a given study, which depends not only on its position in the hierarchy of study designs, but also on its validity. The *validity* of a study refers to the degree that the study design is able to produce final results that are dependable. In other words, are you able to trust the accuracy of a study's findings? Faulty designs that allow outside influences to sway the final results of a study may render it invalid to some degree.

Grades of recommendations are utilized by developers of guidelines to make comments about the appropriateness of various treatment and diagnostic procedures. The resulting recommendations are based on the quantity and quality of evidence that is available for the topic under investigation. The grades of recommendations that are used by SIGN are presented in Table 1.5. The numerical values derived from the SIGN levels of evidence are utilized to assign an A to D estimation of support for the procedures involved.

Articles that are encountered by practitioners using EBC should be critically appraised to establish whether the information they contain should be applied to a given set of clinical circumstances. To do this, the process of critical appraisal is utilized to determine whether the evidence they contain is valid and applicable to the particular circumstances. If it is, then the information can be utilized to make informed clinical decisions. If not, one may entirely reject the information or utilize only the portions of the article that are valid and applicable. Moreover, rating evidence is rarely a black and white process with regard to validity because the studies involved typically represent varying shades of gray. Although very few are extraordinarily valid and a few are awful, the vast majority fall somewhere in between.

Another very important piece of information to consider is that **evidence is almost never definitive**, especially when considering only a single study. The degree of confidence that one may have in evidence that is encountered depends on the strength of the research and how the various pieces of research on that topic are blended together.[53] This is why systematic reviews of the literature that

TABLE 1.5 Grades of recommendations utilized by the Scottish Intercollegiate Guidelines Network

A At least one meta-analysis, systematic review, or RCT rated as 1++ and directly applicable to the target population

or

A systematic review of RCTs or a body of evidence consisting principally of studies rated as 1+ directly applicable to the target population and demonstrating overall consistency of results

B A body of evidence including studies rated as 2++ directly applicable to the target population and demonstrating overall consistency of results

or

Extrapolated evidence from studies rated as 1++ or 1+

C A body of evidence including studies rated as 2+ directly applicable to the target population and demonstrating overall consistency of results

or

Extrapolated evidence from studies rated as 2++

D Evidence level 3 or 4

or

Extrapolated evidence from studies rated as 2+

---

combine all available studies on a particular topic are especially authoritative. The hierarchy of evidence is therefore not inflexible, and a poor-quality study of a design that is normally thought to be at a higher level may be outclassed by a well-done lower-level study. Likewise, evidence is not proof, and although hypotheses and theories may be supported to some extent by evidence, they can never be proven.

In addition to rating the evidence found in journal articles, you should perform similar evaluations of any other matters that have the potential to influence patient care. Examples include the content of professional seminars,[54] therapy equipment being considered for purchase, and even advice from practice management consultants. In this context, one should be concerned with the effectiveness and safety of therapeutic interventions, the dependability of diagnostic methods, and ethical issues.

Relationship of Chiropractic Philosophy to Evidence-Based Chiropractic

In its description of the *chiropractic paradigm*, the Association of Chiropractic Colleges[55] characterized the foundation of chiropractic as follows: "The foundation of chiropractic includes philosophy, science, art, knowledge, and clinical experience." Thus, *philosophy* is well established as one of the keystones of chiropractic. The meaning of chiropractic philosophy, however, is rather divergent among the various factions of the chiropractic profession and is misunderstood by many. Based on personal observation, it appears that most DCs consider chiropractic philosophy to be their fundamental beliefs and underlying principles about the profession. As a result, DCs are often said to *have* a philosophy of chiropractic, which in reality only constitutes a small part of the complete definition of philosophy, which follows:[56]

> 1) Love and pursuit of wisdom by intellectual means and moral self-discipline. 2) Investigation of the nature, causes, or principles of reality, knowledge, or values, based on logical reasoning rather than empirical methods. 3) A system of thought based on or involving such inquiry. 4) The critical analysis of fundamental assumptions or beliefs. 5) The disciplines presented in university curriculums of science and the liberal arts, except medicine, law, and theology. 6) The discipline comprising logic, ethics, aesthetics, metaphysics, and epistemology. 7) A set of ideas or beliefs relating to a particular field or activity; an underlying theory. 8) A system of values by which one lives.

Chiropractic philosophy, then, should be much more than merely a belief system, as depicted in definition 7, and DCs ought to make use of philosophy to its fullest extent. Furthermore, "chiropractic philosophy" is actually a misnomer, since philosophy is an activity that critically considers another subject. A better term would be the *philosophy of chiropractic*.[57]

A belief system taken to an extreme becomes *dogma*, defined as "an authoritative principle, belief, or statement of ideas or opinion, especially one considered to be absolutely true."[56] Some DCs are dogmatic in their beliefs and are reluctant to acknowledge new information, much less change their practices in response to new information. We all have a natural tendency to hold on to our beliefs and resist change, although this is often not a preferred method of dealing with new concepts. Philosophy, on the other hand, is something that when used effectively leads to a willingness to critically examine one's beliefs, drawing near to those that provide evidence of being true and abandoning those that are shown to be false. Surely most DCs would consider themselves to be philosophically minded rather than slaves of dogma, yet many are close-minded, or even argumentative, when challenged about chiropractic concepts such as technique and the vertebral subluxation. Seaman[58] went so far as to say that the chiropractic profession at large is plagued with dogmatism that affects both sides of the political fence. According to Keating and Mootz,[59] dogmatism is the principle barrier to a rational and unifying depiction of the role of chiropractors, as well as the furtherance of chiropractic science. So, rather than being close-minded and dogmatic about new ideas that challenge our old beliefs, we should welcome this evidence and try to incorporate it into our patient care.

The evidence that is utilized in the EBC process is founded on *science* (the observation, identification, description, experimental investigation, and theoretical explanation of phenomena) and the *scientific method* (the principles and empirical processes of discovery and demonstration considered characteristic of or necessary for scientific investigation, generally involving the observation of phenomena, the formulation of a hypothesis concerning the phenomena, experimentation to demonstrate the truth or falseness of the hypothesis, and a conclusion that validates or modifies the hypothesis).[56] Science has been a part of chiropractic since its inception, as evidenced by the title of one of the earliest of the profession's books, published in 1906, *The Science of Chiropractic; Its Principles and Adjustments*.[60] Nevertheless, science was misunderstood and very much neglected in the developing years of the profession.[25] There was a professionwide interest in scientific investigation, but there was a lack of understanding with regard to scientific principles, there were no mechanisms in place to train researchers, and financial resources were very scarce. In recent years, however, chiropractic has made significant headway toward improving its scientific state of affairs, and rather sophisticated chiropractic-related research is currently in progress at colleges and universities worldwide.[61] The findings of this research will facilitate the development of new chiropractic methods of diagnosis and treatment. Current methods of practice will ultimately be tested and those that are established as being valid and effective will continue, whereas those that are not found to be effective will be rejected, not paid for by insurance companies, and possibly barred by licensing agencies.

The point of this section on philosophy and EBC is that they should be complementary to each other and can be used by practicing DCs to provide care that is based on the best available evidence. It should be understood that there are no sacrosanct truths in chiropractic that are never to be questioned. Any conceivable chiropractic-related topic should be open for discussion, and nothing should be exempt from critical investigation. Furthermore, as doctors, DCs have the responsibility to make certain that the care that is provided is likely to be of benefit to patients and to reject harmful or ineffective practices. This will only come about through the open-minded self-evaluation of clinical practices using EBC methods.

References

1. Sackett, D.L., et al. *Evidence-Based Medicine: How to Practice and Teach EBM*. 2nd ed. 2000. Edinburgh: Churchill Livingstone.
2. Leach, R.A. *Evidence-based chiropractic: Critical thinking in the private-practice setting.* J Am Chiropr Assoc, 2005. **42**(1):37–46.
3. Bolton, J.E. *The evidence in evidence-based practice: what counts and what doesn't count? J Manipulative Physiol Ther*, 2001. **24**(5):362–6.
4. Sackett, D.L., et al. *Evidence based medicine: What it is and what it isn't. BMJ*, 1996. **312**(7023):71–2.
5. Straus, S.E., and F.A. McAlister. *Evidence-based medicine: A commentary on common criticisms. CMAJ*, 2000. **163**(7):837–41.
6. Rosenberg, W., and A. Donald. *Evidence based medicine: An approach to clinical problem-solving. BMJ*, 1995. **310**(6987):1122–6.
7. Strauss, S.E. *Evidence-Based Medicine: How to Practice and Teach EBM*. 3rd ed. 2005. Edinburgh and New York: Elsevier/Churchill Livingstone.
8. Kravitz, R.L. *Measuring patients' expectations and requests. Ann Intern Med*, 2001. **134**(9 Pt 2):881–8.
9. Hunink, M.G.M. *Does evidence based medicine do more good than harm? BMJ*, 2004. **329**(7473):1051.
10. Tonelli, M.R. *The limits of Evidence-Based medicine. Respir Care*, 2001. **46**(12):1435–40; discussion 1440–1.
11. McGuirk, B., et al. *Safety, efficacy, and cost effectiveness of Evidence-Based guidelines for the management of acute low back pain in primary care. Spine*, 2001. **26**(23):2615–22.
12. Guyatt, G. *Evidence-based medicine [Editorial]. ACP J Club*, 1991. **114**(A16).
13. Hawk, C., et al. *A randomized trial investigating a chiropractic manual placebo: A novel design using standardized forces in the delivery of active and control treatments. J Altern Complement Med*, 2005. **11**(1):109–17.

References

14. Budgell, B.S. *The placebo, the sensory trick and chiropractic. Chiropractic Journal of Australia*, 2004. **34**(2):58–62.
15. Rosner, A. *Fables or foibles: Inherent problems with RCTs. J Manipulative Physiol Ther*, 2003. **26**(7):460–7.
16. National Institutes of Health. *National Center for Complementary and Alternative Medicine*. 2005. http://nccam.nih.gov. Accessed January 16, 2006.
17. Bolton, J.E. *'Facts' and 'myths' about clinical research. Clinical Chiropractic*, 2004. **7**(3):107–11.
18. Terrett, A.G. *Misuse of the literature by medical authors in discussing spinal manipulative therapy injury. J Manipulative Physiol Ther*, 1995. **18**(4):203–10.
19. Murthy, J.M., and K.V. Naidu. *Aneurysm of the cervical internal carotid artery following chiropractic manipulation. J Neurol Neurosurg Psychiatry*, 1988. **51**(9):1237–8.
20. Terrett, A.G.J. *Current Concepts: Vertebrobasilar Complications Following Spinal Manipulation*. 2001. West Des Moines: NCMIC Group, 140.
21. Bronfort, G., et al. *Efficacy of spinal manipulation and mobilization for low back pain and neck pain: A systematic review and best evidence synthesis. The Spine Journal*, 2004. **4**(3):335–56.
22. Assendelft, W.J.J., et al. *Spinal manipulative therapy for low back pain: A meta-analysis of effectiveness relative to other therapies. Ann Intern Med*, 2003. **138**(11):871–81.
23. Delaney, P.M., and C.E. Fernandez. *Toward an Evidence-Based model for chiropractic education and practice. J Manipulative Physiol Ther*, 1999. **22**(2):114–8.
24. Feise, R. *An inquiry into chiropractors' intention to treat adolescent idiopathic scoliosis: A telephone survey. J Manipulative Physiol Ther*, 2001. **24**(3):177–82.
25. Keating, J.C., Jr., B.N. Green, and C.D. Johnson. *"Research" and "science" in the first half of the chiropractic century. J Manipulative Physiol Ther*, 1995. **18**(6):357–78.
26. Hess, D.R. *What is evidence-based medicine and why should I care? Respir Care*, 2004. **49**(7):730–41.
27. Balon, J.W., and S.A. Mior. *Chiropractic care in asthma and allergy. Ann Allergy Asthma Immunol*, 2004. **93**(2 Suppl 1):S55–60.
28. Troyanovich, S.J., D.D. Harrison, and D.E. Harrison. *Motion palpation: It's time to accept the evidence. J Manipulative Physiol Ther*, 1998. **21**(8):568–71.
29. Seffinger, M.A., et al. *Reliability of spinal palpation for diagnosis of back and neck pain: A systematic review of the literature. Spine*, 2004. **29**(19):E413–25.
30. Tarnow-Mordi, W.O., and M.J.R. Healy. *Distinguishing between "no evidence of effect" and "evidence of no effect" in randomised controlled trials and other comparisons. Arch Dis Child*, 1999. **80**(3):210–11.
31. Busse, J. *User's guide to the chiropractic literature–1A: How to use an article about therapy. J Manipulative Physiol Ther*, 2004. **27**(1):71–2.
32. Shaneyfelt, T.M., M.F. Mayo-Smith, and J. Rothwangl. *Are guidelines following guidelines? The methodological quality of clinical practice guidelines in the peer-reviewed medical literature. JAMA*, 1999. **281**(20):1900–5.
33. Haldeman, S., D. Chapman-Smith, and D.M. Petersen. *Guidelines for Chiropractic Quality Assurance and Practice Parameters: Proceedings of the Mercy Center Consensus Conference*. 1993, Gaithersburg: Aspen Publishers, xli, 222.

34. Lewkovich, G., et al. *An analysis of the ACOEM occupational medicine practice guidelines with recommendations for improvement. J Am Chiropr Assoc*, 2005. **42**(1):29–36.
35. Adams, K., et al. *Ethical considerations of complementary and alternative medical therapies in conventional medical settings. Ann Inter Med*, 2002. **137**(8):660–4.
36. Gordon, J. *Tired of killer 'cures'? The Washington Post*, 2002, HE01, August 20.
37. Keating, J.C., Jr. *Toward a Philosophy of the Science of Chiropractic: A Primer for Clinicians*. 1992. Stockton: Stockton Foundation for Chiropractic Research, 314.
38. Dobbie, A.E., et al. *What evidence supports teaching evidence-based medicine? Acad Med*, 2000. **75**(12):1184–85.
39. Clinicians for the Restoration of Autonomous Practice (CRAP) Writing Group, *EBM: Unmasking the Ugly Truth. BMJ*, 2002. **325**(7378):1496–8.
40. Richardson, W.S., et al. *The well-built clinical question: A key to evidence-based decisions. ACP J Club*, 1995. **123**(3):A12–3.
41. Braunwald, E., et al. *Harrison's Online*. 2005. McGraw-Hill. http://www.accessmedicine.com/home.aspx.
42. Rose, B.D., ed. *UpToDate*. 2005. http://uptodate.com.
43. Shaughnessy, A.F., and D.C. Slawson. *POEMs: Patient-oriented evidence that matters. Ann Intern Med*, 1997. **126**(8):667.
44. Shaughnessy, A.F., and J. Siwek. *Introducing POEMs. Am Fam Physician*, 2003. **67**(6):1196–8.
45. Eddy, D.M. *Clinical decision making: From theory to practice. Anatomy of a decision. JAMA*, 1990. **263**(3):441–3.
46. Shekelle, P.G., et al. *Clinical guidelines: Developing guidelines. BMJ*, 1999. **318**(7183):593–6.
47. Greenhalgh, T. *How to read a paper: Assessing the methodological quality of published papers. BMJ*, 1997. **315**(7103):305–8.
48. Sackett, D.L. *Evidence-based medicine. Spine*, 1998. **23**(10):1085–6.
49. Doig, G.S., and F. Simpson. *Efficient literature searching: A core skill for the practice of evidence-based medicine. Intensive Care Med*, 2003. **29**(12):2119–27.
50. Harbour, R., and J. Miller. *A new system for grading recommendations in evidence based guidelines. BMJ*, 2001. **323**(7308):334–6.
51. West, S., et al. *Systems to Rate the Strength of Scientific Evidence (Evidence Report/Technology Assessment No. 47; AHRQ Publication No. 02-E016)*. 2002. Rockville: Agency for Healthcare Research and Quality, 204.
52. Phillips, B., et al. *Levels of Evidence and Grades of Recommendation*. 2001. Headington, Oxford: Centre for Evidence-Based Medicine, University Department of Psychiatry, Warneford Hospital.
53. Lohr, K.N. *Rating the strength of scientific evidence: Relevance for quality improvement programs. Int J Qual Health Care*, 2004. **16**(1):9–18.
54. Green, B.N., C.D. Johnson, and A. Adams. *Caveat emptor! Evaluate and maximize your technique seminar experience. Topics in Clinical Chiropractic*, 1998. **5**(2):19–26.
55. Association of Chiropractic Colleges. *The Chiropractic Paradigm*. 2003. Bethesda, MD: Association of Chiropractic Colleges.
56. *The American Heritage Dictionary of the English Language*. 4th ed. 2000. Boston: Houghton Mifflin.

57. Coulter, I.D. *Chiropractic: a philosophy for Alternative Health Care*. 1999. Oxford and Boston: Butterworth-Heinemann, 16.
58. Seaman, D. *Philosophy and science versus dogmatism in the practice of chiropractic. J Chiro Humanities*, 1998. **8**(1):55–66.
59. Keating, J.C., Jr., and R.D. Mootz. *The influence of political medicine on chiropractic dogma: Implications for scientific development. J Manipulative Physiol Ther*, 1989. **12**(5):393–8.
60. Palmer, D.D., and B.J. Palmer. *The Science of Chiropractic; its Principles and Adjustments*. 1906. Davenport: The Palmer School of Chiropractic, 1.
61. Haldeman, S. *The evolution of chiropractic—science and theory. FCER Advance*, 2001. **22**(1):3, 6, 19, 22, 25.

CHAPTER

TWO

Types of Evidence

This chapter introduces some of the evidence resources available to EBC practitioners and discusses methods of evaluating their quality. When seeking evidence, there are a number of sources to choose from: articles in scientific journals, textbooks, conference proceedings, advice from colleagues, continuing education seminars, practice guidelines, videotapes, websites, and others. I have denoted only those that (in my opinion) are the most important and trustworthy. The focus of this chapter is on chiropractic resources, to the exclusion of most information relating to other disciplines. This emphasis on chiropractic material is merely for the sake of brevity, not because nonchiropractic resources are thought to be unimportant to EBC practitioners.

Some evidence sources are more important to clinical decision making than others, as shown by the hierarchy of evidence for research designs that was introduced in Chapter 1. To facilitate finding the best and most appropriate EBC information as efficiently as possible, one should determine what the best sources of evidence are prior to beginning the search process. Resources that are less reliable or are lower in the hierarchy of evidence often contain useful information; accordingly, they should not be categorically dismissed. Nevertheless, they should not be the first choice for evidence, and their content should be appraised very carefully prior to using them in clinical decision making.

Peer Review

One of the main criteria that EBC practitioners may use to determine the credibility of health care journals is to ascertain whether *peer review* was utilized. A peer-reviewed journal can be defined as "one that has submitted most of its published articles for review by experts who are not part of the editorial staff."[1] These journals typically have an editorial board made up of experts in the field who have agreed to review submitted manuscripts for quality and importance. The editorial board reviewers typically provide a critique that indicates whether the article should be accepted for publication and any changes that may be necessary. In contrast, articles in trade journals or magazines are typically only reviewed by an editor, who determines whether the topic is of interest to readers and then edits the article with regard to proper grammar and spelling. The peer-review process is generally accepted to be the best method available for ensuring that articles found in biomedical journals are of the highest quality. Because EBC practitioners seek the best evidence possible, nearly all articles that are utilized will have gone through this process. Moreover, practitioners who assume that there is no distinction between reading peer-reviewed versus non-peer-reviewed articles may be the greatest source of error in the EBC process.[2]

Editors of peer-reviewed journals are obliged to publish their peer-review policies in an obvious place within the journal, although some do not.[3] When present, these policies can usually be found in the "Instructions to Authors" section of the journal. *Blinding* (also known as *masking*) of reviewers is one of the more important peer-review policies, which involves the journal's editor removing any traces of the names of the article's authors prior to sending copies out to the reviewers. A study of blinding at a number of medical journals found that the procedure was successful among about 60% of the reviewers involved.[4] Blinding is a crucial step in the review process because most members of editorial boards are published authors themselves and have advanced knowledge about the topic of the submission. Without blinding, reviewers would most likely recognize other published authors, which might bias their opinions.[5] Conversely, if they had never heard of the authors involved, the reviewers might be biased in the opposite direction. Articles are usually sent to two or more reviewers to help ameliorate this and other potential biases. Blinding is generally thought to improve the quality of reviews, although one study showed that it really didn't change their outcomes very much.[6]

Reviewers evaluate articles submitted to journals regarding a variety of issues in an effort to determine whether the involved research is valid and whether the article's conclusions are appropriate. Reviewers are expected to appraise manuscripts critically but constructively and then prepare comments about the manuscript and the related research that will help authors improve their work. Based on the findings of their appraisal, recommendations are made to the journal's editor with regard to the suitability of the manuscript for publication.

Some of the points considered by reviewers during peer review are as follows:

1. The topic of investigation should be important, original, and worth reporting.
2. Allusions to other published research should be accurate.
3. Appropriate research methods should be employed.
4. Data collection and the resulting statistical analysis should be performed correctly.
5. The manuscript's assertions should be logically and clearly stated.
6. The manuscript should be well written and organized.
7. The writing style should be of high quality as expected in scientific publication.
8. Spelling and grammar should be correct.

When one or more of these points are deficient, reviewers have the option to reject the manuscript or require that the authors make corrective revisions. Since two or three reviewers are usually involved in this process, disagreements are common. In these cases, the journal's editor may decide to accept or reject the manuscript based on the conflicting opinions or send it to another reviewer for a tie-breaking review. It has been shown that reviewers trained in epidemiology or statistics are more likely to produce good reviews,[7] so a tie-breaking reviewer might be selected based on his or her advanced knowledge in these areas.

The peer-review process was designed to ensure that information published in scientific journals is accurate and of sufficient quality to be included. This safeguard is not present in trade journals, magazines, seminars, and even textbooks. Consequently, non-peer-reviewed resources will be less reliable and require extra caution when reading them. The process is not flawless, however, and inaccurate information is commonly published in peer-reviewed journals. Because of this situation, all articles utilized in EBC must be critically appraised to verify their validity.

Indexing

High-quality journals are typically indexed by one or more of the major biomedical databases. As a result, this becomes another way to ascertain the credibility of scientific journals. Journals that are not included in these databases may be substandard and their content may accordingly lack validity. *Indexing* is a process whereby certain biomedical journals are included in a list that becomes a part of a database. The databases are designed to facilitate searching for specific articles that are included in the listed journals. There are a number of databases of interest to EBC practitioners, which all have similar criteria regarding which journals they include. In general, to be accepted for inclusion in a biomedical database, journals must be of high quality and incorporate research that is relevant to the database's area of emphasis.

In the case of MEDLINE, the decision to accept or reject a journal for indexing is made by the director of the National Library of Medicine and is based on consideration of both scientific quality and the policy of the library's Board of Regents.[8] Journals that are not peer-reviewed are not typically eligible for inclusion in MEDLINE. Other selection criteria utilized by MEDLINE include the quality of content, the quality of editorial work (e.g., methods of selecting articles and adherence to ethical guidelines), printing and layout quality, whether the journal's audience consists of health professionals, and the geographic coverage. Decisions regarding whether a journal should be indexed may also relate to how long the journal has been publishing and how well it has been able to maintain a consistent publication schedule.

Chiropractic journals, along with those of several other allied health professions (in particular the complementary and alternative health professions) are inadequately covered by MEDLINE. In fact, at the time of this writing, only three chiropractic journals were indexed in MEDLINE: the *Journal of Manipulative and Physiological Therapeutics*, *Chiropractic and Osteopathy*, and *Chiropractic History*. The National Library of Medicine has thus far chosen not to include the other peer-reviewed chiropractic journals. Presumably, only the director of the National Library of Medicine knows the reasons for this omission, although one can surmise that they are probably the same as what has kept chiropractic on the outside of state-funded education, widespread granting of hospital privileges, and many other medical-related programs. Because of this exclusion of chiropractic journals, it is often difficult to locate chiropractic-specific information solely using PubMed/MEDLINE. As a result, other databases must be searched to obtain better results.

Because of the omission of most chiropractic journals by MEDLINE and the need for chiropractic-oriented databases, several others have been created. One such database is the Manual Alternative and Natural Therapy Index System (MANTIS), which primarily includes journals having to do with manipulation and natural therapies. Another is the Index to Chiropractic Literature (ICL), which is more specific to chiropractic journals. Chiropractic literature is also indexed in the Cumulative Index to Nursing and Allied Health Literature (CINAHL), which incorporates peer-reviewed and a few non-peer-reviewed chiropractic journals. The final database to be mentioned, relative to the inclusion of chiropractic journals, is AMED, which is a British database that includes references dealing with several allied medical professions, complementary medicine, and palliative care. A recent study compared the ability of some of these databases to retrieve complementary and alternative care information concerning a spine-related topic and found MANTIS to be superior.[9]

Sources of Evidence

Textbooks are a great information source when background material is needed on a specific topic, although they are usually not very current. The textbook writing and publication process is often protracted. As a result, the information they contain may be several years old by the time the book is published. With this in mind, online textbooks such as *Harrison's Online*[10] are usually a better option when looking for current background information because they are updated frequently.

Conferences are another possible source of information, although they have not been shown very effective at teaching adult learners, especially when they utilize passive educational models.[11] Furthermore, it appears that little or no change occurs in the behavior of practitioners or the outcomes of their patients following this type of learning.[12] Information obtained from colleagues also qualifies as evidence, which may at times be very useful, although it is potentially biased and may be unreliable. In general, it makes sense to obtain the sources that a colleague may have relied on in order to verify the accuracy of his or her interpretation, as well as the validity of the referenced material.

Journal articles are another source of evidence, containing information that is vitally important to the practice of EBC. However, their quantity is overwhelming, with more than 16 million articles being indexed on PubMed alone.[13] Reading only the articles of interest to DCs would be an insurmountable task for even the most dedicated practitioner. There are also several newsletters available that provide synopses of current relevant chiropractic-related research that can be helpful in the quest to stay current. Keep in mind that newsletter synopses may be slanted or inaccurate in relation to the qualifications and veracity of the newsletter's editor.

Publications that are germane to the practice of EBC have contents with varying degrees of trustworthiness. At the pinnacle are journals that are peer-reviewed by blinded experts and are indexed in the more selective databases. This category of journal contains scientific articles that tend to embrace reliable evidence due to the screening process that articles must go through before acceptance. In addition, authors tend to be selective when submitting manuscripts to these types of journals because they know that the article's content will be rigorously scrutinized. Ordinarily, work that does not meet such high standards will instead be submitted to non-peer-reviewed publications. This is not to say that all submissions to non-peer-reviewed publications are of poor quality. In fact, some of these articles are especially useful, although their adherence to scientific rigor may be deficient.

Journals that are peer-reviewed and indexed are considered to be at the high end of the evidence spectrum, whereas those that are neither peer-reviewed nor indexed are considered to be a less desirable form of evidence. These less desirable publications encompass trade journals from the national, state, and local professional organizations; various periodicals that contain news, practice management, and technical information; and "advertorial" publications, which have the potential to contain very biased material.

Journals

In addition to peer review and indexing, high-quality scholarly journals have a number of features that, when present, are indicators that the journal is likely to yield evidence that is trustworthy. In general, scholarly journals have a serious appearance, with few glossy pages or exciting pictures. However, they commonly contain lots of illustrations, graphs, and charts. The articles in these journals are written by experts in the field who are actively conducting research. The language that is utilized assumes a scholarly background on the part of the reader that is germane to the field being covered. Information sources are always cited in the reference section of the articles. The primary function of scholarly journals is to report the results of research being carried out in a particular field of study to other scholars.

Articles that are utilized in EBC originate from either primary or secondary sources. Primary sources include literature that is derived from original research, which provides a firsthand account of the work of the author or authors involved. This is where the researchers who have actually conducted the studies report their findings. Original research represents the most current research or scholarly dialogue on a given subject. Secondary literature, on the other hand, is a synthesis or overview of theories or existing research. Edited books or textbooks may also be classified as secondary literature. Review articles, a common form of secondary literature, summarize the research on a certain topic. They are often written by an expert in the field and typically contain a large number of references.

An inventory of some of the more reliable publications of chiropractic literature is provided alphabetically in Table 2.1. The journals' Internet addresses (also known as Uniform Resource Locators, or URLs) are provided below the description of each journal. Keep in mind that chiropractic journals have historically had a tendency to come and go (as do URLs) and that this list was current as of 2006.

Newsletters

It would be ideal if all practitioners were dedicated enough to read several research journals per month in order to stay current in the field. Realistically, however, many are not willing to take the time and put forth the effort to read this much material, or they may not have the training needed to critique the articles even if they did read them. As an alternative, although not preferred, a realistic way to acquire current information that involves substantially less time and effort is to subscribe to and read professional review newsletters. Newsletters covering chiropractic-related issues are available from a variety of sources, some of which are trustworthy whereas others are not. If at all possible, these publications should not be relied on as the only means of staying current. Another, more constructive,

TABLE 2.1 Chiropractic journals

***Chiropractic History* [Chiropr Hist]:** Published by the Association for the History of Chiropractic, an international organization that was established in 1980 to promote the scholarly recording of the profession's history. Peer-reviewed and indexed in MEDLINE, MANTIS, and ICL.
URL: http://historyofchiropractic.org/historyofchiropractic/chiro_history.html

***Chiropractic Journal of Australia (CJA)*:** Published by the Chiropractors Association of Australia (National) Limited. Published in March, June, September, and December. Indexed by the Australian Medical Index, the British Library Complementary Medicine Index, CINAHL, MANTIS, ICL, and the Australian Public Affairs Information Service.
URL: http://www.chiropractors.asn.au/cjournal/cjamain.htm

***Chiropractic and Osteopathy* [Chiropr Osteopat]:** Edited by Bruce F. Walker, this Open Access journal published by BioMed Central is a continuation of the former journal *Australasian Chiropractic and Osteopathic*. It encompasses all aspects of evidence-based information that are clinically relevant to chiropractors, osteopaths and related health care professionals. Peer-reviewed and indexed in MEDLINE and MANTIS.
URL: http://www.chiroandosteo.com

***Clinical Chiropractic*:** The official journal of the College of Chiropractors (United Kingdom). It endeavors to provide authoritative information to clinical chiropractors to aid in the development of their professional career, clinical skills, and performance to deliver optimal patient care. Published quarterly by Elsevier. Peer-reviewed and indexed by CINAHL and ICL.
URL: http://intl.elsevierhealth.com//journals/clch/Default.cfm

***Journal of the American Chiropractic Association (JACA) Online*:** An official journal of the American Chiropractic Association. Peer-reviewed and published monthly, *JACA* is dedicated to the advancement of chiropractic health care principles and practice. Research papers and scholarly work are published in the Research and Science section. Indexed in MANTIS, CINAHL, ICL, and SPORTDiscus.
URL: http://www.amerchiro.org/publications/jaca_index.cfm

***Journal of the Canadian Chiropractic Association (JCCA)*:** Published since 1957, *JCCA* is published quarterly by the Canadian Chiropractic Association "as a medium of communication between the Association and its members and is a forum for fair comment and discussion of all matters of general interest to the chiropractic profession and the association." *JCCA* is peer-reviewed and indexed by CINAHL, MANTIS, British Library Complementary Medicine Index, ICL, and PASCAL (1998), and selectively in SPORTDiscus.
URL: http://www.jcca-online.org/

Journal of Chiropractic Education (JCE): The official journal of the Association of Chiropractic Colleges, it is published twice a year. Its mission is to promote excellence in chiropractic education through the publication of research and scholarly articles concerned with educational theory, methods, and content relevant to the practice of chiropractic. Peer-reviewed and indexed in MANTIS, CINAHL, and ICL.
URL: http://www.datatrace.com/medical/JCE_body.htm

Journal of Chiropractic Humanities: Published by the National University of Health Sciences, the primary purpose of this journal is to foster learned debate and interaction within the chiropractic profession regarding the uses of philosophical and sociological scholarship in advancing the chiropractic tenets. Peer-reviewed and indexed in MANTIS, CINAHL, and ICL.
URL: http://www.journalchirohumanities.com

Journal of Chiropractic Medicine: Formerly known as the *Journal of Chiropractic Technique*, this journal is devoted to providing a forum for the chiropractic profession to disseminate information dedicated to the developing primary care emphasis within the profession. Peer-reviewed and indexed in MANTIS and ICL.
URL: http://www.journalchiromed.com/

Journal of Clinical Chiropractic Pediatrics (JCCP): Published quarterly by the International Chiropractors Association, Council on Chiropractic Pediatrics. *JCCP*'s primary focus is the clinical care of mothers and children. Peer-reviewed and indexed in MANTIS and ICL.
URL: http://www.chiropractic.org

***Journal of Manipulative and Physiological Therapeutics (JMPT)* [J Manipulative Physiol Ther]:** Published by the National University of Health Sciences. Dedicated to the advancement of chiropractic health care, *JMPT* provides the latest information on current developments in therapeutics, as well as reviews of clinically oriented research and practical information for use in clinical settings. Peer-reviewed and indexed in MEDLINE, MANTIS, Current Contents/Clinical Medicine, and ICL.
URL: http://journals.elsevierhealth.com/periodicals/ymmt

Journal of Vertebral Subluxation Research (JVSR): Publishes contributions relevant to the vertebral subluxation and other variables that may affect the condition. Articles dealing with the anatomical, physiological, biomechanical, philosophical, clinical, epidemiological, legal, theoretical, administrative, technical, and practice realms that relate to the progressive model of vertebral subluxation, are within the domain of its publication content. *JVSR* is peer-reviewed and indexed in MANTIS and ICL.
URL: http://www.jvsr.com/index.asp

Note: Journals are listed in alphabetical order. Brackets indicate MEDLINE abbreviations.

approach is to use the newsletters as an introduction and guide to pertinent articles. The selected articles can subsequently be retrieved for thorough reading and evaluation.

Some newsletters are of a very high quality and some are substandard, so it is important to examine their quality before making a decision about which ones to subscribe to. First, evaluate the qualifications of the newsletter's editorial board to see if some of the acknowledged experts in the field are represented. Be wary if there is no editorial board, if there is only one editor, or if the members of the board are unknown to you or lack credentials. A second area of concern involves newsletters that are sponsored by technique proponents, practice management companies, or manufacturers of chiropractic-related products. Although none of these areas of concern should be considered an absolute reason for nonsubscription, they are red flags that require further investigation. For instance, *Back into Research* is listed in Table 2.2 as a newsletter useful to EBC, yet there is only one editor (James M. Cox, DC, DACBR) and he is a proponent of a chiropractic technique. However, Dr. Cox is a well-known and respected author who would certainly be considered an expert in the field, the newsletter has a long track record, and sample copies are provided that allow potential readers to verify its veracity. Table 2.2 provides an alphabetical list of a few of the better newsletters of interest to chiropractors that you may want to consider.

Websites

Table 2.3 lists some websites that DCs who are involved in EBC should find helpful. Keep in mind, however, that most of these are medical resources, so antichiropractic biases may exist. As an example, a comment on manipulation as a treatment for neck pain that was offered by Paul Shekelle, MD in the *ACP Journal Club* asserted "Because neck manipulation has no proven benefit compared with mobilization and has been associated with serious, albeit rare, adverse events, neck manipulation cannot be recommended and should be avoided."[14] In effect, Dr. Shekelle denounced one of the primary interventions utilized in chiropractic in favor of mobilization, based only on observations that vertebral artery dissection and stroke occur in some people after receiving neck manipulation. There are several reasons that this opinion is erroneous. First, no studies capable of determining whether a cause-and-effect relationship exists between neck manipulation and stroke have ever been carried out. Studies thus far have only been observational,

Websites

TABLE 2.2 Newsletters useful to EBC

The Back Letter: Published by Lippincott Williams & Wilkins, *The Back Letter* is a monthly newsletter that delivers evidence-based information needed to stay current regarding the diagnosis and treatment of spinal problems and back pain. It is written in consultation with Sam W. Wiesel, MD, and an eminently qualified editorial board, one-third of whom have chiropractic degrees.
URL: http://www.lww.com/product/?0894-7376

The Chiropractic Report: Published by Chiropractic Report, Inc., of Toronto, Canada, *The Chiropractic Report* is an international review of professional and research issues published six times per year. It has an international interdisciplinary editorial board and is the largest subscription-based publication in the chiropractic profession. Its purpose is to provide chiropractors and others in the health care system the most important new information relevant to chiropractic and to provide chiropractors with a tool for promoting referral of patients who can benefit from chiropractic care.
URL: http://www.chiropracticreport.com

Chiropractic Research Review: A 12-page monthly newsletter that reviews chiropractic-related research papers from more than 100 scientific journals. Published by Dynamic Chiropractic and National Chiropractic Mutual Insurance Company. Features articles that review the latest research, covering a broad range of topics applicable to chiropractic practice, including clinical chiropractic, musculoskeletal health, pediatrics, diagnostics, sports/fitness, women's health, senior health, general health, and nutrition.
URL: http://www.chiropracticresearchreview.com

The Week in Chiropractic: Published by the Foundation for Chiropractic Education and Research (FCER), *The Week in Chiropractic* is a news and research bulletin especially for chiropractors. It provides information on chiropractic and health care in general, plus capsule summaries of current research. Free via e-mail. Also available from FCER at the same URL is the free ***FCER Advance*** **magazine**. Published quarterly, it contains news, articles, interviews, and research information of interest to the chiropractic professional.
URL: http://www.fcer.org/subscribe.htm

and many times observed relationships are merely coincidental rather than causative. Just because one event follows another event does not mean that the first one caused the second. Indeed, it is thought that many of the implicated patients were actually experiencing symptoms of vertebral artery dissection (unilateral neck pain, headache, etc.) and that this is what prompted them to seek chiropractic care. Second, it is inappropriate to discard cervical manipulation based on existing evidence that has to do with the "observation" that many of these patients had predisposing factors that may have been contributory (e.g., ultrastructural connective tissue abnormalities, elevated homocysteine levels, and recent infection).[15]

TABLE 2.3 Websites useful to EBC

AccessMedicine (C): Published by McGraw-Hill, this resource is updated daily and contains the full text, graphics, images, and illustrations of the most recent editions of world-class medical references. *Includes Harrison's Online, Current Medical Diagnosis and Treatment, Fitzpatrick's Color Atlas Online*, and several others.
URL: http://www3.accessmedicine.com

ACP Journal Club (C): Published by the American College of Physicians, the *ACP Journal Club* site contains the cumulative contents of the journal's bimonthly print edition since its inception in 1991. The content is carefully selected from over 100 clinical journals through reliable application of explicit criteria for scientific merit, followed by assessment of relevance to medical practice by clinical specialists. Commentary by ACP authors provides clinical recommendations.
URL: http://www.acpjc.org

Centre for Evidence Based Medicine (F): Produced by the University of Toronto, this website was designed to help develop, disseminate, and evaluate resources that can be used to practice and teach EBM for undergraduate, postgraduate, and continuing education for health care professionals from a variety of clinical disciplines.
URL: http://www.cebm.utoronto.ca

Centre for Reviews and Dissemination (F): Established in January 1994 by the University of York in the United Kingdom. Aims to provide research-based information about the effects of interventions used in health and social care.
URL: http://www.york.ac.uk/inst/crd

Chiropractic Resource Organization (F): A nonpartisan Internet site that is both for chiropractors and maintained by chiropractors. The website is sectioned into projects with chiropractors volunteering to be responsible for the information contained in each section.
URL: http://www.chiro.org

Clinical Evidence (C): Published by the BMJ Group, *Clinical Evidence* is an international source of the best available evidence for effective health care. Informed decision making is promoted by summarizing what's known—and not known—about nearly 200 medical conditions and over 2,000 treatments.
URL: http://www.clinicalevidence.com

eMedicine.com (F): The largest and most current clinical knowledge base available to physicians and health professionals. Nearly 10,000 physician authors and editors contribute to the eMedicine clinical knowledge base, which contains articles on 7,000 diseases and disorders. Content undergoes four levels of physician peer review plus an additional review by a PharmD. eMedicine.com, Inc., is a privately held company.
URL: http://www.emedicine.com

***Gray's Anatomy of the Human Body* (F):** The Bartleby.com edition of *Gray's Anatomy* features 1,247 engravings—many in color—from the classic 1918 publication, as well as a subject index with 13,000 entries.
URL: http://www.bartleby.com/107

Websites 51

***The Cochrane Library* (C):** Published on a quarterly basis, *The Cochrane Library* provides current dependable information on the effects of interventions in health care. *The Cochrane Library* is designed to provide information and evidence to support decisions taken in health care and to inform those receiving care. Includes systematic evidence reviews that are updated periodically by the Cochrane Group. Reviewers discuss whether adequate data are available for the development of EBM guidelines for diagnosis or management. *The Cochrane Library* is published by Wiley InterScience and is available on a subscription basis.
URL: http://www.thecochranelibrary.org

***The Merck Manual of Diagnosis and Therapy* (F):** Produced by Merck & Company, Inc., one of the world's largest pharmaceutical companies, the *Merck Manual* is a searchable online textbook that covers subjects that are relevant to internal medicine.
URL: http://www.merck.com/mrkshared/mmanual/home.jsp

National Guideline Clearinghouse (NGC) (F): A public resource for evidence-based clinical practice guidelines. NGC is an initiative of the Agency for Healthcare Research and Quality (AHRQ), part of the U.S. Department of Health and Human Services.
URL: http://www.guideline.gov

PubMed Central (PMC) (F): PMC is a digital archive of life sciences journal literature, developed and managed by the National Center for Biotechnology Information at the U.S. National Library of Medicine. PMC provides unrestricted access to the electronic literature, where free full-text articles may be retrieved. There is a growing tendency to publish material online only, to the exclusion of print, and PMC targets these journals.
URL: http://www.pubmedcentral.gov

TRIP Database (C): Produced by TRIP Database, Ltd., its aim is to allow health professionals to easily find the highest-quality material available on the Web. The TRIP Database has the world's largest explicit collection of evidence-based articles, clinical guidelines, and medical images. Query-answering services are available that allow users to ask clinical questions, which are then answered by specialists.
URL: http://www.tripdatabase.com

***UpToDate* (C):** This privately owned resource is specifically designed to quickly and easily answer the clinical questions that arise in daily practice so that it can be used right at the point of care. *UpToDate* is an official educational program of a number of major medical associations, including the American College of Rheumatology.
URL: http://www.uptodate.com

Note: Websites are notorious for changing their Internet addresses periodically. As a result, the URLs provided may be incorrect; in this case, simply search the Internet using the website's name (printed in bold in the table). Sites are listed in alphabetical order. F, free access; C, charge for access.

Then again, even if there was an established cause-and-effect relationship in this area, the incidence rate is so low that neck manipulation would still be considered a safe treatment. This issue is complicated and controversial, but is certainly a good example of medical bias against chiropractic. Moreover, DCs should be wary of this bias against chiropractic and manipulation that may be present within any source that is derived from medical authors.[16]

Regrettably, at this time there are no websites created specifically for DCs that have rigorous screening methods in place like some of the established medical websites do (e.g., the *Cochrane Library*[17] or *UpToDate*[18]). The Chiropractic Resource Organization is a useful nonprofit website that contains a large amount of material relevant to EBC, although the content of the various sections is at the discretion of volunteer DCs, who are responsible for developing and maintaining their assigned section. Other than volunteering for the task, contributing DCs apparently are not required to meet any eligibility criteria in order to head a section. Some of the content is derived from peer-reviewed journals, but much of it is merely shared information from other DCs. I hesitate to mention this website as a resource for EBC because of these limitations; accordingly, the website is listed in Table 2.3 with a caveat to check the sources of its subject matter for accuracy. Even considering its limitations, however, it is a worthwhile Internet resource for chiropractors.

Evaluating Health Websites

There is no screening or censorship on the Internet; as a result, many websites contain false or misleading information. This is especially true of health-related websites, which can range in quality from abysmal to extraordinary. Consequently, the truism "caveat emptor" (let the buyer beware) applies when considering information from this nearly inexhaustible source. Refer to the appendices for a *health information websites evaluation checklist* that will facilitate appraising them. A number of other tools are available to evaluate Internet health resources, although none of them (including this one) has been established as being effective.[19] When considering health information from the Internet, keep in mind that anyone with a computer and an Internet connection can publish a website. A beautifully constructed and professional looking website may signify a talented webmaster, but not necessarily reliable health information. This especially applies to many commercial websites, which may offer health information that is biased toward a product or service that is marketed by the owner of the site.

The Internet has provided extensive access to health information for professionals, as well as the public. This is a positive step, on the one hand, since it has a great potential to advance knowledge and improve communication among decision makers. On the other hand, it has created a number of problems, including patient harm.[20] Due to its enormity, the Internet can be confusing, and finding useful health information may be time-consuming. Even when found, the information is often of questionable validity and may be contradictory. Erroneous information derived from the Internet could possibly negatively affect a person's health because of resulting incorrect decision making.[21]

The University of Maryland's Center for Integrative Medicine provides some general direction to assist with the evaluation of health websites, especially those dealing with complementary and alternative medicine.[22] Essentially, the same standards used to assess the value of printed health information apply to the Internet. The standards of evaluation that they have proposed are as follows:

- *Authorship*: The affiliations and qualifications of authors should be provided.
- *Attribution*: References and sources of information for the website's content should be provided, along with pertinent copyright information.
- *Disclosure*: The ownership and sponsorship of health websites and discussion forums should be fully disclosed and prominently displayed. Furthermore, any advertising, underwriting, commercial funding arrangements, or other potential conflicts of interest (including financial remuneration for links to other websites) should be disclosed.
- *Currency*: The dates on which the website's content was posted or updated should be provided.

As with other less desirable sources of information, one should be wary of any information derived from the Internet that fails to meet these standards. The information would have to be validated by comparison with other sources that are already established as being reliable.

The Health on the Net Foundation is an organization that has established a code of conduct for medical and health websites, as well as providing accreditation to those that qualify. The Health on the Net Foundation's code of conduct[23] mentions eight principles of compliance, which can also be used for appraising these sources (Table 2.4).

TABLE 2.4 Health on the Net Foundation's code of conduct for medical and health websites

1. *Authority:* Any medical or health advice provided and hosted on this site will only be given by medically trained and qualified professionals unless a clear statement is made that a piece of advice offered is from a nonmedically qualified individual or organization.
2. *Complementarity:* The information provided on this site is designed to support, not replace, the relationship that exists between a patient/site visitor and his or her existing physician.
3. *Confidentiality:* Confidentiality of data relating to individual patients and visitors to a medical/health website, including their identity, is respected by this website. The website owners undertake to honor or exceed the legal requirements of medical/health information privacy that apply in the country and state where the website and mirror sites are located.
4. *Attribution:* Where appropriate, information contained on this site will be supported by clear references to source data and, where possible, have specific HTML links to that data. The date when a clinical page was last modified will be clearly displayed (e.g., at the bottom of the page).
5. *Justifiability:* Any claims relating to the benefits/performance of a specific treatment, commercial product or service, will be supported by appropriate, balanced evidence in the manner outlined in principle 4.
6. *Transparency of authorship:* The designers of this website will seek to provide information in the clearest possible manner and provide contact addresses for visitors that seek further information or support. The webmaster will display his or her e-mail address clearly throughout the website.
7. *Transparency of sponsorship:* Support for this website will be clearly identified, including the identities of commercial and noncommercial organizations that have contributed funding, services or material for the site.
8. *Honesty in advertising and editorial policy:* If advertising is a source of funding, it will be clearly stated. A brief description of the advertising policy adopted by the website owners will be displayed on the site. Advertising and other promotional material will be presented to viewers in a manner and context that facilitates differentiation between it and the original material created by the institution operating the site.

Source: Health on the Net Foundation. HON code of conduct (HONcode) for medical and health websites. 2004. http://www.hon.ch/HONcode/Conduct.html. Adapted from Health on the Net Foundation. All information (including graphics and website design) contained on the www.hon.ch site is copyright © Health On the Net Foundation and shall remain the property of the Health On the Net Foundation.

Be cautious of websites that present an overly optimistic report on a given topic. You should be concerned whether the authors have considered the negative issues, which are a part of all forms of treatment. The same could be said about overly bleak reports that ignore positive research findings and only point out the associated ineffectiveness and harm of a treatment. Chiropractic itself has been an ongoing target of criticism by several antichiropractic websites that offer a great deal of dismal information about this profession.[24,25] Interestingly, the authors of these websites violate many of the same evidentiary principles that they criticize the chiropractic profession for violating. These include reliance on anecdotal information, sweeping generalizations, passing on half-truths, and pointing to rare and extreme practices. Chiropractic patients will no doubt be exposed to websites such as these and, as a result, ask questions that may be difficult to answer without preparation.

Anatomy of a Scholarly Article

Scientific scholarly articles are typically divided into sections with the following headings: *Introduction*, which tells why the study was carried out; *Materials and Methods*, how the study was carried out; *Results*, what the study found; *Discussion*, what the results might mean; *Conclusions*, why is it important; and *References*, a list of the evidence used to support statements made in the article.[26] These sections are usually preceded by an abstract and a list of a few of the article's key words. An acronym that is often used to denote the Introduction, Materials and Methods, Results, and Discussion sections of a scientific paper is IMRaD.[27]

The article may include subheadings to break up the content and make it more comprehensible when sections are especially long. Common subheadings that may be used deal with such things as technical information, selection of participants, and statistics. The previously mentioned format is typical for experimental and observational studies, although case reports, literature reviews, and editorials often utilize alternate formats. We can then refer to the *anatomy of a scholarly article* as including these five headings, plus an abstract and the References section (Table 2.5).

Each of the sections of a research article should contain specific components to ensure that the article's purpose is achieved. An article would be considered flawed if any of its anatomy were missing or if the individual pieces of anatomy were incomplete. Following is a brief description of what is commonly included in the various sections of research articles, although these requirements may vary somewhat from journal to journal.

The first section is the *abstract*, which provides a brief summary of the article and is usually limited to a few paragraphs. The abstract should not be confused

TABLE 2.5 Anatomy of a scholarly article

Abstract
Introduction
Materials and methods
Results
Discussion
Conclusions
References

with the Introduction section of an article: An abstract is a summary of the entire manuscript, whereas the introduction develops the problem being presented and states the purpose of the article. The abstract is a very important element in an article because it informs readers about what they should expect if they continue and read the entire article. Abstracts are provided along with citations when literature searches are carried out at several biomedical databases, including PubMed. By reading only the abstracts, numerous articles can be reviewed very quickly to determine if they are worthwhile before obtaining a full-text copy and investing the time required to read the entire article.

Many journals utilize *structured abstracts*, which contain subheadings and subsections, rather than simply paragraphs as seen in traditional abstracts.[28] Subheadings in structured abstracts include items such as "Background," "Objectives," "Methods," "Results," and "Conclusions." Structured abstracts are usually longer and are considered more informative and accessible than traditional narrative abstracts. They are judged to be more useful by authors, and readers like them because they make it easier for them to select suitable articles more quickly.[29]

The *Introduction* section provides a rationale for the research that is being presented and states the purpose of the article. It also provides a brief review of the literature that highlights the most prominent works of other researchers regarding the topic under investigation. The purpose of this review is not to deliver a complete exposition of the topic, but to convey the context of the research. The introduction should stimulate a reader's interest. Thus, if it is uninteresting, the reader may want to consider going on to another article as an alternative.

The next section, *Materials and Methods* (sometimes simply entitled *Methods*), deals with details of how the study was carried out. This section covers how subjects (humans or animals) were selected and assigned to groups, and describes any equipment that was utilized, any drugs and chemicals used (including dosage and route of administration), and the procedures involved in the study. The experimental design that was utilized should be fully described as well. The Methods section should be comprehensible enough so that other researchers can reproduce the work and compare results if desired. The study's methods should also be justified by providing references or, if novel, a complete description and rationale. Research involving human participants or animals requires a statement about how ethical standards were dealt with, and because the anonymity of study participants is essential, patient names or any other identifiable labels should not be included. (It is highly unlikely that a manuscript that included patient names would ever pass through peer review.) How the data was analyzed and details about the statistical significance of the findings are also included in the Methods section.

The *Results* section is where the findings of the study are reported in a comprehensive and convincing manner, often using tables, illustrations, and graphs. Data that were collected are summarized, and the main findings are presented. One thing to look for when reviewing this section is the failure of authors to report data that are contradictory to the study's hypotheses. Omissions of data that were at odds with the rest of the study can often be detected by observing and comparing the total numbers of participants reported in subsections that otherwise should agree. This problem may be present if totals do not correspond. Tables incorporated in this section are at times rather complex and difficult to interpret. However, some may contain inaccurate data, which is often the result of transcription errors; hence, they should be reviewed for accuracy along with the rest of the article. Any problems with the data (e.g., small sample size or possible selection biases) should be acknowledged by the authors. Statements given in this section should be supported by the data using appropriate statistical tests. Statistical findings do not actually "prove" anything; rather, they point out how likely the study's results are to be correct. Science overall does not "prove" things; rather, it observes and reports them. Rigid assertions based on a study's findings are therefore inappropriate and should not be present in a research article.

The *Discussion* section should highlight new or important features of the study and discuss how the study's results compare with previously published data. The authors will at this point state whether the data supported the study's hypothesis. The text should not merely repeat the results of the study; rather, it should discuss and interpret them. Relevant work of other authors is often reported concerning how it relates to the current investigation. Implications of the study's findings should be presented, along with any known limitations and possible alternate explanations that may be relevant. Authors typically make suggestions about how readers could utilize the information presented, although practitioners' needs are quite variable and you will have to determine how applicable the suggestions are to your particular circumstances.

Conclusions should be directly related to and fully supported by the data that was presented. Often included in the conclusion is a statement about the importance of the study's findings and what it adds to the existing literature. It is appropriate for authors to accentuate the strengths of their study in order to impart an awareness of this importance to readers. Recommendations for future related research are commonly made. Frequently, there is no *Conclusions* section per se, in which case the study's conclusions will be incorporated into the *Discussion* section.

The *References* section should be complete and accurate, consisting only of relevant citations that were actually utilized and appropriately cited throughout the paper. References used to support statements in research articles typically must be derived from journals, as opposed to books and other lower forms of evidence. This is because information found in journals is almost always more current and, when based on peer-reviewed sources, more accurate. Be alert for the unethical practice of authors representing the ideas of others as being their own and accordingly not providing references for nonoriginal material. This practice may be difficult to identify, but can be recognized by comparison of the text with the works of other authors.

Articles that do not adhere to the "anatomy of a scholarly article" layout that was previously mentioned should be regarded as being suspicious. They will accordingly require careful appraisal to establish their validity prior to using them as evidence.

Red Flags for Untrustworthy Information

There are a number of *red flags* for untrustworthy health information that one should be aware of while collecting EBC evidence. Sometimes referred to as *junk science*, untrustworthy information can be characterized as the use of scientific methods for purposes other than the pursuit of truth. Another related term, *pseudoscience*, refers to any body of knowledge thought to be scientific or supported by science that does not adhere to the scientific method. Regardless of what it is called, untrustworthy information should be recognized and avoided in the interest of optimal patient care. Table 2.6 lists common red flags that should help you to identify untrustworthy information as it is encountered in journal articles and other sources of evidence.

Other red flags include feeble referencing that is insufficient or outdated; a journal that is peer-reviewed, but whose peer reviewers are obviously biased (e.g., they may have a vested interest in products or techniques advocated in the articles); and articles that are written by authors with a stake in the advertising that appears in the same issue of the journal. No doubt there are other red flags, but the main thing to keep in mind as you read the literature is that research is supposed to be presented in a totally unbiased manner. Anything that appears to deviate from this position is suspect and should be scrutinized for factors that would influence authors or journal editors to perform in a prejudiced manner.

The Food and Nutrition Science Alliance[30] has produced a list of red flags designed to help identify information that qualifies as junk science, which is reproduced in Table 2.7. Although it is specifically designed for evaluating sources of nutrition-related science, most of the red flags are applicable to the appraisal of any health information.

Appraising Evidence

The steps involved in appraising journal articles are somewhat variable, depending on which type of research design was utilized. Accordingly, specific appraisal

TABLE 2.6 Red flags for untrustworthy information

- Journal is not peer-reviewed.
- Writing quality is substandard.
- Author has a personal agenda.
- Article has an advertising tone.
- Article format is incorrect.
- References are insufficient or outdated.
- Journal is not indexed.
- Printing and layout are ostentatious.
- Article has a testimonial function.
- Conflicts of interest exist.

TABLE 2.7 The Food and Nutrition Science Alliance's 10 red flags of junk science

- Recommendations that promise a quick fix
- Dire warnings of danger from a single product or regimen
- Claims that sound too good to be true
- Simplistic conclusions drawn from a complex study
- Recommendations based on a single study
- Dramatic statements that are refuted by reputable scientific organizations
- Lists of "good" and "bad" foods
- Recommendations made to help sell a product
- Recommendations based on studies published without peer review
- Recommendations from studies that ignore differences among individuals or groups

Source: Food and Nutrition Science Alliance. Junk science: Scientists issue 10 red flags for consumers [News release]. 1995. Chicago: Author.

tactics will be provided in subsequent chapters of this book to correspond with the various research designs that are presented. Some general appraisal strategies apply across all of these designs, however. These strategies correspond to the various sections of an article's anatomy. For example, when appraising the *abstract*, notice whether the purpose and results of the study are correctly and adequately described. The abstract should also be evaluated for the presence of obvious biases. The *Introduction* section should be examined to see if the purpose of the study is conveyed plainly and rationally. A suitable literature review should be presented in the introduction that adequately covers the topic, and deficiencies in this area should be sought out.

There are several items to consider when evaluating the *Methods* section of an article. First, look for a description of what research design was utilized and determine whether it was adequately implemented. Second, look for a description of the population and samples involved in the study and look for potential biases. Third, determine whether the data collection methods that were employed were adequately described and whether they were appropriate for the condition under investigation.

The *Results* section should be assessed to determine whether the data presented was reported in enough detail so that the results could be effectively interpreted. The demographic characteristics of the groups involved should be presented and summarized. The statistical procedures utilized for analyzing the data should be described and should be appropriate for the type of data involved. The *Discussion* section should follow from and be supported by the data that were presented in the Results section. Accordingly, look for unreasonable and unsupported statements in this section that do not logically flow from the study's data. Additionally, conclusions should be in agreement with the predetermined objectives of the study. Newly developed hypotheses at this point in an article will likely be the result of a "fishing expedition"[31] rather than planned research.

An article's *references* should also be included in the appraisal process, since flaws here can negatively affect the overall trustworthiness of the article. References should be assessed with regard to their appropriateness for the study. If a reference does not directly relate to the topic it points to in the article, it should not be listed. However, there should be enough references to support all of the statements that were made. Articles referred to in this section should be of high quality and from respected evidence sources. A common flaw to look for in the References section involves the authors misrepresenting the findings of the referenced studies.

After working through these appraisal steps, try to form an overall impression about the trustworthiness of the article. Then determine its applicability to the clinical circumstances that prompted you to read the article in the first place, whether in relation to a question about a specific patient or your practice in general. Based on the appraisal and the article's applicability, make a decision about whether it is something that you want to rely on as evidence. Be advised that this decision will rarely be clear-cut; rather, it will be a continuum ranging from acceptable to not acceptable. As a result, it is common to accept certain portions of an article and reject others. In fact, it is very rare to encounter an article that can be unconditionally accepted.

References

1. International Committee of Medical Journal Editors. *Uniform requirements for manuscripts submitted to biomedical journals. Ann Intern Med*, 1997. **126**(1):36–47.
2. Leach, R.A. *Evidence-based chiropractic: Critical thinking in the private-practice setting. J Am Chiropr Assoc*, 2005. **42**(1):37–46.
3. Colaianni, L.A. *Peer review in journals indexed in Index Medicus. JAMA*, 1994. **272**(2):156–8.
4. Cho, M.K., et al. *Masking author identity in peer review: What factors influence masking success? PEER Investigators. JAMA*, 1998. **280**(3):243–5.
5. Godlee, F., C.R. Gale, and C.N. Martyn. *Effect on the quality of peer review of blinding*

reviewers and asking them to sign their reports: A randomized controlled trial. JAMA, 1998. **280**(3):237–40.
6. Justice, A.C., et al. *Does masking author identity improve peer review quality? A randomized controlled trial. PEER Investigators. JAMA*, 1998. **280**(3):240–2.
7. Black, N., et al. *What makes a good reviewer and a good review for a general medical journal? JAMA*, 1998. **280**(3):231–3.
8. National Library of Medicine: *Journal selection for Index Medicus/MEDLINE* [Fact sheet]. 2004. Bethesda: Author.
9. Murphy, L.S., et al. *Spinal palpation: The challenges of information retrieval using available databases. J Manipulative Physiol Ther*, 2003. **26**(6):374–82.
10. Braunwald, E., et al. *Harrison's Online.* 2005. McGraw-Hill. http://www.accessmedicine.com/home.aspx.
11. Mazmanian, P.E., and D.A. Davis. *Continuing medical education and the physician as a learner: Guide to the evidence. JAMA*, 2002. **288**(9):1057–60.
12. Davis, D., et al. *Impact of formal continuing medical education: Do conferences, workshops, rounds, and other traditional continuing education activities change physician behavior or health care outcomes? JAMA*, 1999. **282**(9):867–74.
13. National Center for Biotechnology Information. *PubMed overview.* 2004. http://www.nebi.nim.nih.gov/entrez/query/static/overview.html.
14. Shekelle, P. *Cervical spine manipulation was not better than mobilization for improving outcomes in neck pain. ACP J Club*, 2003. **138**(2):48.
15. Brandt, T., and C. Grond-Ginsbach. *Spontaneous cervical artery dissection: from risk factors toward pathogenesis. Stroke*, 2002. **33**(3):657–8.
16. Terrett, A.G. *Misuse of the literature by medical authors in discussing spinal manipulative therapy injury. J Manipulative Physiol Ther*, 1995. **18**(4):203–10.
17. The Cochrane Collaboration. *The Cochrane Library.* http://www.cochrane.org/reviews/clibintro.htm.
18. Rose, B.D., ed. *UpToDate.* http://uptodate.com.
19. Gagliardi, A., and A.R. Jadad. *Examination of instruments used to rate quality of health information on the Internet: Chronicle of a voyage with an unclear destination. BMJ*, 2002. **324**(7337):569–73.
20. Crocco, A.G., M. Villasis-Keever, and A.R. Jadad. *Two wrongs don't make a right: Harm aggravated by inaccurate information on the Internet. Pediatrics*, 2002. **109**(3):522–3.
21. Jadad, A.R., et al. *The Internet and evidence-based decision-making: A needed synergy for efficient knowledge management in health care. CMAJ*, 2000. **162**(3):362–5.
22. Center for Integrative Medicine. *Complementary Medicine Resources for Health Professionals and Researchers.* 2005. Baltimore: University of Maryland School of Medicine, Center for Integrative Medicine.
23. Health on the Net Foundation, *HON code of conduct (HONcode) for medical and health Web sites.* 2004. http://www.hon.ch/HONcode/Conduct.html.
24. Barrett, S. *Quackwatch.* http://www.quackwatch.org.
25. Barrett, S. and S. Homola. *Chirobase.* http://www.chirobase.org/.
26. International Committee of Medical Journal Editors. *Uniform Requirements for Manuscripts Submitted to Biomedical Journals: Writing and Editing for Biomedical Publication.* 2004. http://www.icmje.org/.

27. Sollaci, L.B., and M.G. Pereira. *The introduction, methods, results, and discussion (IMRAD) structure: A fifty-year survey.* J Med Libr Assoc, 2004. **92**(3):364–7.
28. Nakayama, T., et al. *Adoption of structured abstracts by general medical journals and format for a structured abstract.* J Med Libr Assoc, 2005. **93**(2):237–42.
29. Hartley, J. *Current findings from research on structured abstracts.* J Med Libr Assoc, 2004. **92**(3):368–71.
30. Food and Nutrition Science Alliance. *Junk science: Scientists issue 10 red flags for consumers [News release].* 1995. Chicago: Author.
31. Swaen, G.G., O. Teggeler, and L.G. van Amelsvoort. False positive outcomes and design characteristics in occupational cancer epidemiology studies. *Int J Epidemiol*, 2001. **30**(5):948–54.

CHAPTER THREE

Literature Searching

Journal articles are the primary source of evidence for EBC practitioners; therefore, it is essential to know how to find articles that suitably address clinical questions that arise. However, finding journal articles that will effectively provide answers to these clinical questions can sometimes be a daunting task. For example, PubMed, undoubtedly the best known of the biomedical databases, contains bibliographic citations and corresponding abstracts from more than 4,800 biomedical journals, a total of more than 15 million citations at the time of this writing. Because of the enormous size of PubMed, if a practitioner were to indiscriminately attempt to retrieve citations from this database to answer a particular question, it would most likely take years to locate one or two applicable studies. For this reason, PubMed, along with all of the other comparable literature cataloging systems, utilizes search and retrieval schemes to make the process easier and quicker. Articles pertaining to a specific topic can be searched for among the millions of possibilities by using focused search strategies. Accordingly, this chapter presents some of the basic search strategies that are essential to EBC, along with a description of the more appropriate databases.

Before delving into the subject of literature searching, the chapter presents a brief overview of databases and how they are searched. Basically, a database is a compilation of data that has been organized in such a way that it is quick and easy to search and retrieve specific information using a computer. The biomedical databases that we deal within EBC contain bibliographic data regarding articles from scientific journals. One way to think of a database is as an electronic filing system that can quickly be accessed by a computer. When equipped with an Internet connection, this access can be from a remote source. Databases are organized by *fields* (single bits of information), *records* (collections of fields), and *files* (groups of records). Figure 3.1 shows an example record from PubMed with the various fields labeled. Each of the labeled components represents a particular field of the record. The unlabeled PMID field represents the number assigned to the record by PubMed.

To search a database, one enters specific terms that correspond to the various fields of a record. For example, the citation in Figure 3.1 can be searched for by using one or more of the authors' names, any of the terms found in the title, or the journal volume and issue numbers. The search can be narrowed down by entering combinations of data found in the various fields of a given record. Hence, if one of the authors' names was queried along with the journal name and volume number, more than likely only one citation would result and would represent the particular article that was being searched for. On the other hand, if only one of the terms in the title were to be queried, many citations (sometimes thousands) would be retrieved. After a successful search is achieved, the corresponding citations can be selected and retrieved from the database. Details about search strategies that involve limiting as well as expanding operations are covered later in this chapter.

The Databases

It is imperative to understand how to search biomedical databases for evidence, but it is equally important to know which databases to search.[1] There are a number of

FIGURE 3.1 **Typical record from a PubMed citation.**

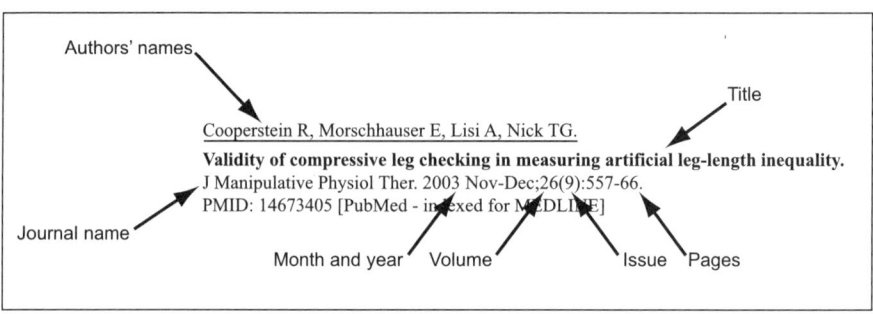

databases that include biomedical information, and familiarity with several of them is vital to successfully practice EBC. Table 3.1 simply contains a list of databases presented in order of their usefulness to EBC practitioners. Additional material is presented later that will help you decide which one is appropriate for a given situation. The last three listed databases deal with homeopathic, herbal, and nutritional matters. They are included because the use of these interventions is common among chiropractors, and appropriate evidence should be accessible when needed. The URL, or Web address, is provided for each of the listed databases. These URLs may change over time, in which case you will have to search the Internet to find the new Web address. You are urged to explore these databases in order to familiarize yourself with them.

A database not listed in Table 3.1 that you may want to consider is the Physiotherapy Evidence Database (PEDro). It consists of clinical practice guidelines, systematic reviews, and randomized controlled trials that specifically deal with physical therapy treatments. Maher[2] points out that PEDro contains evidence that is relevant not only to physical therapy but also to the chiropractic profession. However, this database may not index important information that is available through PubMed, and sometimes the citations do not include the abstracts.[3] The URL for PEDro is http://www.pedro.fhs.usyd.edu.au.

When searching for information about chiropractic and other complementary and alternative medicine procedures, it is almost always necessary to utilize more than just one database. A study that compared the effectiveness of searching a number of databases regarding the topic of the reliability of spinal palpation procedures found that MANTIS yielded the highest number of citations, and PubMed yielded almost half as many.[4] Another study found searching MANTIS to be faster and more complete for chiropractic information than other databases.[5] On the other hand, PubMed/MEDLINE was found to be more efficient than CHIROLARS (the previous name of MANTIS) or ICL for searching for chiropractic-related literature. In head-to-head search comparisons, however, MEDLINE retrieved the highest proportion of relevant citations and was less expensive than the other two.[6] Incidentally, MEDLINE is the online counterpart of *Index Medicus*, which is an extensive index of scientific biomedical literature that is compiled by the National Library of Medicine (NLM). PubMed provides free Internet access to this vast collection of information.

One thing to keep in mind about MEDLINE is that it only includes material from medical journals. Thus, if information related to the social sciences or

Chapter 3 Literature Searching

TABLE 3.1 Databases

PubMed (F): PubMed includes over 15 million (and growing) citations for biomedical articles dating back to the 1950s. These citations are from MEDLINE and additional life science journals. MEDLINE itself has nearly 13 million records from 1966 to the present. PubMed includes links to many sites providing full-text articles and other related resources. PubMed is a service of the National Library of Medicine.
URL: http://PubMed.gov

Manual Alternative and Natural Therapy Index System (MANTIS) (C): MANTIS addresses all areas of alternative medical literature. It covers health care disciplines not significantly represented in the major biomedical databases and includes references from more than 1,400 journals, with preference given to peer-reviewed journals. MANTIS began including the full text of alternative medical journals in the fall of 1999. Produced by Action Potential, it has become the largest index of peer-reviewed articles for several disciplines, including chiropractic, osteopathy, homeopathy, and manual medicine.
URL: http://www.healthindex.com

Cumulative Index to Nursing and Allied Health (CINAHL) (C): The CINAHL database, produced by CINAHL Information Systems, covers nursing and allied health literature from 1982 to the present. It includes citations from 2,593 journals, of which 1,798 include author abstracts. Journals cover nursing, allied health, biomedicine, alternative and complementary medicine, consumer health, and health sciences librarianship.
URL: http://www.cinahl.com

Index to Chiropractic Literature (ICL) (F): ICL indexes all chiropractic peer-reviewed journals cover to cover, and others topically, using terms from the MeSH database and CHIROSH (*Chiropractic Subject Headings*). ICL is indexed by the Chiropractic Library Consortium (CLIBCON), which is a group of health science librarians from chiropractic colleges throughout the world whose goal is to improve access to the chiropractic literature.
URL: http://www.chiroindex.org

AMED (C): The AMED database is produced by the Health Care Information Service of the British Library. It includes resources in three subject areas: (1) several professions allied to medicine, (2) complementary medicine, (3) palliative care. AMED covers relevant references to articles from around 596 journals, many not indexed by other biomedical sources. It is available in a variety of formats from print to online.
URL: http://www.bl.uk/collections/health/amed.html

CAM on PubMed (F): CAM on PubMed is a subset of the PubMed database that was created through a partnership between the National Center for Complementary and Alternative Medicine and the National Library of Medicine. CAM on PubMed uses a feature to locate citations with a predetermined CAM search criterion. This feature can be utilized directly from PubMed by choosing "Limits" and then "Complementary Medicine" from the Subsets menu. Currently there are over 270,000 citations in the CAM subset of PubMed from 1966 forward.
URL: http://www.nlm.nih.gov/nccam/camonpubmed.html

The Databases

CAMLINE (F): CAMLINE is an evidence-based complementary and alternative medicine website designed for health care professionals as well as the public. CAMLINE provides search capabilities and information on the safety and efficacy of CAM products, therapies, and practitioners.
URL: http://camline.org

The Cochrane Library (C): Consists of eight regularly updated evidence-based databases, all of which are concerned with the effects of interventions in health care. *The Cochrane Library* is designed to provide information and evidence to support decisions taken in health care and to inform those receiving care. The Cochrane database of systematic reviews is full text, whereas most of the other databases contain primarily citations and abstracts. Published on a quarterly basis.
URL: http://www.thecochranelibrary.org

The Hom-Inform Database (F): A database of indexed literature on the subject of homoeopathy with key terms and some abstracts. Produced by the British Homoeopathic Library at Glasgow Homoeopathic Hospital.
URL: http://hominform.soutron.com

HerbMed (F): HerbMed is an interactive, electronic herbal database that provides hyperlinked access to the scientific data underlying the use of herbs for health. It is an impartial evidence-based information resource for professionals, researchers, and the general public, project of the nonprofit Alternative Medicine Foundation. HerbMedPro is an enhanced version of HerbMed that is available for subscription and licensing. The public site has information on 75 herbs; HerbMedPro has an additional 93 herbs.
URL: http://www.herbmed.org

International Bibliographic Information on Dietary Supplements (IBIDS) (F): IBIDS provides access to bibliographic citations and abstracts from published, international, and scientific literature on dietary supplements. IBIDS contains over 730,000 citations on the topic of dietary supplements from four major database sources: biomedical-related articles from MEDLINE, botanical and agricultural science from AGRICOLA, worldwide agricultural literature through AGRIS, and selected nutrition journals from CAB Abstracts and CAB Health.
URL: http://ods.od.nih.gov/databases/ibids.html

Phytotherapies.org (F): A resource for herbal practitioners. It includes editorial content, articles, and an extensive searchable and hyperlinked herbal database on current herbal therapeutics. Sponsored by Herbworx Corporation.
URL: http://www.phytotherapies.org

Note: Databases are listed by order of usefulness to EBC practitioners. F, free access; C, charge for access.

humanities is being sought, the appropriate social science and humanities indexes will need to be searched. Also, consumer-oriented periodicals that include information on medical topics are not listed in MEDLINE. These types of articles would have to be searched for in general periodical indexes.

Databases can be searched (or *queried*) using *keywords*, *text words*, or *subject headings*. When searching using keywords or text words, PubMed looks for the words entered in each of the possible fields of a record (e.g., author, title, abstract, and journal). Text word searching may utilize any word or number present in the article's title, abstract, or assigned MeSH terms to locate applicable citations. Medical subject heading (MeSH) searches use specific terms that are found in the NLM MeSH list. These MeSH terms are assigned by the NLM to describe the subject of a journal article and are included in all articles catalogued by MEDLINE.

Some databases provide links directly to full-text articles, whereas others only offer the citations (i.e., author, title, journal name, date, volume, issue, and page numbers), often with the article's abstract. When only the citations are provided by the database, you will need to obtain the text of the articles directly from the publisher or from a biomedical library at a chiropractic college or other health-related school. These libraries are excellent resources for obtaining articles, since they have many of the journals on site or have online access to websites where the full text of the articles may be acquired. If you live too far from an acceptable biomedical library, documents found on PubMed can be ordered through their Loansome Doc program. Users of this service must first establish an agreement with a library that uses DOCLINE, and then can order articles using links provided during PubMed searches. Information about how to use Loansome Doc to order full-text articles, and a list of participating libraries, can be found at the following Internet address:

http://www.nlm.nih.gov/loansomedoc/loansome_home.html

Searching Essentials

As previously noted, there are many biomedical databases and in order to thoroughly explore your topic, you should be capable of searching several of them. Fortunately, common searching methods are involved with all of them, so once you have learned the steps involved in searching one, the others are reasonably

Searching Essentials

straightforward to use. PubMed is presented as the primary focus of this section, although basic differences between it and MANTIS are also mentioned. Each of the databases has unique features that one should become familiar with before using them; consequently, nearly all of them provide tutorials or help sections to facilitate learning. The material in this section is difficult to comprehend without actually seeing it in action; thus, it is very helpful to go to the PubMed website while reading to try out the various steps of database searching as they are presented.

Figure 3.2 is a screenshot of the PubMed home page with labels and arrows pointing to some of its more important features. The features bar contains links to some helpful PubMed features; of particular interest is the Limits tab, which links to a page where limiting query parameters can be set. The query box is where search terms are typed before initiating searches. The Search drop-down list will typically be left in its default position, which allows PubMed to be the object of

FIGURE 3.2 PubMed home page.

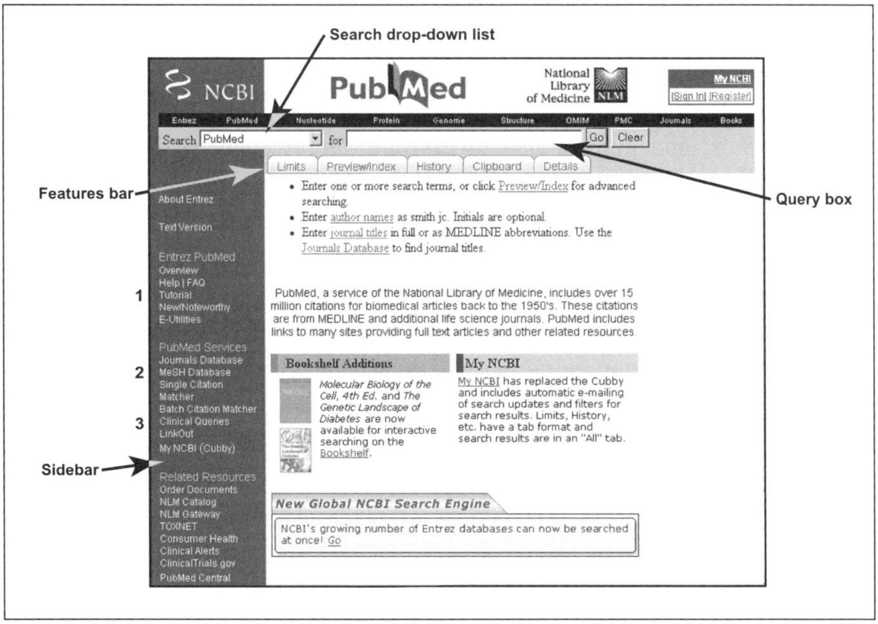

Source: Courtesy of National Library of Medicine.

the search. Another useful item located on this drop-down list permits searching of the MeSH database directly from the PubMed home page. The number 1 in the figure indicates a link to the PubMed tutorial, which is really quite good; I highly recommend that you take the time to work through it. Number 2 identifies a link to the MeSH Database, which contains the specific vocabulary used to index many of the articles included in PubMed, as well as tools to help you use MeSH terms in your searches. This topic is more thoroughly covered later in this chapter. Number 3 indicates the Clinical Queries link, where searches can be created that are specifically designed to answer clinical questions. Topics can be searched from the Clinical Queries page by clinical study categories or targeted to only find systematic reviews.

The MANTIS database has a High Clinical Relevancy option (Figure 3.3) that is comparable to PubMed's Clinical Queries link in that it searches for articles with high clinical relevance. Searching MANTIS with the High Clinical Relevancy option selected limits the results of the search to articles that deal with clinical trials or case reports involving humans.

PubMed searches can be accomplished several different ways, using methodologies that range from simple to complex. Simple searches, sometimes referred to as the *basic search* mode, may involve merely entering a few search terms in the query box and clicking Go. Complex searches utilize a choice of functions and operators in addition to the search terms. *Stopwords*, such as *the*, *and*, *because*, *thus*, and quite a few others, are simply ignored during PubMed searches because they so common that they are found in too many records. Consequently, you can enter them if you like, but they will not add or detract from the search results.

Once a query has been completed, PubMed will present a list of the resulting citations that were retrieved (Figure 3.4). The full record of a single citation can be viewed by clicking on the author's name, which will show the document in the default citation format. Several full records can be viewed at once by selecting the checkboxes in front of the authors' names for the desired citations and selecting one of the drop-down menu choices to display the records in a desired format. When checkboxes are selected while browsing through multiple pages of records, PubMed will keep track of what was checked and display them all when requested.

One fairly straightforward PubMed search tactic is to use limits, which is achieved by clicking the appropriate tab on the features bar and making selections

Searching Essentials 73

FIGURE 3.3 MANTIS Advanced Search page.

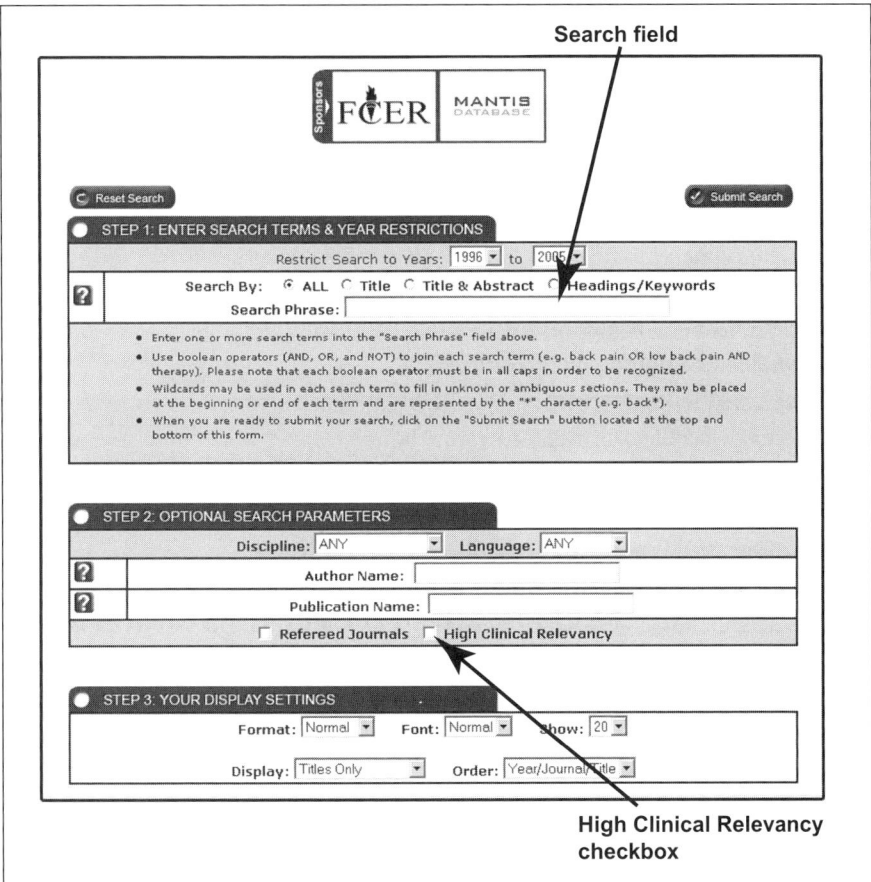

Source: Reproduced with permission from Action Potential, Inc., The MANTIS Database.

from the various drop-down menus presented (Figure 3.5). The use of limits while searching PubMed allows you to set frequently used parameters for your query to retrieve more relevant citations. This feature limits the search results so that only articles that meet these limiting criteria will be retrieved. Thus, using the drop-down menus and changing the Publication Type field to Clinical Trial and the Human or Animal field to Human will retrieve only articles dealing with clinical trials that involve humans. For example, typing neck manipulation into the

FIGURE 3.4 PubMed results page showing 2 of 435 retrieved citations. To view the default citation format, click the authors' names or the checkbox and click the Display button.

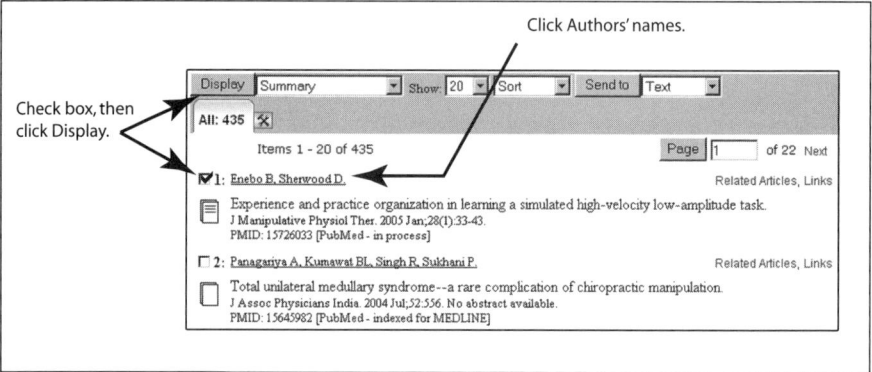

Source: Courtesy of National Library of Medicine.

FIGURE 3.5 The drop-down menus that appear after clicking the Limits tab on the PubMed features bar.

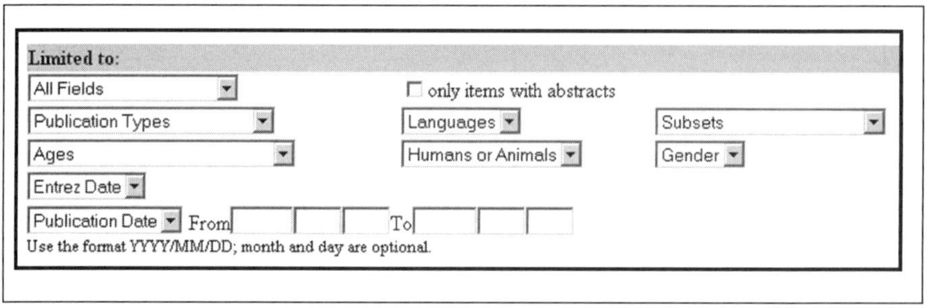

Source: Courtesy of National Library of Medicine.

PubMed query box and searching without using limits produces 979 citations.* Alternatively, using the same search terms but changing the Publication Type field to Clinical Trial and the Human or Animal field to Human produces only 151 citations. To go one step further, if quotation marks are placed around the

---

*Search terms and phrases appear in boldface in this discussion.

search terms, which will limit the search to the specific phrase *neck manipulation*, only 2 citations are retrieved. This limiting strategy facilitates practicing EBC because only 2 articles will have to be considered after the search rather than 979.

Other possible selections located in the Limits drop-down menus are also helpful. Of particular interest is the Publication Types menu, which allows you to limit searches to include only meta-analyses, RCTs, case reports, editorials, and so forth. The next section, "Advanced Strategies," discusses the use of field tags, which are more complicated to use than limits, but often quicker. Bear in mind, however, that much of the more complicated field tag searching can be accomplished using limits. MANTIS includes a number of similarly functioning drop-down menus and several radio buttons that are also capable of limiting searches (Figure 3.6).

One of the primary reasons for creating foreground questions, as mentioned in Chapter 1, is to help generate search terms. Using one of the foreground questions presented in Chapter 1 as an example, specific search terms will now be selected. The question is as follows: *Is manipulation effective at reducing back and leg pain in a middle-aged female patient with lumbar spinal stenosis and concomitant radicular pain, or are any alternative methods more favorable?* The first step in selecting search terms is to identify the major concepts that are present in the clinical question.[7] In this case, the major concepts are "manipulation," "back and leg pain," and "lumbar spinal stenosis." These concepts are used to select the terms needed to initiate a literature search that will be created purposely to answer the clinical question. The selected terms can be searched individually or combined in several different ways using advanced strategies. If search terms are too general, such as using **spine** as a keyword in a biomedical database, the result will be far more citations than one can reasonably deal with. The solution

FIGURE 3.6 **The PubMed search bar, which includes the query box, and the features bar, which includes tabs linking to additional search features.**

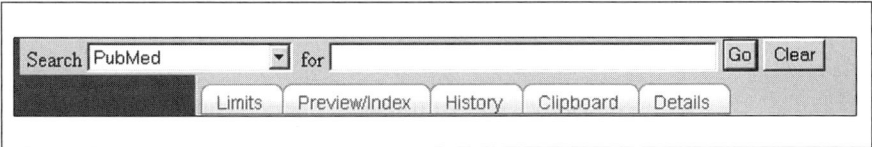

Source: Courtesy of National Library of Medicine.

is to link the term with another specific concept that will limit the results. This may make the search too specific, however, and very few or possibly no citations may be found. In this case, one should try alternate terms to search a somewhat broader subject.

Advanced Strategies

When searching a large database such as PubMed, many queried terms will produce hundreds or even thousands of citations. With this many possibilities, it becomes necessary to sort through scores of titles and abstracts to find a few pertinent articles. Thus, procedures that are capable of creating more focused searches can be very useful. In addition to using limits, as was previously described, *Boolean operators* and *field tags* are more advanced strategies that greatly enhance the process of finding relevant articles.

Boolean Operators

Boolean operators (sometimes referred to as *logical operators*) combine search terms in ways that can either narrow or broaden searches, depending on which Boolean operator is used. They include AND, OR, and NOT and should always be capitalized. These operators work the same in the MANTIS database as they do in PubMed.

The Boolean operator AND combines terms in such a way that only articles that contain *both* terms will be retrieved in a search. Thus, AND *limits* or *narrows* a search. For example, if one searches PubMed using the term **neck**, 102,193 citations will be retrieved from the database. Similarly, if the term **pain** is used in a search of PubMed, 289,566 records can be found. But if the two terms are combined using the Boolean operator AND, and another search is performed, only 7,632 citations will be retrieved. This is still a very large number of citations to evaluate for relevance to a clinical question; hence, another limiting search of terms would be necessary. An example would be combining **"chiropractic manipulation"** with the previous terms, again using AND. The PubMed query box for this would be as follows:

> neck AND pain AND "chiropractic manipulation"

This query generates 48 citations, a much more manageable number. It should be

Advanced Strategies 77

noted that search results are listed in order of relevancy, with the most relevant listed first.[8]

Figure 3.7 illustrates via Venn diagram what happens when several terms are searched using the AND operator. In effect, only articles that contain all three terms will be retrieved. The terms involved can be single words or phrases, as long as quotation marks are placed around phrases. At this point, I recommend that you go to a computer where you can access PubMed and reconstruct the searches that were covered so far in order to clarify and reinforce the process. Do not be surprised if your results are different from mine, however, because new citations are added to PubMed continually.

Another Boolean operator that *limits* the breadth of searches is NOT. When used to combine search terms, NOT retrieves only citations that include the first term, eliminating those that also include the second term. NOT should be used to exclude the retrieval of certain terms from a search. Thus, when **"neck pain" NOT manipulation** is searched, citations of all articles dealing with neck pain except those that also include manipulation will be retrieved.

FIGURE 3.7 **Combining three terms with the AND operator returns only citations that include all three terms.**

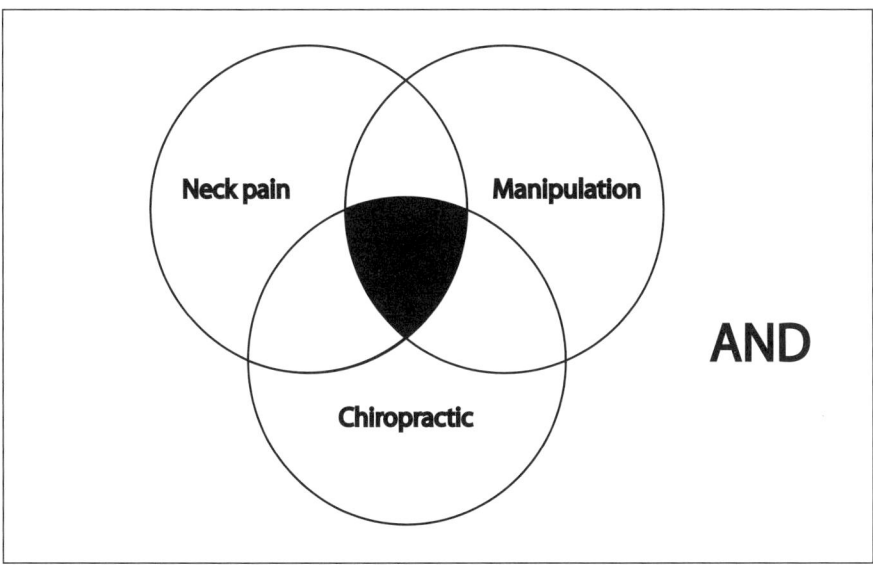

The OR operator *expands* searches by retrieving all articles that contain either one of the terms being queried. In other words, searching two terms with OR will return all documents that contain either the first term or the second term, or both. For example, if the terms **"neck pain"** and **manipulation** were combined using OR (i.e., **"neck pain" OR manipulation**), all instances of *neck pain* plus all instances of *manipulation* would be retrieved. The use of the OR operator is especially helpful when searching for either of two versions of a word (e.g., **manipulation OR adjustment**) (Figure 3.8).

It is sometimes advantageous to control the order PubMed uses to process search terms, which is normally from left to right.[8] This order can be changed by enclosing terms and Boolean operators (if any) in parentheses, a process called

FIGURE 3.8 **Diagrams representing searches for topic 1 (light gray) and topic 2 (white) using various Boolean operators. The dark gray areas are the search results associated with the specified Boolean operator.**

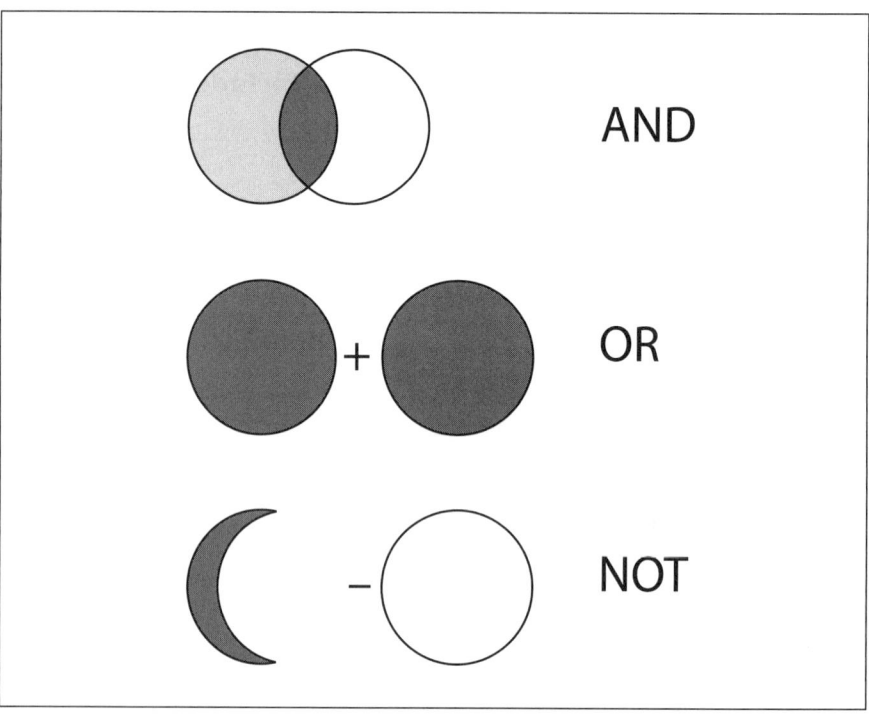

nesting. Terms within the parentheses are processed first and then integrated into the remainder of the search strategy. A search that utilizes nesting might look something like this:

> carpal tunnel syndrome AND (treatment NOT surgery) OR prognosis

Instead of processing **carpal tunnel syndrome** first, PubMed would begin with **treatment NOT surgery**, then proceed to the terms to the left, and finally go on to **prognosis** with the operator OR.

If terms are queried without the use of Boolean operators, the AND operator is automatically placed between the concepts that are entered. Thus, when **headache chiropractic** is queried, it is translated to **headache AND chiropractic** and only those records where each term is present will be displayed. More specifically, the full search strategy utilized by PubMed can be viewed by clicking the Details tab on the features bar. There, in the *Query Translation* box, you can see that the actual syntax for this search was

> ("headache"[MeSH Terms] OR headache[Text Word]) AND ("chiropractic"[MeSH Terms] OR chiropractic[Text Word])

You can observe the query translation of any PubMed search by clicking the Details tab after the initial search has been completed. This PubMed feature is often helpful in figuring out the next step to pursue when searches do not retrieve useful citations.

Field tags can be used to refine search strategies by forcing a given search term to consider specific search fields. The use of PubMed field tags is optional, since searching with limits accomplishes practically the same results. Field tags are not available with MANTIS. On the other hand, you may find field tags to be more adaptable than limits when searching PubMed.

To use this feature, simply enter a search term in the query box and qualify it with the appropriate search field tag. Table 3.2 lists some of the more common PubMed search field tags that are applicable to EBC. Field tags should always be placed within brackets after search terms, although the number of spaces between the search term and the field tag does not matter. Also, it does not matter whether uppercase or lowercase letters are used. As an example, to find articles by an author named Smith using the Author Name field tag, type **smith [au]** in the

TABLE 3.2	Common PubMed field tags
Affiliation [AD]	Page Number [PG]
All Fields [ALL]	Publication Type [PT]
Author Name [AU]	Volume [VI]
Journal Title Abbreviation [TA]	Issue [IP]
Language [LA]	Subset [SB]
MeSH Terms [MH]	Text Words [TW]
Publication Date [DP]	Title Words [TI]

query box. Only citations of articles authored by Smith will be returned. Unfortunately, there are more than 100,000 of them, so additional qualifiers will be needed. Adding the author's initials is helpful. For instance, adding **TS** to **Smith** limits the results of the search to 69 citations. Search terms with field tags may be combined, but when they are, Boolean operators are required (e.g., **Smith [AU] AND 2004 [DP]**).

Brief descriptions of the field tags listed in Table 3.2 follow.

- **Affiliation [AD]:** The institutional affiliation and address of the article's lead author.
- **All Fields [ALL]:** Searches all PubMed fields.
- **Author Name [AU]:** When searching for an author's name, the correct format is to type the last name and the first one or two initials without using commas or periods (e.g., triano jj).
- **Journal Title [TA]:** The name of the journal or its abbreviated form.
- **Language [LA]:** The language that was utilized to write the article.
- **MeSH Terms [MH]:** Searches the National Library of Medicine's controlled vocabulary of biomedical terms.
- **Publication Date [DP]:** The date that the article was published, using the format yyyy/mm/dd [DP] (e.g., **2005/12/02 [DP]**). A date range can be specified by placing a colon between two dates (e.g., **2002/01/01:2004/12/31 [DP]**).
- **Page Number [PG]:** The first page number of the article is all that is required.

- **Publication Type [PT]:** Allows you to specify the type of study referred to in the article (e.g., randomized controlled trial, review, case report).
- **Volume [VI] and Issue [IP]:** The volume and issue of the journal containing the article being searched can be assigned using these field tags.
- **Subheadings [SH]:** Can be used with MeSH terms to help clarify certain attributes about a subject, producing citations that have to do with that attribute. Examples of subheadings include Adverse Effects, Diagnosis, and Therapy.
- **Subset [SB]:** Search will be restricted to articles that only deal with a specified category. The use of subsets allows you to limit searches to a particular section of PubMed. Of interest to chiropractors is the Complementary and Alternative Medicine (CAM) subset, which can be typed in the query box along with the search term (e.g., **manipulation AND CAM [SB]**).
- **Text Words [TW]:** Searches all words and numbers in the title and abstract, MeSH terms, subheadings, and others.
- **Title Words [TI]:** Searches any words or numbers in the title of an article.

PubMed uses a feature called *automatic term mapping* when unqualified terms (those without search tags) are entered in the query box. The entered terms are matched against the MeSH translation table, the journals translation table, the full author translation table, and the author index, in that order. If the entered term matches a MeSH term from the MeSH translation table, it will be searched as a MeSH term and also as a text word. Thus, when **"intervertebral disc herniation"** is searched in PubMed, the term is first handled as a text word, and then it is translated into the MeSH term "intervertebral disk displacement." The journals translation table produces the journal title abbreviation when the full title of a journal is entered. For example, when a search is performed using **"Journal of Manipulative and Physiological Therapeutics,"** it will be translated to the journal abbreviation "J Manipulative Physiol Ther." The full author translation table retrieves full author names, if available, but is only available for articles published from 2002 forward. Terms can be entered in natural or inverted order when using full author searching. For instance, **John J Triano** would be equivalent to **Triano John J**. It is not necessary to include authors' middle initials, but if they are used, only citations that included those initials will be retrieved. It is not necessary to use a comma following the last name, but it is a nice option when trying to distinguish the last name from the first. For example, it would be difficult for PubMed to distinguish the first from the last name given a name like James John. The author index is searched by PubMed if no matches are located after completion of the preceding automatic term mapping steps.

Truncation and Wildcards

Truncation is another helpful feature available with many databases that permits searching for multiple uses of the same root word. For example, the root "manipulat" can be developed into the words *manipulate*, *manipulates*, *manipulation*, and *manipulative*. If one were to search using only **manipulate**, all of the other words just listed would be excluded, including the plural form. Truncation (sometimes called a *wildcard search*) permits searching using the root word plus an asterisk to retrieve all instances of the word with its variant suffixes (Table 3.3). Wildcards effectively complete indefinite sections of search terms and are represented by the "*" character, which for truncations is positioned at the end of search terms. The search engine of the chosen database will search for all terms that begin with the letters immediately preceding the asterisk. In our example, **manipulat*** would be typed into the query box, which would incorporate all of its variant forms as search terms.

TABLE 3.3 Common PubMed Operators

Boolean operators: Combine search terms in ways that narrow down or broaden searches.

AND	Only articles that contain both terms will be retrieved.
OR	All articles that contain either one of the query terms will be retrieved.
NOT	Retrieves only citations that include the first term, eliminating those that also include the second term.

"Term": Searches for the exact phrase inside quotation marks.

Truncation: Searches the root of a word for variant endings. For example, enter **analy*** to search for *analyze, analytic, analytical,* and so on.

Wildcard: Substitute an asterisk for a letter to search for variant spellings. For example, enter **analy*e** to search for *analyze* or *analyse*.

Wildcards can also be positioned within a word so that they replace a letter that is variable or absent. For example, a search using the term **an*emia** will search for both *anemia* and the British version, *anaemia*. If using truncation or wildcards produces too many terms for PubMed to process efficiently (usually more than 600), the search will be abbreviated and an error message to that effect will be displayed.

Phrase Searching

Phrase searching is carried out by placing all of the terms that make up a particular phrase within quotation marks. This action forces PubMed to search for the specific phrase rather than individual terms. Phrase searching can be very helpful in finding targeted citations that contain a precise phrase, and for forcing PubMed to consider certain divided terms as one. For example, PubMed will not recognize that **grade 3 spondylolisthesis** is all one term and will search for each word separately, yielding 102 citations. However, if quotation marks are placed around the phrase, **"grade 3 spondylolisthesis,"** only 1 citation will be retrieved. It is usually best to place terms in quotes only when a search has failed to find anything due to a word grouping failure. This is because phrases that are not indexed exactly like the group being searched for will result in a "Quoted phrase not found" error being returned.

MeSH Terms

Medical subject headings (MeSH) is a standardized list of medical vocabulary terms that has been developed by the National Library of Medicine for indexing medical literature. All records in MEDLINE have several MeSH terms assigned to them that correspond to the major topics of the indexed articles. MeSH headings are assigned by NLM indexers, who look at articles and then list the most specific headings that properly describe the topic under consideration. There may be up to 15 headings assigned to any given article. When there are no suitable headings available to describe the topic, the closest general heading is used.

Utilizing MeSH terms is not mandatory when constructing search strategies, but it is valuable because it facilitates searching. Citations are searchable using any word that appears in the title, abstract, or elsewhere in the citation entry, but using of the vocabulary terms listed in MeSH, as opposed to simply searching by keywords, will narrow down the search and help provide focused results.

MANTIS has a *controlled supplemental vocabulary* list that is similar to and functions together with MeSH terms, although the controlled supplemental vocabulary list consists of search terms that are specific to complementary and alternative medicine.

There are several ways to find suitable MeSH terms. The most direct method is to utilize PubMed's thesaurus tool by selecting MeSH from the drop-down list located next to the Search button on the PubMed home page. After that, terms entered into the PubMed query box and searched will produce a list of the appropriate MeSH terms or alternative suggestions, or both. Once the desired MeSH term has been selected, PubMed can be searched as usual using the term plus the MeSH field tag ([MesH] or [MH]). When the MeSH field tag is used, only the MeSH field of the target records will be searched. Searches using MeSH terms but not the MeSH field tag will search text words as well.

Another way to find suitable MeSH terms is to display the *citation format* of an exemplar article for the topic being investigated. The citation format can be viewed by selecting Citation from the drop-down list adjacent to the Display button located at the bottom of the page of all retrieved records. This format provides the complete list of MeSH terms that were assigned to the article by the NLM. One or more of these terms can then be selected to locate similar articles. A final way is to carry out a free-text search and then look to see how it was translated by PubMed's automatic term mapping, search rules, and syntax to identify the related MeSH headings. For example, after searching PubMed for **lumbar strain** and clicking the Details tab, a *query translation* box appears containing the actual terms and field tags used by PubMed to perform the search. In this case, the query translation box contents would be as follows:

lumbar[All Fields] AND (("sprains and strains"[TIAB] NOT Medline[SB])
    OR "sprains and strains"[MeSH Terms] OR strain[Text Word])

The All Fields tag indicates that all of the possible PubMed fields will be searched, TIAB searches for words or numbers that are included in the title or abstract, and the Text Word tag generates a search of almost all of the fields where text can be located.

The MeSH database can be accessed directly by clicking the MeSH Database link located in the left-hand sidebar of PubMed's home page. Using the tools that are provided, a PubMed search can be created that utilizes MeSH terms exclusively. Searching from this page produces a list of suitable MeSH terms that become the building blocks of the intended PubMed search. One should make selections from the list of MeSH terms by clicking the box next to the desired term. Checked terms can then be sent to the search box with an appropriate Boolean operator by clicking the Send To button. Figure 3.9 shows the MeSH search page and the results of a MeSH query of **lumbar strain**.

The MeSH terms that are listed after querying can be expanded by clicking on them or checking the boxes next to them and clicking the Display button. At this point, any of the listed subheadings can be selected to add them to the search. If none of the presented MeSH terms satisfies your requirements, review the suggested alternates and select one if applicable. If you are satisfied, however, click the Send To button to send the selected term or terms to the search box, where you can either continue to build the search by adding more terms or click the Search PubMed button to perform the search. Additional terms sent to the search box can include the AND, OR, or NOT operators by using the Send To dropdown menu.

A handy field tag that can be used to limit searches to articles in which a particular MeSH term is a major topic is [MAJR], or MeSH Major Topic. For instance, searching the MeSH term **scoliosis** retrieves 11,152 PubMed citations,

FIGURE 3.9 Results of searching the MeSH database for lumbar strain.

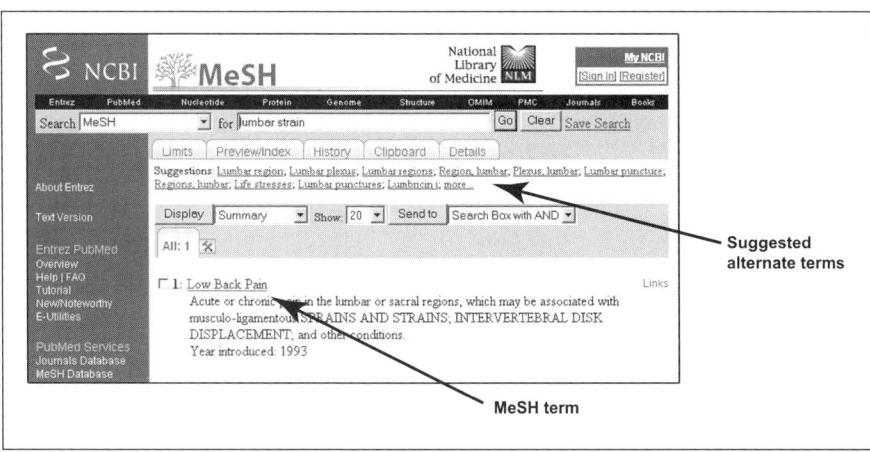

Source: Courtesy of National Library of Medicine.

whereas searching **scoliosis [majr]** returns 6,406. Without the MeSH Major Topic tag, many of the citations are for articles in which scoliosis is a less important topic, and you most likely would not want to consider them in the search. With the tag, however, the search is more focused and the involved articles more relevant. Then again, 6,406 is still a huge number of citations to consider, so other limiting tactics would definitely be helpful.

Earlier in this chapter, the major concepts "manipulation" and "lumbar spinal stenosis" were formulated based on a foreground question. We will now craft an example search using these concepts that finds and then uses MeSH terms. Please go to PubMed and try this search yourself as the steps are presented. Start from the PubMed home page and click the MeSH Database link located on the left. From the MeSH web page, search for **lumbar spinal stenosis**. You should see a "No items found" message, which indicates there are no corresponding MeSH terms. Now remove **lumbar** from the query box and search **spinal stenosis**. Only one term should be found and it exactly matches the search term, so mark the checkbox to the left and send it to the search box by selecting "search box with AND" from the send to drop-down menu. Now type **manipulation** into the query box and search for MeSH terms. Quite a few potential terms will appear this time, some of which have nothing at all to do with manipulating skeletal articulations. Select "Manipulation, Chiropractic" and then set the send to drop-down menu to "Search box with AND." Click to combine it with the previous MeSH term. Now, click the Search PubMed button below the search box to perform the search.

Search Filters

The *Clinical Queries* link on the left sidebar of PubMed's home page opens a page that allows clinicians to search using search filters that will only retrieve articles dealing with either systematic reviews, therapy, diagnosis, etiology, or prognosis. Select the desired radio button specify the type of filter from the list that is to be used, and then enter search terms in the text box at the bottom of the page. The only categories of articles that will result from the search will coincide with the filter type that is utilized (Table 3.4).

Summary

Learning how the biomedical literature is organized within databases and getting acquainted with the fundamental search strategies presented in this chapter is

TABLE 3.4   PubMed searching: Basics

Enter last name and initials to search by *author* (e.g., **jones ts**).

Use double quotation marks to search by *phrase* (e.g., **"low-back exercise"**).

Click on the MeSH Browser link in the sidebar to search by *subject*.

To search for *journals*, enter complete journal titles (e.g., **"Journal of Manipulative and Physiological Therapeutics"**) or MEDLINE abbreviations (e.g., **"J Manipulative Physiol Ther"**). Click on Journals Database to find journal titles, if needed.

Searches can be combined by performing several searches, then clicking on History and following the instructions.

---

essential to becoming proficient at EBC. In fact, literature searching is one of the most important skills one should develop to progress in this area. A great deal of time can be wasted, and information needed to answer clinical questions ultimately may not be found, when unskillful search strategies are utilized. Unfortunately, however, there are no literature searching rules (i.e., cookbook approaches) available to help formulate searches; hence, you will have to experiment with the various search tools to become skilled.

Practitioners new to evidence-based methods can easily become discouraged and fall back into outmoded practice routines if they have to struggle too much while finding evidence. Accordingly, please take whatever time is needed to learn this material, realizing that your proficiency level will improve with every search that you carry out. It will probably take quite a bit of effort to carry out literature searches at first, but that too will improve with practice. As a final point, no matter how proficient a literature searcher you become, a good librarian at a biomedical library can be an invaluable asset to help you construct profitable searches.

References

1. Gore, G. *Searching the medical literature. Inj Prev*, 2003. **9**(2):103–4.
2. Maher, C. *User's guide to the chiropractic literature-1A: How to use an article about therapy [Comment]. J Manipulative Physiol Ther*, 2004. **27**(1):70–1.
3. Busse, J. *User's guide to the chiropractic literature-1A: How to use an article about therapy [Author reply]. J Manipulative Physiol Ther*, 2004. **27**(1):71–2.
4. Murphy, L., et al. *Spinal palpation: The challenges of information retrieval using available databases. J Manipulative Physio Ther*, 2003. **26**(6):374–82.

5. Curl, D., and C. Shapiro. *Literature searching by a field doctor: A comparison of manual versus computerized methods. Chiropractic Technique*, 1993. **5**(1):15–22.
6. Aker, P.D., et al. *Searching chiropractic literature: A comparison of three computerized databases. J Manipulative Physiol Ther*, 1996. **19**(8):518–24.
7. Crumley, E., and T. Klassen. *Searching for the evidence: The process involved. Paediatrics & Child Health*, 2002. **7**(8).
8. Stave, C.D. *Field Guide to MEDLINE: Making Searching Simple*. 2003. Philadelphia: Lippincott Williams & Wilkins, ix.

CHAPTER FOUR

Biostatistics Basics

Many otherwise rational individuals practically flee in terror when the term *biostatistics* is mentioned, much less when faced with reading a chapter on the topic. Face it, biostatistics is based on statistics, which is in turn based on mathematics, and it is all terribly difficult. I can certainly empathize, because it was something I struggled to learn. Accordingly, I will endeavor to present biostatistics in such a way that it is as straightforward as possible, yet understandable to you the reader. This chapter has intentionally been presented as a basic introduction to this very expansive and complex field. However, fundamental concepts are covered that should prepare you to not only understand but also be able to critique biostatistical matters that will be found in the research-related articles that are encountered in evidence-based chiropractic (EBC). Mathematical calculations are presented only in enough detail to understand the basic concepts. The reader is referred to computer programs such as Microsoft Excel, SAS, or SPSS to perform computations if so desired. Be advised that certain aspects of biostatistics will not be covered in this material, but there are plenty of excellent statistics books available if you want more, such as *Fundamentals of Biostatistics* by Rosner[1] and *Statistics* by Witte and Witte.[2] Another book that is not as comprehensive, but is straightforward in presenting material of interest to doctors, is *High-Yield Biostatistics* by Glaser.[3]

Several frequently misunderstood statistical terms should be mentioned before delving into this topic. The term *data* is plural for *datum* and refers to the measurements or observations of a variable. A *variable* is a characteristic that can be observed or manipulated and can take on different values. When referring to summary data from a population, these characteristics are known as *parameters*, and when referring to summary data from samples, they are known as *statistics*. There are also different kinds of variables. *Independent variables* temporally precede dependent variables and are often manipulated by the researcher. They represent whatever treatment or intervention is used in a study. *Dependent variables* are whatever is measured as an outcome in a study whose values depend upon the independent variable.

Populations and Samples

Populations are typically thought of as the total number of inhabitants in a given geographical area. However, in research, *population* refers to the larger group from which a sample is drawn. Examples of some populations are lower back patients in a chiropractic practice and whiplash patients presenting to an emergency room. It is generally not practical to include all members of a population in research projects; instead, a representative sample is selected and only those members are included in the study. Accordingly, a *sample* is a subset of a population that is selected for a given study.

Members of a sample are often randomly selected, which produces samples that have an advantage over the nonrandom variety in that they are more likely to be representative of the population from which they were drawn. This means that members of the sample group will have characteristics similar to the persons included in the original population. *Random samples* are generated by selecting persons from a population so that each individual has the same probability of being selected. A random sample only includes a partial subset of the population, but participants are selected in such a way as to ensure that the sample is representative of the entire population. *Nonrandom samples* are predisposed to being biased regarding variables such as age, gender, condition severity, and socioeconomic status and are frequently nonrepresentative.

In research it is often necessary to make inferences about the population from which a sample has been taken. One would be more confident when making inferences about a population based on information derived from a sample, if random sampling was involved. However, random selection is seldom carried out in health care research; instead, a process of *randomization* (also known as *random assignment*) is utilized. Randomization is covered more thoroughly in Chapter 5, but briefly it involves starting with a nonrandom sample and then assigning study participants to either treatment or nontreatment groups in such a way that each person has an equal chance of being assigned to either of the groups. This is often accomplished by mechanical means, such as a coin toss or drawing numbers from a hat, or in any other way that gives each of the sample members the same likelihood of being selected for assignment to one of the study groups.

Descriptive Statistics

The most basic form of statistics is known as *descriptive statistics*, which is a branch of statistics that lays the foundation for more complex statistical methods and can be distinguished from inferential statistics, whereby hypotheses may be tested. Descriptive statistics summarize various aspects of a collection of data from a sample or a population in such a way that it is easier to read and comprehend. Common descriptive statistical measures include the mean, median, and standard deviation, with which you are surely familiar. Articles in scientific journals provide these statistics concerning the demographics and baseline measurements of patients involved in the studies that are presented.

Descriptive statistics characterize the *shape*, *central tendency*, and *variability* of a set of data. When referring to the shape of data, the frequencies of the values of observations are described. When represented graphically, a frequency distribution takes on a particular shape that provides important information about the underlying data. Measures of central tendency include the mean, median, and mode, which give information about where the middle of the data lies. The variability of data is the degree to which values are spread above and below the central values. The variability of data is sometimes referred to as *dispersion*.

As an example, descriptive statistics can be used to depict the number of visits provided to patients in a hypothetical study that is presented in Table 4.1.

The distribution of this set of values can be evaluated by counting the frequency of occurrence of each of the listed values. Hence, there are five 2s, seven 3s, six 4s, and so on. One way to represent this distribution is to simply list the values along with their frequency of occurrence; another way is to represent them in a graph (Figure 4.1).

92 Chapter 4 Biostatistics Basics

TABLE 4.1 Hypothetical study of total visits

Case No.	Total Visits	Case No.	Total Visits
1	7	15	6
2	2	16	4
3	2	17	3
4	3	18	5
5	4	19	4
6	3	20	5
7	5	21	3
8	3	22	6
9	4	23	6
10	6	24	4
11	2	25	3
12	3	26	2
13	7	27	2
14	4	28	6

FIGURE 4.1 Frequency distribution and matching histogram of the Total Visits hypothetical data presented in Table 4.1.

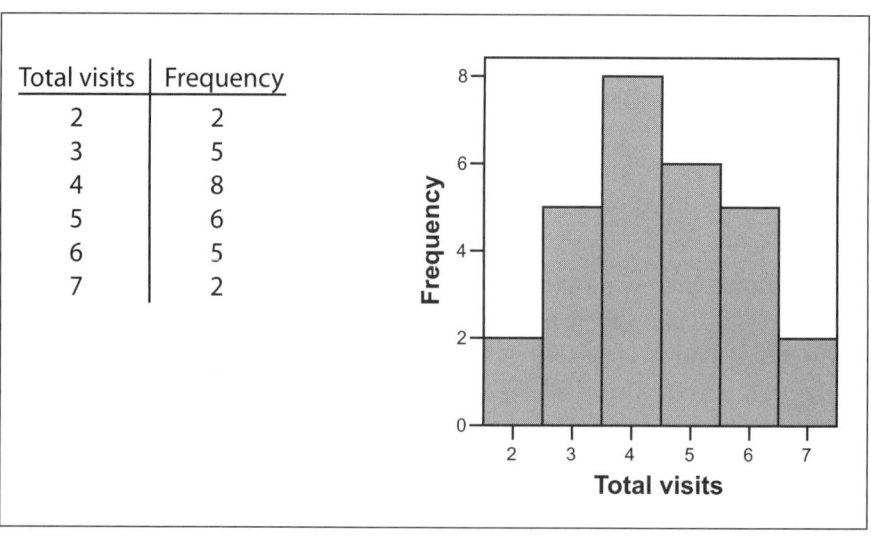

Descriptive Statistics

The graph illustrated in Figure 4.1 is called a *histogram*, which is similar to a bar chart, except without spaces between the bars. In reality, a histogram is a type of bar chart. However, histograms are used to visually depict frequency distributions of continuous data (data that can take on any value within an interval), whereas bar charts are used for categorical information (e.g., male or female; mild, moderate, or severe). The term *discrete data* is used in contrast to *continuous data* and refers to data that is derived from observations that are separate and distinct; for instance, patients in a study receiving manipulation. Each patient is separate and distinct, because patients cannot be divided (you cannot have 0.5 patient). Categorical data are also considered to be discrete.[4]

In addition to frequencies, the percentages at which each of the values occurs in a distribution and cumulative percentages help describe the data even more. Cumulative frequency tables are typically provided by statistics software packages and frequently appear in research papers (Table 4.2). Ranges of values will also sometimes be presented; in this case, the lowest value is 2 and the highest is 7.

Measures of Central Tendency

The *mean* (also known as *average*) is the most commonly used descriptive statistic (or parameter when referring to a population), with which you are no doubt already quite familiar. Essentially, all values of a series of numbers are added together, and then divided by the number of elements. This operation is represented by the following formulas:

TABLE 4.2 **Cumulative frequencies**

Value	Frequency	Percentage	Cumulative Percentage
2	5	17.9	17.9
3	7	25.0	42.9
4	6	21.4	64.3
5	3	10.0	75.0
6	5	17.9	92.9
7	2	7.1	100.0
Total	28	100.0	—

Chapter 4 Biostatistics Basics

Mean of a sample: $\overline{X} = \dfrac{\Sigma X}{n}$

Mean of a population: $\mu = \dfrac{\Sigma X}{N}$

where $\overline{X}$ ("X bar") refers to the mean of a sample, and μ refers to the mean of a population, ΣX is a command that adds all of the X values. *n* is the total number of values in the series of a sample, and *N* is the same for a population.

Technically speaking, the mean should be referred to as the *arithmetic mean*, in contrast to the geometric mean. However, by convention, just plain *mean* denotes the arithmetic mean. Do not worry about what the geometric mean is, because you will rarely encounter it when reading clinical research journals.

The *mode* is simply the most frequently occurring value in a series. In the Total Visits example (Table 4.1), the most frequently occurring number of visits was 3 (there were seven occurrences of this value), making it the mode. This is obvious on the corresponding histogram, where the modal value is represented by the highest bar.

Another measure of central tendency is the *median*, which is the value that divides a series of values in half when they are all listed in order. When there is an odd number of values in a series, the median is simply the middle value. When there is an even number of values, count from each end of the series toward the middle and then average the two middle values. There are 28 values in the Total Visits example, so the median is calculated by placing all of the numbers in order, counting 14 in from each end of the series to find the middle two values, and then averaging these values:

2,2,2,2,2,3,3,3,3,3,3,3,3,4,4,4,4,4,4,4,5,5,5,6,6,6,6,6,6,7,7
↑↑

Middle two values

Median = (4 + 4)/2 = 8/2 = 4.0

At this point, you are probably wondering why there are three different ways of measuring central tendency (i.e., where most of the data are). It is because

Descriptive Statistics

there are different types of data that must be analyzed by specific methods designed to deal with each of the data types. This is true not only regarding calculations of central tendency, but also regarding the more advanced statistical tests that will be discussed later in this chapter. Moreover, it is fairly common for researchers to make mistakes in this area, which can result in the reporting of inaccurate findings. One of the main factors regarding the choice of the appropriate statistical test has to do with what level of measurement was utilized with the data, which is covered in the next section.

Levels of Measurement

There are four *levels of measurement*, each one having specific rules for the operation and interpretation of associated data. Comprehending and applying these rules is imperative in determining how the data should be analyzed and which statistical test should be used in a given study. The four levels of measurement are *nominal*, *ordinal*, *interval*, and *ratio*.

The *nominal* scale of measurement involves data that are coded in the form of a number, name, or letter that is assigned to each category or group that is involved (i.e., categorical data). Examples include gender (e.g., male or female), job category (e.g., managerial, clerical, or blue-collar), and hair color (e.g., black, brunette, blonde, or red). Nominal measurement is also known as the *classificatory scale* because individuals or objects are classified into categories. A numerical code is often assigned to the various categories to facilitate analysis. For instance, the job category example just mentioned could be coded as follows: 0 = managerial, 1 = clerical, and 2 = blue-collar. The only permissible mathematical operation that is appropriate for nominal data is counting of the categories (e.g., 25 males and 30 females).

Ordinal measurement also involves categories, but the data is rank-ordered. In other words, the data can be listed in a meaningful order. Ranking in the military is a good example (e.g., Lieutenant, Captain, Major, Colonel, General). Rating the severity of pain as being mild, moderate, or severe is a common use of ordinal measurement. An important consideration about ordinal values is that they only represent position of order, not quantity. Therefore, the spacing between steps may not be uniform (e.g., a lieutenant plus a captain does not equal a general). As a result, no mathematical operations are possible. Imagine if you will, dividing 15 patients in severe pain by 10 in mild pain to derive 1.5 patients in moderate pain. It just doesn't work or even make sense. As with categorical data, however, the incidence of each value can be depicted.

The next level of measurement is the *interval* scale, which has several distinctive properties. One property requires that interval measurements exhibit equal intervals, and another requires them to be ordered. Thus, interval measurements are like ordinal data in that they can be placed in a meaningful order. An interval scale does not have a true zero, however. The classic example is the Fahrenheit scale, where 0° does not correspond to an absence of heat, so it does not represent a measurement of true zero. The Kelvin scale, on the other hand, does have a true zero that corresponds to an absence of heat; therefore, it would not be considered an interval measurement. Height, weight, and age qualify as interval measures, but also qualify at the next higher level of measurement, which is ratio. The mathematical operations permitted with interval data include addition and subtraction.

The *ratio* scale involves the most advanced level of measurement, which can accommodate most types of arithmetic operations. In this level of measurement, there are equal intervals and a true zero. An example is measurement of cervical range of motion, where no movement corresponds to zero degrees and the difference between 10 and 20 degrees is the same as the difference between 40 and 50 degrees. The Kelvin scale, which did not meet the criteria of interval measurement, is another ratio scale example. As you read scientific literature, there are some questions that can be posed to help you determine if a measurement qualifies as being ratio. First, does the measurement of zero represent an absence of the characteristic being tested? Second, do differences between consecutive measured numbers represent equal amounts of the characteristic?

Spend a little time to learn these levels of measurement, because their misapplication is common, yet very important for you to identify when appraising articles. A useful mnemonic is *NOIR*, which is helpful to not only remember the names of the levels, but also their order:

Nominal
Ordinal
Interval
Ratio

With an understanding of the various levels of measurement, take a look at Table 4.3, which presents the mathematical operations that are permitted and the appropriate measures of central tendency.

This presentation of dscriptive statistics has been light regarding the mechanics of performing the various calculations, since virtually all statistical programs will analyze data very quickly and produce accurate descriptive statistics without the user understanding the mechanisms involved in the actual calculations. However, readers who are interested in learning more about this topic, possibly because they plan to undertake a research project of their own in the future, are referred to one of the biostatistics textbooks listed in this chapter's reference section. Table 4.4 contains the descriptive statistics that correspond to the Total Visits example, which were easily produced in Microsoft Excel, a very common program that is part of the Microsoft Office suite. Thus, if you decide to verify figures for a study that you are reviewing, you most likely already have the software that is capable of performing the calculations.

The Shape of Data

The fact that data has a shape is very important to statistics. This shape can be seen when looking at a histogram of the frequency distribution of a given set of

TABLE 4.3 **Permissible mathematical operations and best measure of central tendency to correspond with the levels of measurement**

Measurement Scale	*Permissible Mathematical Operations*	*Best Measure Central Tendency*
Nominal	Counting	Mode
Ordinal	Greater or less than operations	Median
Interval	Addition and subtraction	Symmetrical: Mean Skewed: Median
Ratio	Addition, subtraction, multiplication, and division	Symmetrical: Mean Skewed: Median

TABLE 4.4 Descriptive statistics of the Total Visits example

Mean	4.07
Standard error	0.30
Median	4.0
Mode	3.0
Standard deviation	1.59
Sample variance	2.51
Kurtosis	−1.02
Skewness	0.35
Range	5
Minimum	2
Maximum	7
Sum	114
Count	28

data. Figure 4.2 is a histogram representing the ages of a group of individuals. Each bar represents an age category (e.g., ranging from age 20 to 30 years), and the heights of the bars correspond to how many people are in each category. Notice how the distribution is fairly symmetrical, with most of the ages falling in the middle of the distribution (say, between 30 and 60 years) and progressively fewer cases toward the extremes at either end of the age scale. This phenomenon is true with regard to much biological data and is what gives rise to the *normal curve* (also known as the *bell-shaped curve*). The area beneath a normal curve is said to have a normal distribution (or *Gaussian distribution*), which has some properties that are very helpful in statistics. These properties are as follows:

1. A normal distribution is symmetric about its mean.
2. The highest point of the overlying normal curve is at the mean.
3. As one moves away from the mean in either direction, the height of the curve decreases, approaching, but never reaching, zero (Figure 4.3).

In a normal distribution, the various measures of the location of its center are equivalent, where the mean, median, and mode are all equal and in the same position (Figure 4.4). Conversely, these measures of central tendency have dissimilar positions in *skewed distributions* (Figure 4.5). This is because data are not distributed symmetrically in skewed distributions. Instead, scores tend to congregate toward one end of the distribution. while a relatively small number of extreme

Descriptive Statistics

FIGURE 4.2 Histogram of ages with most values falling in the middle of the distribution.

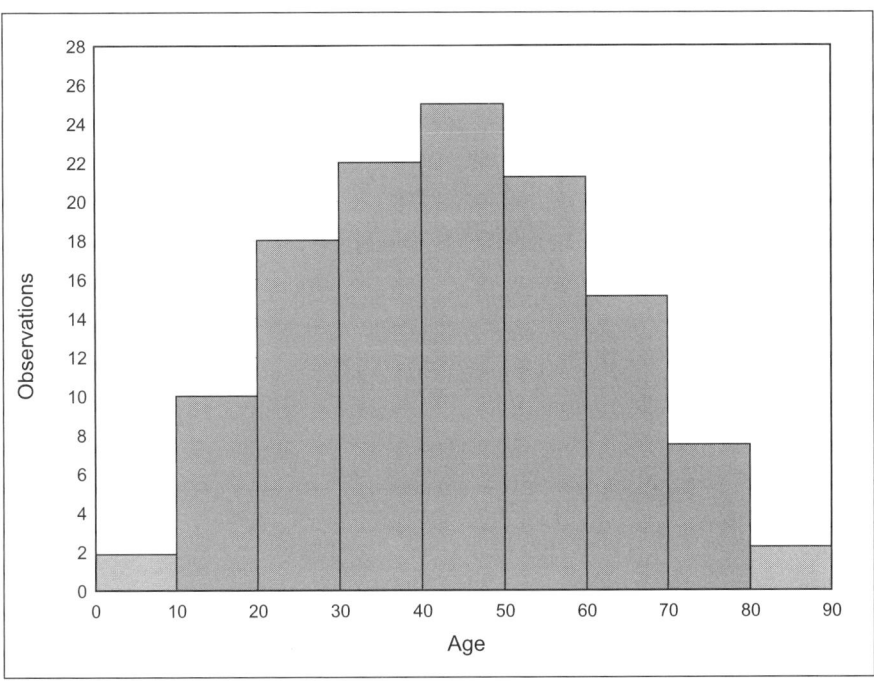

FIGURE 4.3 Properties of a normal distribution.

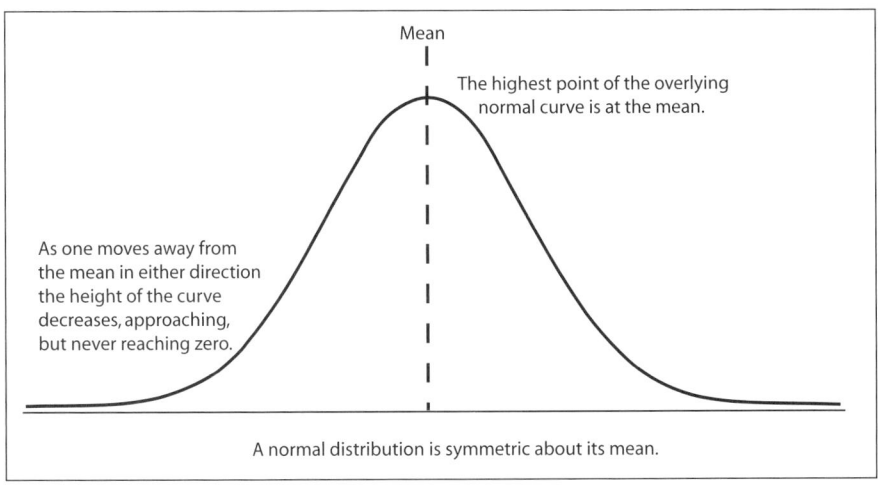

FIGURE 4.4 In a normal distribution, the mean, median, and mode are all equal in the same position.

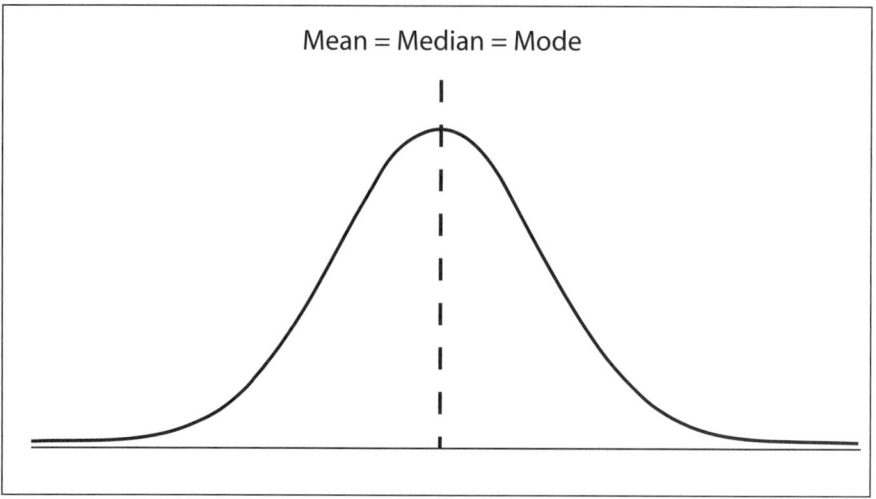

values are located in the farthest extent of the opposite end. Skew is always to the direction of the longer tail: to the right if positively skewed, and to the left if negative.

The distribution of family income is a good example of a skewed distribution, where relatively few very wealthy families skew the distribution to the right (positively skewed), thus raising the mean income. On the other hand, a few very wealthy people will have little effect on the median in this type of distribution, making it a preferred measure of central tendency for skewed distributions. Since the mean estimates the central point of a distribution, it is better not to use it as an estimate of the average score for a skewed distribution. Having said this, it is not uncommon for researchers to report means and standard deviations of skewed data. The median, on the other hand, will be the central point of any distribution, since 50% of the values fall above and 50% below it. Therefore, the median works better than the mean to describe the center of skewed distributions. Authors reporting on the findings of health care research should comment on the normality of their data so readers are able to determine which measures and which statistical tests would be appropriate.

Descriptive Statistics | 101

FIGURE 4.5 Positively skewed distributions have tails extending to the right, whereas negatively skewed distributions have tails extending to the left. The mean is influenced the most and is drawn toward the tail of the distribution.

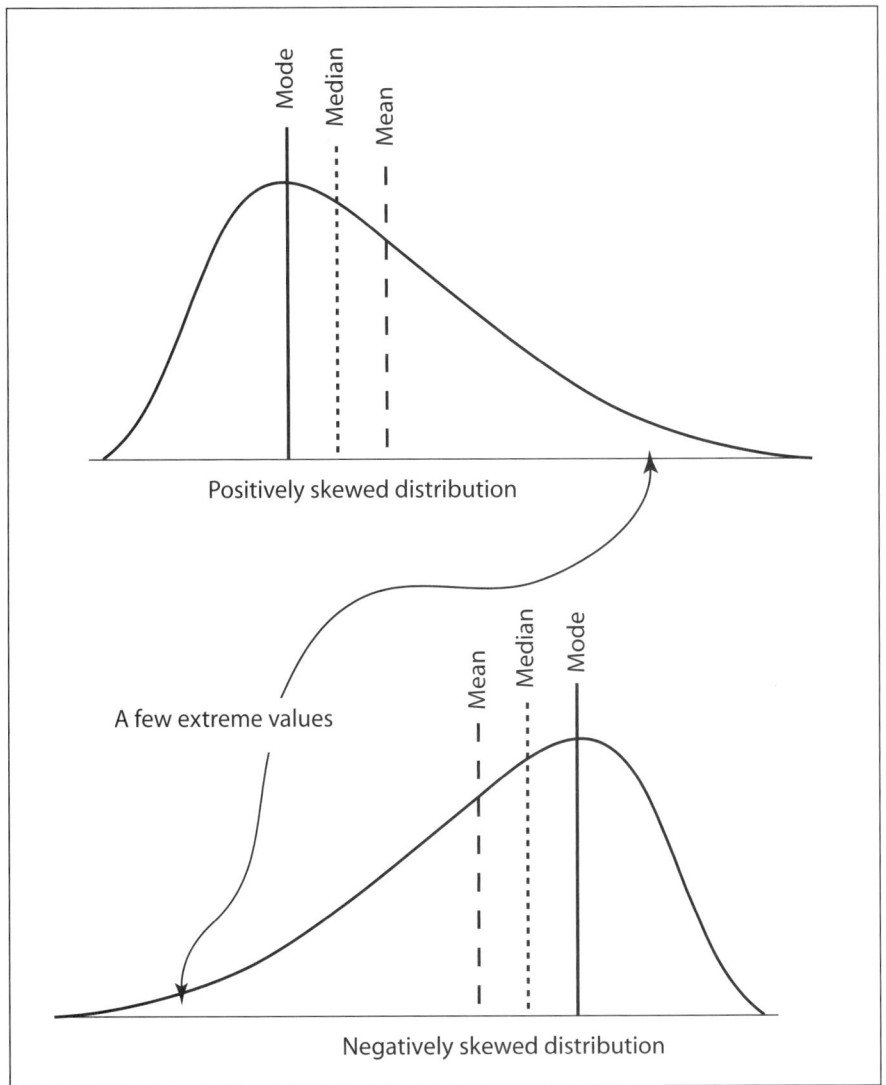

An additional property of normal curves states that about 68.3% of the area under the curve is within 1 standard deviation (defined shortly) of the mean, about 95.5% is within 2 standard deviations of the mean, and about 99.7% is within 3 standard deviations of the mean (Figure 4.6). Furthermore, 95% of the normal distribution (a proportion that is frequently encountered in research) is within 1.96 standard deviations of the mean. These proportions will correspond to the number of observations in a study that is made up of normal data.

The theory of the normality of data not only applies to descriptive statistics, but also is very important when statistical analyses involving hypothesis testing are carried out. That subject is addressed later in this chapter, but for now, the concepts of *variance* and *standard deviation* will be introduced. In brief, the standard deviation has to do with the variability of a set of data. Consider another

FIGURE 4.6 Most observations (approximately 68%) in a normal distribution are within 1 standard deviation above and below the mean, while very few (less than 5%) are more than 2 standard deviations away from it in either direction.

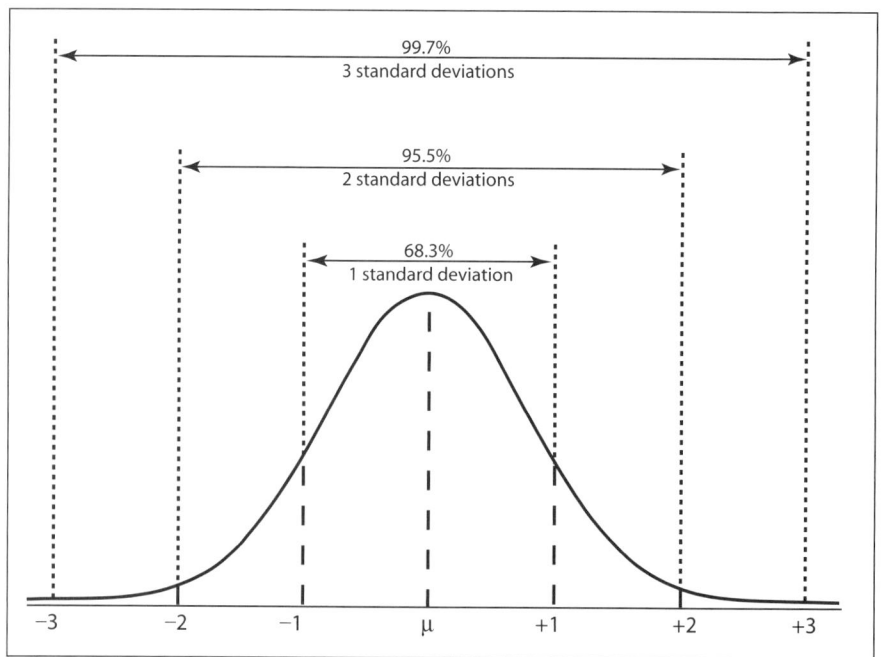

hypothetical study involving 10 participants, where the mean age was 40 years. However, some participants were older and some were younger; 40 was just the average age. Figure 4.7 shows these ages in a column on the left and spread out along an *x*-axis on the right. The amount that the ages are spread out along the *x*-axis is referred to as the *dispersion* or *spread* of the data. There are two measures of the spread of data, *variance* and *standard deviation*, which correspond to the amount that the data deviates from the mean.

To calculate *variance*, the distance that each of the values has deviated from the mean in either the positive or negative direction is considered. Since the objective is to find the average amount of dispersion of the data, intuitively one would add up each of the distances by which the values deviate above and below the mean and then divide by the number of values. This is problematic, however, because adding deviations above and below the mean always equals zero (Figure 4.8). The solution is to first square the distances from the mean, which cancels any negative signs, and then calculate the average of the squared distances (Figure 4.9). This value represents the *variance* (S^2), the average squared dispersion from the mean. In the example, S^2 is 200, which is confusing since the mean age was 40. To resolve this problem, take the square root of the variance, which

FIGURE 4.7 Ages of 10 study participants presented in a column (left) and spread out along an *x*-axis (right).

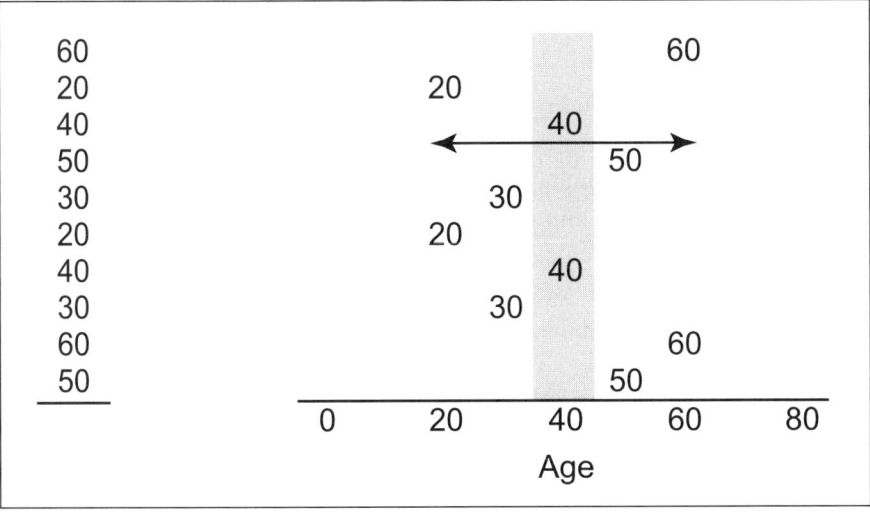

Chapter 4 Biostatistics Basics

FIGURE 4.8 The distances the scores in the age study deviate above and below the mean.

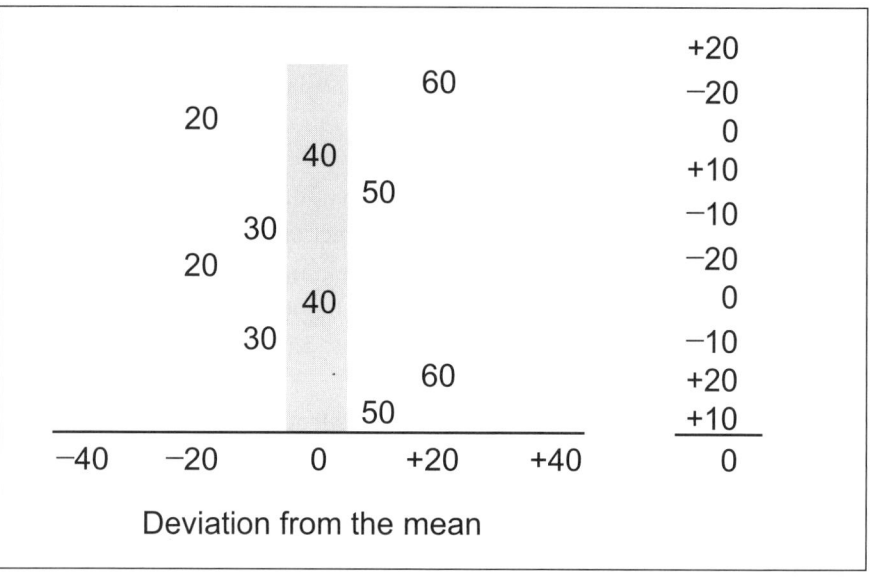

generates the *standard deviation* (S for a sample and σ for a population). The result is in the original, more understandable, units of measurement and represents the approximate average amount that observations deviate above or below the mean.

The following few paragraphs cover the formulas used to calculate variance and standard deviation, although there are many computer programs available that will do it for you, including Microsoft Excel. Nevertheless, some practitioners may want the formulas in order to work through the calculations for themselves. The definition formula is based on the method of calculation shown in Figure 4.9 and represents intuitively how the standard deviation is derived. The definition formulas for calculating S and σ are as follows (note that S^2 and $σ^2$ use the same formulas, but without the square root sign). The formula on the left is used with sample data, and the one on the right with populations.

$$S = \sqrt{\frac{\sum(X - \bar{X})^2}{n}} \quad \text{or} \quad σ = \sqrt{\frac{\sum(X - μ)^2}{N}}$$

FIGURE 4.9 Variance (S^2) is the mean of all deviations from the mean, and standard deviation (S) is the square root of S^2.

$$
\begin{aligned}
+20^2 &= 400 \\
-20^2 &= 400 \\
0& \\
+10^2 &= 100 \\
-10^2 &= 100 \\
-20^2 &= 400 \\
0& \\
-10^2 &= 100 \\
+20^2 &= 400 \\
+10^2 &= 100 \\
\hline
& 2000
\end{aligned}
$$

$$S^2 = \frac{2000}{10} = 200$$

$$S = \sqrt{200} = 14.1$$

where $\bar{X}$ ("X bar") refers to the mean of a sample, and μ refers to the mean of a population. $\Sigma(X - \bar{X})$ is an operation that adds up the differences between the sample mean and the X values. n is the total number of values in the series of a sample, and N is the same for a population. σ represents the standard deviation of a population.

The definition formulas are cumbersome to use in practice, especially when a lot of data is involved. The computational formula, on the other hand, is much easier to work with and is as follows:

$$S = \sqrt{\frac{n \sum X^2 - \left(\sum X\right)^2}{n^2}}$$

The sample formulas presented earlier are only appropriate when applied to descriptive statistics, not inferential statistics. This is because an adjustment is required to accurately represent the variability in the population where a parameter must be estimated. This adjustment is accomplished by changing n to $n - 1$

in the denominator for the sample definition formula and changing n^2 to $n(n-1)$ for the sample computational formula. Thus, when the standard deviation (S) of a sample is used to estimate the standard deviation (σ) of a population, the following formula should be used. Notice that a lowercase *s* is used to denote this estimate of σ.

$$s = \sqrt{\frac{n\sum X^2 - (\sum X)^2}{n(n-1)}}$$

The standard deviation represents the average amount of dispersion for a given set of data, so it follows that data that are more spread out will result in relatively higher standard deviations, whereas data that have a narrow spread will have relatively lower standard deviations (Figure 4.10).

It is often desirable to compare the means of two or more groups to determine whether they are equal. This is done in hypothesis testing when the mean outcome of an active treatment group is compared with a control group. The difference between the means is important in this situation, but equally important is the amount of variance or the standard deviation. It is helpful to visually observe the means of two groups that are placed side by side with their respective normal curves in place (Figure 4.11). If the distributions overlap too much, it is difficult to perceive that the group means are really different. One could say they more or less blend together. Another thing that is helpful in understanding the properties of normal curves is to visually observe an overlay of the curves of several normal distributions that have the same mean, but different standard deviations (Figure 4.12). Notice that wide distributions have large standard deviations, and narrow distributions have small standard deviations.

Corresponding to the number of standard deviations above or below the mean, a given score that is above or below the mean for a distribution of scores is its *z-score* (Figure 4.6). A raw score in a distribution can easily be converted to a *z*-score by subtracting the mean from the raw score and then dividing the difference by the standard deviation (SD). The formulas for calculating *z*-scores are as follows:

$$z = \frac{X - \mu}{\sigma} \text{ for a population}$$

$$z = \frac{X - \mu}{S} \text{ for a sample}$$

Descriptive Statistics 107

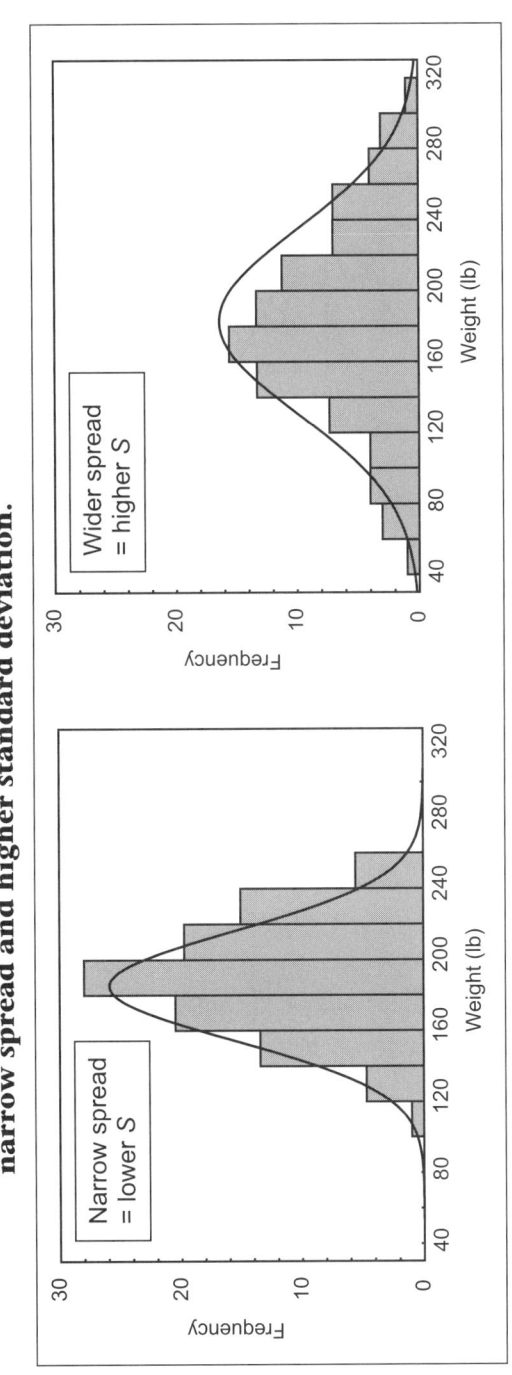

FIGURE 4.10 The distribution on the left has a narrow spread with a correspondingly low standard deviation, whereas the one on the right has a comparatively narrow spread and higher standard deviation.

FIGURE 4.11 The means of two groups are compared. They have different means but equal standard deviations.

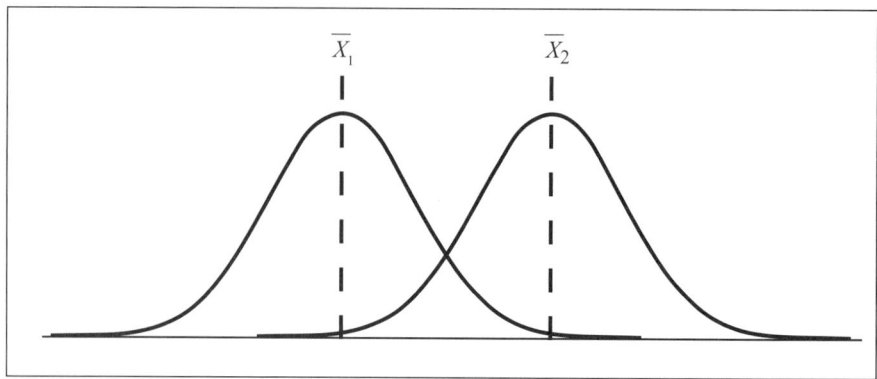

FIGURE 4.12 Three groups having the same mean but different standard deviations are superimposed to illustrate the fact that the value of a standard deviation affects the shape of normal curves.

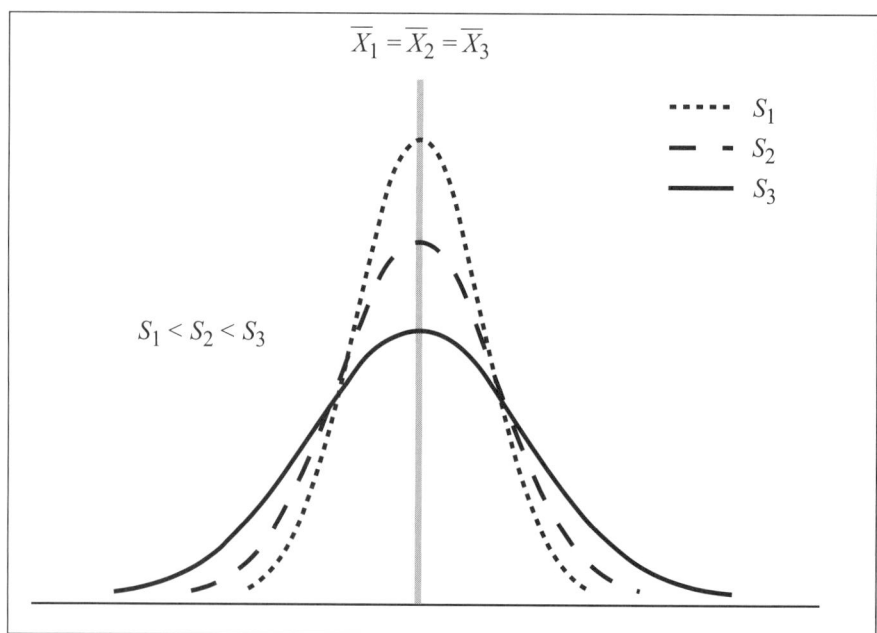

This conversion process is often called *standardization* because the resulting distribution of z-scores will always have a mean of zero and a standard deviation of 1, and the area under the curve can be standardized to equal 1. Once the z-score has been calculated for a given raw score, the proportion of scores that are higher or lower can be determined by referring to a z-table rather than having to use calculus.

As an example, the mean of the cervical range of motion scores for 50 patients was 40 degrees, with a standard deviation of 10. If one of the participant's range of motion was 55 degrees, what is the corresponding z-score and, based on that z-score, what is the percentage of individuals with higher scores?

Figure 4.13 shows the normal curve that corresponds to the 50 participants, and the z-score has been calculated to be 1.5. The area under the curve can be determined based on the z-score by referring to a z-table (Table 4.5), which can be found in just about any statistics book or online. Z-tables provide the proportions of the area under a normal curve for various values of z. The proportions listed in Table 4.5 correspond to the area extending from z to the limit of the left tail. Notice that the proportion corresponding to $z = 1.5$ is 0.9332, and, since $1 - 0.93 = 0.067$, 6.7% of scores were found to be 55 degrees or higher.

Inferential Statistics

The branch of statistics that is concerned with using data from a sample to make inferences about a population is referred to as *inferential statistics*. Statistical tests that allow inference enable the researcher to use a smaller number of observations to make generalizations about the entire population from which the sample was taken. Because of time and financial constraints, it is rarely feasible, or even possible, to test each person in a population, making statistical inference an essential component of research. For example, a researcher may want to determine how effective cervical manipulation is for the entire population of sinusitis patients by testing only a small sample, instead of the entire population of patients.

If repeated random samples are taken from a given population, the sample means will not all have the same value. For instance, consider a sample of 10 lower back pain patients derived from a population of chiropractic patients who were assessed for lifting capacity, having a mean score of 55 pounds. If another sample of the same size from the same population were tested, the mean would likely be different—possibly very different. Repeating this process many times

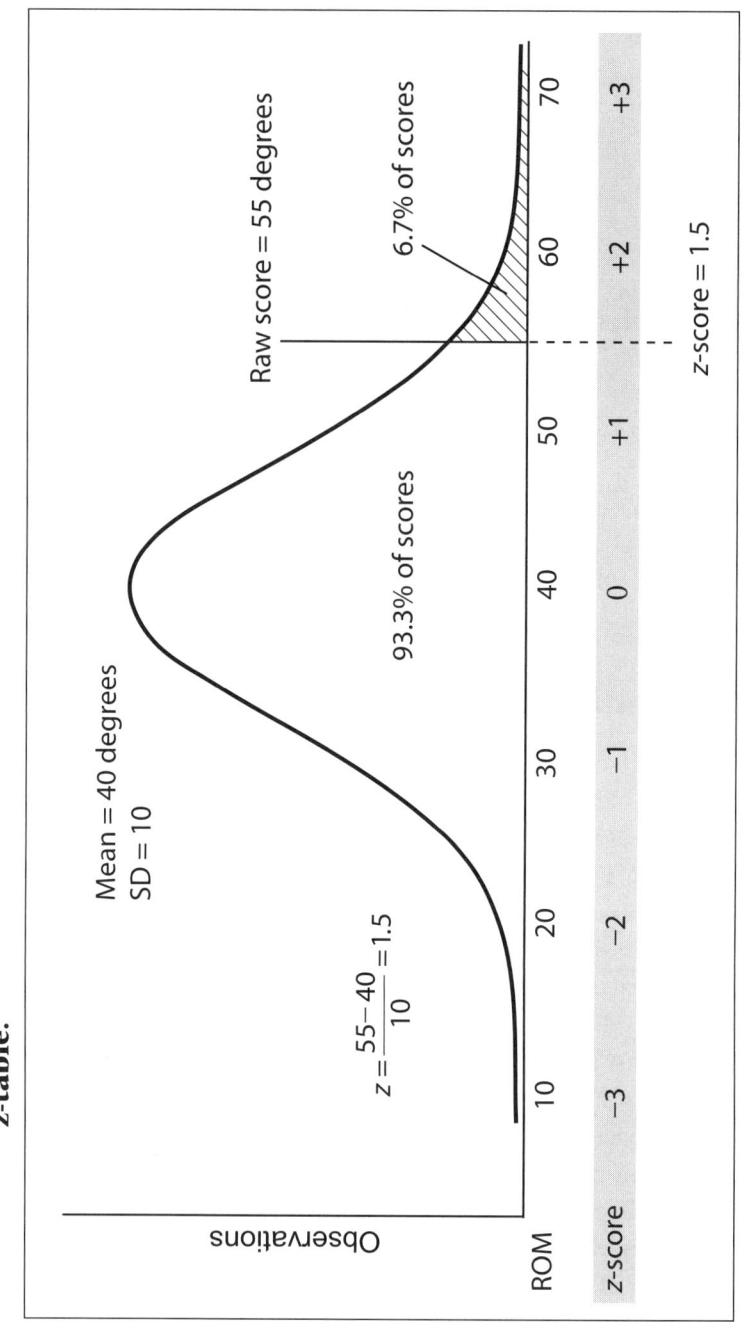

FIGURE 4.13 A raw score of 55 degrees is converted to a z-score of 1.5, which permits one to find the proportion of individuals with higher scores after referring to a z-table.

TABLE 4.5 Partial z-table (to z = 1.5) showing proportions of the area under a normal curve for different values of z

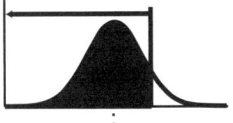

z	0.00	0.01	0.02	0.03	0.04	0.05	0.06	0.07	0.08	0.09
0.0	0.5000	0.5040	0.5080	0.5120	0.5160	0.5199	0.5239	0.5279	0.5319	0.5359
0.1	0.5398	0.5438	0.5478	0.5517	0.5557	0.5596	0.5636	0.5675	0.5714	0.5753
0.2	0.5793	0.5832	0.5871	0.5910	0.5948	0.5987	0.6026	0.6064	0.6103	0.6141
0.3	0.6179	0.6217	0.6255	0.6293	0.6331	0.6368	0.6406	0.6443	0.6480	0.6517
0.4	0.6554	0.6591	0.6628	0.6664	0.6700	0.6736	0.6772	0.6808	0.6844	0.6879
0.5	0.6915	0.6950	0.6985	0.7019	0.7054	0.7088	0.7123	0.7157	0.7190	0.7224
0.6	0.7257	0.7291	0.7324	0.7357	0.7389	0.7422	0.7454	0.7486	0.7517	0.7549
0.7	0.7580	0.7611	0.7642	0.7673	0.7704	0.7734	0.7764	0.7794	0.7823	0.7852
0.8	0.7881	0.7910	0.7939	0.7967	0.7995	0.8023	0.8051	0.8078	0.8106	0.8133
0.9	0.8159	0.8186	0.8212	0.8238	0.8264	0.8289	0.8315	0.8340	0.8365	0.8389
1.0	0.8413	0.8438	0.8461	0.8485	0.8508	0.8531	0.8554	0.8577	0.8599	0.8621
1.1	0.8643	0.8665	0.8686	0.8708	0.8729	0.8749	0.8770	0.8790	0.8810	0.8830
1.2	0.8849	0.8869	0.8888	0.8907	0.8925	0.8944	0.8962	0.8980	0.8997	0.9015
1.3	0.9032	0.9049	0.9066	0.9082	0.9099	0.9115	0.9131	0.9147	0.9162	0.9177
1.4	0.9192	0.9207	0.9222	0.9236	0.9251	0.9265	0.9279	0.9292	0.9306	0.9319
1.5	0.9332	0.9345	0.9357	0.9370	0.9382	0.9394	0.9406	0.9418	0.9429	0.9441

would produce a distribution of sample means that, if repeated enough times, would take on a normal shape; if repeated an infinite number of times (theoretically), it is called a *sampling distribution*.

In actuality, it would not be practical to sample a population again and again, yet it would be useful to know the true mean of the population. The population mean can be inferred from the sample, however, by using the sample mean as a reasonable estimate, often referred to as the *point estimate*. The spread of means around the mean in a sampling distribution is referred to as the *standard error* or *standard error of the mean*, which can be estimated from the sample. Whereas standard deviation refers to the spread of scores around a sample mean, the spread of the means in a sampling distribution is known as the standard error of the mean. The standard error (SE) may be calculated by dividing the standard deviation of the sample by the square root of the number of units in the sample:

$$SE_m = S/\sqrt{n}$$

Accordingly, the standard error estimate will be higher when the sample's standard deviation is large or when the sample size is small. Conversely, it will be lower when the standard deviation is small or the sample size is large. A smaller standard error is preferable because it allows more precise generalizations from samples to populations.

Confidence Intervals

An important feature of a sampling distribution is that its shape becomes normal as the size of the sample becomes larger, even if the population from which the samples were obtained was not normally distributed. As a result, the symmetrical properties of the normal distribution can be utilized, including the property concerning the proportion of the area under the curve. Moreover, about 68.3% of the sample means will be within 1 standard error of the mean, about 95.5% within 2 standard errors, and about 99.7% within 3 standard errors. Samples become more representative of the population, and their means closer to the population means, when samples are larger.

A *confidence interval* (CI) is an estimated range of values that is likely to contain the population parameter that is being estimated (e.g., the mean). The probability that this range of values contains the population parameter is typically set at 95%, although 99% and 90% are occasionally encountered; hence, the "95% confidence interval" is commonly used. This means that if repeated samples are drawn from a population, and a confidence interval is calculated for each sample, then 95% of the intervals are likely to contain the population mean. In other words, once a confidence interval for a mean is calculated, one can have 95% confidence—or in yet other words, 95% probability—that the true mean value lies within that calculated interval.

The CI of a mean can be calculated with reference to the normal distribution as follows (Figure 4.14):

1. Find the z-scores that correspond to the percentage specified for the confidence interval by referring to a z-table to find the z-score that corresponds to the area under the standard normal distribution that includes 95% of all values (e.g., $z = \pm 1.96$ for a 95% CI). This z-score is so common in health care research that it can be memorized.
2. Multiply the z-scores by the standard error of the mean.
3. Add the product of the positive multiplication to the sample mean to find

FIGURE 4.14 Ninety-five percent confidence interval (shaded area).

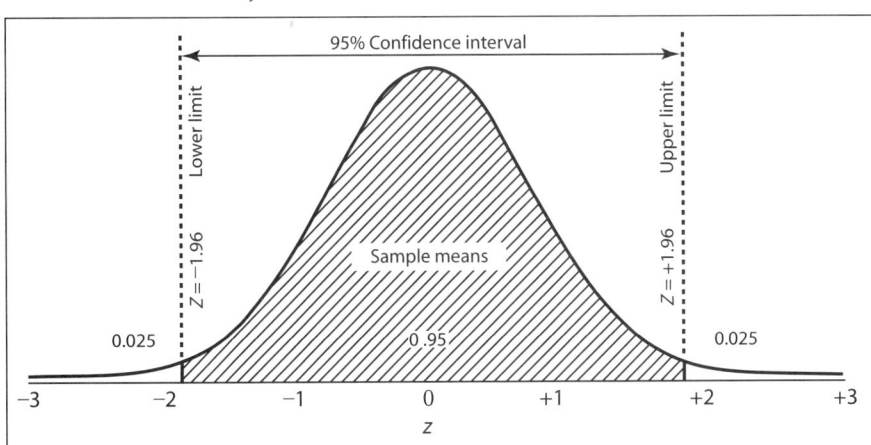

the upper limit of the CI, and then subtract the negative product to find the lower limit of the CI.

For example, the mean age of a random sample of 25 neck pain patients is 39 years, and the standard deviation is 12 years. To find the 95% CI for this group, first find the corresponding z-scores using a z-table, which is $z = \pm 1.96$. Second, find the standard error using the formula given previously, which is $12/\sqrt{25} = 2.4$, and then multiply 2.4 by ± 1.96, which equals ± 4.7. The third step is to add and subtract ± 4.7 to the mean to determine the upper and lower bounds of the CI, respectively (i.e., 95% CI = 34.3 to 43.7 years).

This discussion has only dealt with CIs using the normal distribution; however, they are also used with chi-square and t-distributions, which will be discussed later in this chapter. In addition to using CIs to estimate the mean of a population, they can be helpful to describe differences between means, differences in proportions, relative risk, or odds ratios.[5] For instance, a CI could be calculated for the difference between the mean cholesterol levels of a group of patients who followed a vegetarian diet and those of another group of meat eaters.

Most important for understanding inference and testing of differences between groups, there is a tight relationship between the size of the sample, the size of the data variation (standard deviation or variance), and the CI. The smaller the sample, the larger the CI, because the chance of getting it wrong is greater; the larger the sample size, the smaller the CI, because the chance of estimating it correctly is greater. Similarly, the larger the variation in the data (standard deviation or variance), the larger the CI, because greater variation leads to greater uncertainty.

Hypothesis Testing

A *hypothesis* is an assumption that appears to explain certain phenomena, which must be tested to see whether it is true. An example is a researcher's claim that chiropractic manipulation is better than standard medical treatment for the treatment of migraine headaches. The *research hypothesis* in this case states that chiropractic is a better treatment than standard medical care for migraine headache. A research hypothesis is also known as the *alternative hypothesis* and is denoted H_1. The research hypothesis is not tested directly in hypothesis testing; rather, the *null hypothesis* (denoted H_0) is tested first, and then, depending on the outcome of this test, there is either support for or against the research hypothesis. Hypothesis testing is achieved by comparing the means of the experimental groups to determine if they are significantly different. At times the difference between groups may appear real, but one cannot be sure whether this difference is the result of chance until it has been tested using statistical methods. Chance plays a part in hypothesis testing in relation to random sources of error. For example, by chance the experimental groups, which are supposed to be equivalent before the experimental intervention, may actually have been dissimilar before the intervention begins and therefore any differences found following the intervention may not actually be related to the effectiveness of treatment.[6]

The null hypothesis assumes there is no difference between the groups being tested, and the research hypothesis is adopted only if the null hypothesis proves to be unlikely. Since the null hypothesis asserts there is no difference between the means, the idea is to reject it on the grounds that it is very unlikely to be true. In health care research, it typically must be at least 95% *unlikely* that the null hypothesis is true before it can be rejected. This logic is similar to the "innocent until proven guilty" concept utilized in our legal system. Researchers assume that the null hypothesis is "innocent" until it has been proven, with at least 95% certainty, that it is guilty. When the null hypothesis is found guilty, it is then rejected and the research hypothesis can be accepted as being true.

A null hypothesis that deals with the comparison of the means of two groups can be written in notation form as follows: $H_0 : \mu_1 = \mu_2$. This expression states that the null hypothesis is such that the means of two groups are considered to be the same. The research hypothesis, on the other hand, states that the means are different and therefore one of the groups will have a superior outcome as compared with the other. The notation form of a research hypothesis that compares the means of two groups is: $H_1 : \mu_1 \neq \mu_2$. The form of notation for the research and null hypotheses may vary from that just given, but they will always be in opposition to each other.

Consider a hypothetical study that compares two groups of lower back pain patients managed with either chiropractic or usual medical care. The increase in mean range of motion (ROM) following treatment is the outcome measure. The research hypothesis (H_1) is that patients who receive chiropractic care will have greater gains in ROM than those who receive usual medical care. Conversely, the null hypothesis (H_0) states that there will be no difference between the groups after treatment. The results of this hypothetical study demonstrated that the mean gain for chiropractic patients was 20 degrees, while the medically treated patients only gained 15 degrees. The group that received chiropractic care at first glance appears to be superior. However, to be confident that the observed difference is enough to conclude that it probably did not occur by chance, a statistical test must be carried out. Statistical tests are covered in the next section, but at this point it is only necessary to understand that if the difference between means is considered real after the statistical test, it is then said to be *statistically significant*. In this hypothetical case, one can say that chiropractic care was superior to usual medical care in the treatment of lower back pain and that the difference between the mean outcomes for ROM was statistically significant.

Statistical significance is a term that indicates that a study's results are unlikely to be the result of chance at a specified probability level. That the results are not due to chance would lead to rejection of the null hypothesis and acceptance of the research hypothesis. The specified probability level is referred to as *alpha* (α), which is the probability that randomization alone would have led to the measured difference between the experimental groups. Thus, the alpha value is the probability of incorrectly rejecting a null hypothesis. Typically, it must be at least 95% unlikely that the null hypothesis is true before it can be rejected. In other words, there is a 5% chance that the null hypothesis will be rejected when it is actually true. Accordingly, probability (P) values must be equal to or less than 5% in order for the results of a study to reach a level of statistical significance. This 5% or less level of significance is the alpha level and is commonly notated as $P \leq 0.05$. Be careful, though, because the level of significance is not the same as a *P* value. The level of significance (i.e., alpha level) must be set before the study begins. The *P* value, on the other hand, is calculated after the study has been completed, using its resulting data. The level of significance represents the value at which a calculated *P* value would be considered small enough to say that the study's findings were probably not due to chance. If it is indeed smaller, the result is considered to be statistically significant. The null hypothesis would be rejected and the research hypothesis supported. Resulting *P* values above 0.05 would not be considered statistically significant, and the research hypothesis would not be supported.

When a 0.05 level of significance is attained, it means that the likelihood that the experiment's conclusion was a mistake is less than or equal to 5%. At that rate, there is a 1:20 probability that there would be different results if a similarly conducted experiment were repeated 20 times. This is important to consider when researchers perform a lot of different statistical tests on their data, a practice that is sometimes referred to as "fishing."[7] This practice increases the possibility of at least one of the tests incorrectly reaching statistical significance, leading to rejecting a null hypothesis that is actually true. This kind of mistake is referred to as a *type I error*, which is also known as *alpha error* because the probability of making a type I error is equal to the value of α. On the other hand, a *type II error* occurs when the null hypothesis is actually false, yet is mistakenly not rejected. This type of error is also known as *beta error* because the probability of making a type II error is equal to the value of β. Figure 4.15 shows the possible outcomes when making decisions about null hypotheses.

There is a rationale as to why the alpha level is generally set at 0.05 in health care research rather than something smaller or larger. It has to do with the trade-off between the likelihood of a given study producing a type I error versus a type II error. Since a type I error is the probability of rejecting a H_0 when it was actually true, one might ostensibly think that it would always be better to use a smaller alpha level, like 0.01, for example. Moreover, a smaller alpha level would decrease the chance of mistakenly rejecting the H_0. On the other hand, this reasoning must also take into account the effect that setting alpha very low has on the likelihood of a type II error occurring, because the smaller the alpha level is, the greater the likelihood is that a false H_0 will not be rejected when it actually should be. In other words, as the alpha level becomes smaller, the likelihood of making a type I error decreases while the likelihood of making a type II error increases (Figure 4.16). Thus, the widely used 0.05 alpha level is an

Inferential Statistics

FIGURE 4.15 Consequences of a decision to accept or reject true and false null hypotheses.

		Actual state of the null hypothesis	
		True H_0	False H_0
Decision	**Reject H_0**	Type I error (alpha error)	Correct decision
	Fail to reject H_0	Correct decision	Type II error (beta error)

FIGURE 4.16 As alpha becomes smaller, the likelihood of making a type I error decreases and the likelihood of mking a type II error increases. As alpha becomes greater, the opposite is true.

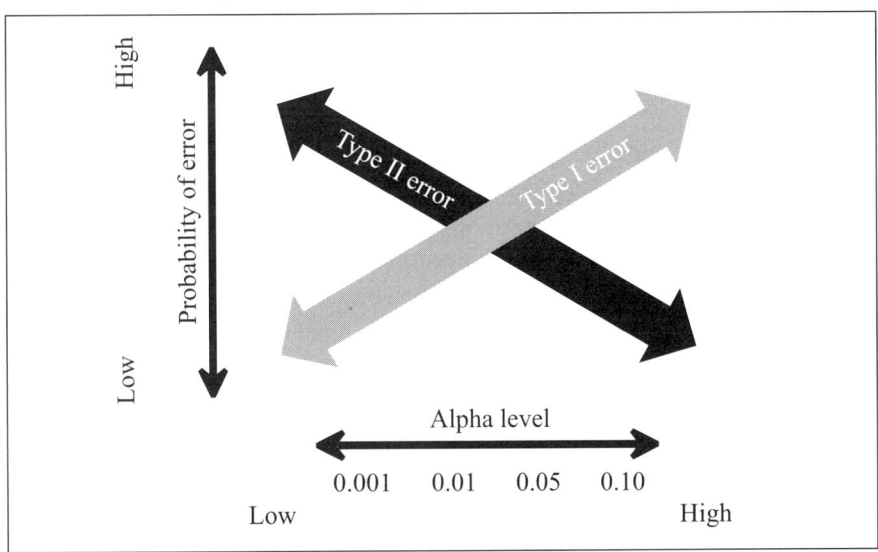

acceptable compromise between the possibilities of making type I and type II errors, which is why it is so commonly used in health care research.

The 0.05 confidence level has been reported in the literature for years and has been accepted as a realistic compromise for the point at which the null hypothesis should be rejected. However, the 0.05 cutoff point is somewhat illogical, because, in reality, 0.049 is not that much different from 0.051, yet one would be considered significant whereas the other would not. Consequently, this type of statistical testing may not always be able to detect the true outcome of a study.[8]

Another issue is the mistaken idea that if means are different at a 0.05 confidence level, then that difference is "less significant" than values that are different at a 0.01 confidence level. Values are statistically significant or not; it is not possible to be "more statistically significant."

Power is a term that expresses the probability of correctly rejecting a false H_0 and is related to β error. As you know, β error occurs when a false H_0 is mistakenly not rejected, so it follows that power is equal to $1 - \beta$. The power of a test is influenced by the size of the sample and the amount of the difference between group means—the bigger the better in both cases—as well as by the value of alpha. On the other hand, there is a point at which increasing the sample size provides little statistical advantage but comes at a monetary expense for having a larger group. Researchers typically strive to achieve a power value of 0.80 in the studies they design. Power can also be calculated after a study has been completed (post hoc) to determine if enough subjects were included. If low power is detected during post hoc power analysis and $\mathbf{H_0}$ was not rejected, there may be a case for repeating the study using a larger sample.

Hypothesis testing can also be carried out using confidence intervals (CIs) rather than *P* values. In fact, many biostatisticians advocate the use of CIs in place of *P* values because they convey more information than *P* values alone. Accordingly, their use is increasing in the health care literature. Hypothesis testing with CIs involves determining whether the value specified as the difference between group means in the null hypothesis is included in the CI that would result if the means of numerous samples were compared in a study. Recall that the null hypothesis states that there is no difference between group means; therefore, this difference will always be zero. If this value (zero) *is* contained in the 95% CI, the null hypothesis *should not be* rejected. Conversely, if the value (zero) *is not* contained in the 95% CI, the null hypothesis *should be* rejected.

Guyatt and associates[9] described the "estimation" approach to interpreting study results using CIs. They pointed out that information is contained in the CI that permits one to determine whether the result of a study is strong or weak, and whether it is definitive. If the lower limit of a CI is above the minimum level of clinical significance, then the trial is positive and definitive. On the other hand, if the lower limit is only a little below this minimum level, the trial is considered positive, but larger studies are needed to confirm the results. Referring to the upper limit of a CI, if it is below the minimum level of clinical significance, the trial is negative and definitive. If the CI of a negative result crosses the minimum level of clinical significance a small amount, then studies with larger samples are needed to make the determination definitive.

In clinical situations, findings found to be statistically significant may not always be clinically significant. *Clinical significance* (also known as *practical significance*) has to do with whether the statistically significant findings of a study really matter in a clinical situation. If a study's results are trivial in terms of practical implications, it may not apply, or have limited application, to clinical practice. The potential for conflict between statistically significant and clinically significant findings increases as sample sizes get larger. If the sample size is big enough, sometimes very small differences between treatment groups can produce P values that point to statistical significance. For example, if a study concluded that there was a statistically significant difference of mean lumbar range of motion scores between groups in a lower back pain study, but the difference only amounted to 2 degrees, this would not be of importance to clinicians because measuring range of motion in the clinical setting is not accurate enough to detect such small changes.

Statistical Tests Commonly Encountered in Research

The purpose of this brief discourse on statistical tests is to enable practitioners to better understand the mechanisms used by researchers as they evaluate and then draw conclusions from data in scientific articles. Nonetheless, there are quite a few other statistical tests that may occasionally be encountered when reading articles relating to EBC, as can be seen in Table 4.6. The emphasis in this section is on understanding concepts, while mathematics is purposefully deemphasized.

TABLE 4.6 Statistical tests that may be encountered in EBC

t-Test on means
Two-group *t*-test, equal group sizes, equal SD
Two-group *t*-test, unequal group sizes, equal SD
Two-group *t*-test, equal group sizes, unequal SD
Matched-pairs *t*-test
One-sample *t*-test
Nonparametric versions of *t*-tests
    Mann-Whitney *U*-test
    Wilcoxon test

Analysis of variance (ANOVA) (F-test comparing more than two means)
ANOVA, fixed effects: Single-factor designs
ANOVA, fixed effects: Multi-factor designs
ANOVA, planned comparisons
Analysis of covariance (ANCOVA)

F-test for multiple correlation and regression
One predictor set
Two predictor sets

Other F-tests
Multivariate analysis of variance (MANOVA)
Multivariate analysis of covariance (MANCOVA)
Repeated measures designs

Chi-square tests
Goodness-of-fit test
Test of independence

Note: SD, standard deviation.

Statistical tests are utilized to determine the probabilities of the relationships that are present in studies (i.e., the probability that a relationship may be due to chance alone). Some of the tests that are commonly encountered in the process of reading scientific articles are the *t*-test, analysis of variance (ANOVA), and chi-square.

The t-Test

The *t*-test (also known as Student's *t*-test) was developed by W. S. Gossett (1876–1937), who wrote under the pseudonym "Student." The *t*-test is used to determine whether the means of two groups are statistically different from each other. However, the results of a *t*-test are not entirely black and white. The results actually indicate that the means are probably different, or, if the study fails to show an effect, that the means are probably the same. Thus, *t*-tests deal in probabilities rather than absolutes, and there will always be a chance for type I or type II errors to occur.

In order to infer that the differences between the means of two groups are statistically different using a *t*-test, one must not only consider the actual differences between the means but also the amount of variability of the groups' scores (Figure 4.17). Similar to what was previously mentioned in the section on normal

FIGURE 4.17 **The means in examples A and B are equal, but the variability of the groups differs. The difference between means would be more likely to reach statistical significance in example B because of the narrow spread.**

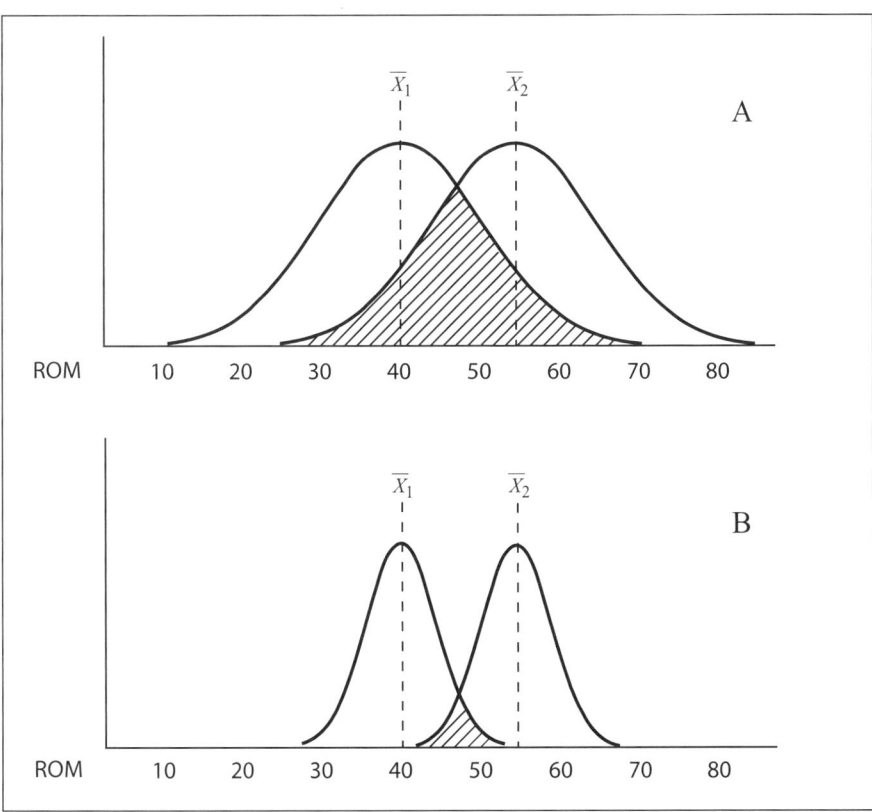

curves, large amounts of variability of group data in comparison to the difference between means clouds the issue, making it more difficult to see a clear difference.

Some assumptions should be met to legitimately carry out *t*-tests. The first assumption is that the data should be derived from a normal population, and the second is that the groups being compared should have equal variances. However, it is common to see violations of these assumptions in research; one should not be too concerned unless they are substantial. In general, these violations are minimized when the sample size is sufficiently large, at about 30 subjects. There are alternatives to the *t*-test that can be used to account for these violations, such as the *t*-test for unequal variances, or nonparametric tests such as the Mann-Whitney *U*-test or the Wilcoxon test.

If the means of two groups are found to be statistically different via a *t*-test, then H_0 is rejected and H_1 is accepted. The *t*-test can also be carried out on a single group by comparing the mean of a study with a known value. For instance, the mean from a cervical range of motion study could be compared with recognized normal values.

The *t*-test produces a test statistic, termed the *t-score* or *t-ratio*, that is similar to a *z*-score, but the *t*-distribution and a corresponding *t*-table are used instead of the *z*-table. The *t*-distribution is used when the SD of the population is estimated from sample data because it is unknown, as is the case with nearly all health care research. The *t*-distribution represents the theoretical result of taking infinite samples of a given size from a population and calculating *t*-scores (i.e., the distribution of standard deviations) on each of them. The *t*-score is used to identify the *P* value by way of a *t*-table, which, unlike a *z*-table, considers the number of subjects in the groups (Table 4.7). The term *degrees of freedom* (*df*) is used to signify the number of subjects in each group minus 1, and minus 2 if there are two groups. Table 4.7 lists the *df* to the left of the *t*-scores, but it is truncated at 15, whereas most *t*-tables include at least 100 degrees of freedom. Eventually *t*-distributions become approximately normal when many subjects are included in the groups.

The *t*-ratio is determined by dividing the difference between the means of the involved groups by the variability of the data. Variability, in this situation, is represented by the *standard error of the difference* ($S_{\bar{x}_1-\bar{x}_2}$) rather than the standard deviation. This is because here variability has to do with the distribution that would result from repeatedly calculating the standard deviation of the differences between the means of two groups after taking repetitive samples from the source population. The equation for calculating the *t*-score is as follows:

TABLE 4.7 Partial *t*-table showing critical values for *t* (to 15 *df*)

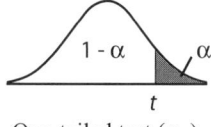
One-tailed test (α_1)

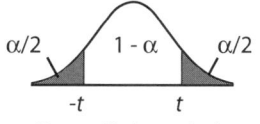
Two-tailed test (α_2)

	α_1	0.10	0.05	0.025	0.01	0.005	0.001	0.0005
df	α_2	0.20	0.10	0.05	0.02	0.01	0.002	0.001
1		3.078	6.314	12.710	31.82	63.66	318.30	636.62
2		1.886	2.920	4.303	6.965	9.925	22.330	31.60
3		1.638	2.353	3.182	4.541	5.841	10.210	12.92
4		1.533	2.132	2.776	3.747	4.604	7.173	8.610
5		1.476	2.015	2.571	3.365	4.032	5.893	6.869
6		1.440	1.943	2.447	3.143	3.707	5.208	5.959
7		1.415	1.895	2.365	2.998	3.499	4.785	5.408
8		1.397	1.860	2.306	2.896	3.355	4.501	5.041
9		1.383	1.833	2.262	2.821	3.250	4.297	4.781
10		1.372	1.812	2.228	2.764	3.169	4.144	4.587
11		1.363	1.796	2.201	2.718	3.106	4.025	4.437
12		1.356	1.782	2.179	2.681	3.055	3.930	4.318
13		1.350	1.771	2.160	2.650	3.012	3.852	4.221
14		1.345	1.761	2.145	2.624	2.977	3.787	4.140
15		1.341	1.753	2.131	2.602	2.947	3.733	4.073

$$t = \frac{\overline{X}_1 - \overline{X}_2}{S_{\overline{X}_1 - \overline{X}_2}} \quad \text{or simply:} \quad t = \frac{\text{The difference between group means}}{\text{Variability of the data}}$$

The *t*-test formula is effectively a signal-to-noise ratio, where the difference between the group means is the signal, and the variability of the data is the noise.[10] In order to reach statistical significance, the effect of the treatment must cause a large enough difference between the means (the numerator), and the variability of the data must be small enough (the denominator), to produce a *t*-score that is larger than the critical value of *t*. After calculating a *t*-score and allowing for the *df* and the level of alpha that was set, one would refer to the *t*-table to see if the calculated *t* is greater than or equal to the critical value listed in the table. If it is larger, then the results are statistically significant.

Notice in Table 4.7 that one-tailed and two-tailed tests are mentioned, with the one-tailed version having alpha all in one tail and the two-tailed version having alpha split between the tails. These figures correspond to whether the test involved is *directional* or *nondirectional*. Hypotheses can be directional or nondirectional as well, depending on the research question that is being asked. A hypothesis is *directional* if, prior to conducting the analysis, the researcher specifies that the scores of one group will be higher (or lower) than the other group. In a directional hypothesis, one is interested in either an increase or a decrease in the dependent variable, but not both. For instance, in a study investigating alcohol consumption and reaction time, one would only expect reaction time to decrease, and there would be no interest in the results of the test going in the other direction. Thus, a directional hypothesis would be appropriate.

In a nondirectional hypothesis, a researcher is interested in knowing if the scores are different, but no predictions are made about whether either of the scores will be higher or lower than the other. As an example, in a study comparing chiropractic care to standard medical care for the treatment of lower back pain, the results could go either way. Chiropractic care might be better or medical care might be better. Even though the research hypothesis may state that chiropractic care will be superior, it is still possible that standard medical care would end up in the best position. Therefore, the researcher is interested in considering outcomes in either direction, and a two-tailed, nondirectional test would be used.

In a nondirectional test, alpha is split between the two tails of the distribution, whereas alpha is all in one tail in a directional test. As a result, it is much easier to reach statistical significance using a directional test than a nondirectional test. For this reason, researchers are sometimes tempted to use a directional test when they really should not. In order for a researcher to make a statement that one set of scores will be higher than the other, the opposite direction must be of no interest. This type of statement can rarely be made in chiropractic research because it is usually possible for the test to go either way.

An example of how the *t*-test is reported in the literature can be found in an article by Kuhn and colleagues.[11] The researchers used a paired *t*-test to determine that the quadriceps femoris angle (Q-angle) was significantly reduced after the insertion of full-length flexible orthotics. The reduction was 2.5 degrees

(t (39) = –7.31, P < 0.01) on the left, and 2.3 degrees with a two-tailed matched sample (t (39) = –9.25, P < 0.01)) on the right. The elements that should be included when reporting test statistics are as follows:

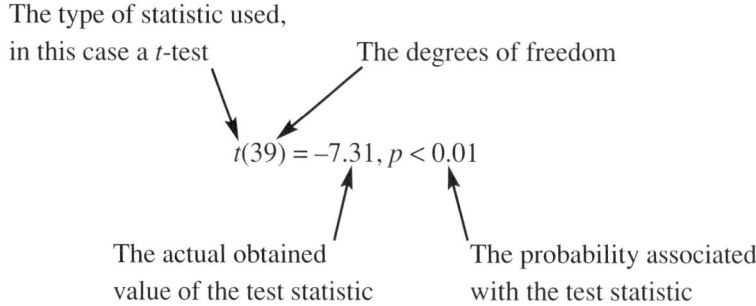

The style of reporting may vary somewhat, but the main information that should be provided should consist of the statistic used, the degrees of freedom of the actual analysis, the obtained value of the statistic, and the probability of the results (the P value).

Table 4.8 contains data from a hypothetical study comparing chiropractic care with standard medical care for the treatment of lower back pain. The improvements that the hypothetical study participants gained in their lumbar range of motion scores are listed. These data can be analyzed with a t-test using Microsoft Excel or another brand of statistics software to perform the calculations.

Microsoft Excel easily produced Table 4.9 from the hypothetical study data. Notice that statistics for both the one-tailed and two-tailed results were generated and that the critical value of t is much less for the one-tailed version. Since the t-score is larger than the critical values, the results would be considered statistically significant and the H_0 would be rejected. One could then say that chiropractic care significantly improved ROM compared with medical care in this study (t (14) = 7.90, p = 0.00029). Notice in Table 4.7 that the critical value of t for a two-tailed test with 14 degrees of freedom is 2.145, which is the same as what was generated by computer and shown in Table 4.9.

Under similar circumstances, some researchers may use the directional test because they presume that chiropractic care will produce a better outcome. However, since it is possible that medical treatment may be superior, a nondirectional

TABLE 4.8 Hypothetical study comparing the mean improvements in lumbar range of motion of lower back pain patients receiving chiropractic care versus standard medical care

Chiropractic Care		Standard Medical Care	
Case No.	ROM Gain (Degrees)	Case No.	ROM Gain (Degrees)
DC1	17	MD1	12
DC2	12	MD2	8
DC3	12	MD3	4
DC4	13	MD4	5
DC5	9	MD5	7
DC6	13	MD6	5
DC7	15	MD7	9
DC8	18	MD8	4

Note: ROM, range of motion.

TABLE 4.9 Output from Microsoft Excel t-test for hypothetical chiropractic versus medical care study

	Chiropractic Care	Medical Care
Mean	13.625	6.750
Variance	8.554	7.929
Observations	8	8
Pooled variance	8.241	
df	14	
t-statistic	4.790	
$P(T \leq t)$ one-tail	0.00014	
t critical one-tail	1.760	
$P(T \leq t)$ two-tail	0.00029	
t critical two-tail	2.145	

Note: t–test is two-sample, assuming equal variances.

test is required. To use a directional test, there must be good reason for the researcher to propose that the results will only go in one direction (Table 4.10).

Another form of *t*-test is the *paired t-test*, which is utilized when the samples are *dependent*. In dependent (paired) samples, the same subjects are in each of the study groups or are matched with other subjects regarding one or more characteristics. Paired *t*-tests are used to compare the means of the same or related subjects over time or in differing circumstances. For instance, repeated measures studies compare measurements obtained initially and then at follow-up evaluations. In this case, subjects are tested in a before and after situation across time, with some intervention occurring in between, such as chiropractic manipulation. Another instance in which the paired *t*-test is appropriate is when subjects are paired, such as twins, or when subjects are very much alike in some respects. The assumptions of the paired *t*-test are that the observed data are from the same subjects or from matched subjects and are drawn from a population with a normal distribution.

Analysis of Variance

When more than two groups are involved in a study, ANOVA must be used to compare their means. Intuitively, one would think that a *t*-test could simply be repeated for as many groups as are involved in the study, but this increases the probability of committing a type I error (rejecting a true null hypothesis). ANOVA can only compare one outcome variable and is sometimes referred to as a *univariate* (one-variable) analysis.

To perform the ANOVA test, the mean and standard deviation for each of the study groups must be calculated, just like in the *t*-test. ANOVA will then provide

TABLE 4.10 Steps involved in the *t*-test

1. After collecting the data, calculate the means and standard deviations of the groups.
2. Calculate the *t*-ratio.
3. Check to see if the calculated *t* is statistically significant on a *t*-table.
4. If t is greater than the critical value of *t* (typically at the 0.05 level), it is significant.
5. One can then conclude that the group means are different.

Remember: Big *t*-value → Small *P* value → Significance.

information about three things. First, it shows whether there are any significant differences among the group means. This information is provided by the *F-ratio*, which is to some extent similar to the *t*-ratio. Second, it tells whether any of the particular groups differ from each other by means of *comparison tests*. Third, it tells whether the differences are relatively big or small. *Measures of explained variance* provide this information.

The F-ratio compares the variance between the groups with the variance within the groups. Thus,

$$F = \frac{\text{Variance between groups}}{\text{Variance within groups}}$$

The *within-group variance* is related to sampling error and ordinary differences between the subjects. For instance, the diastolic blood pressure of a group of 30 people will normally vary considerably. This variability will contribute to the within-group variance and is the same as the variance that was previously discussed in this chapter. *Between-group variance*, on the other hand, is due to the differences between the groups that are attributable to the inequality of the means (Figure 4.18). Not unlike the *t*-ratio, if the F-ratio is small, then the groups are probably not significantly different from each other, but if it is big, then two or more of the groups would be considered significantly different from each other.

The F-ratio avoids the type I error problem because it is an overall test. An F-ratio that is statistically significant means that there are differences between some of the groups, but it does not specify which particular groups differ. That is why comparison techniques are used, which compare the individual group pairs (pairwise comparison). Some of the names of comparison tests that one might encounter in health-care-related articles are Tukey, Scheffé, and Bonferroni. The Tukey-Kramer test is appropriate if groups are of unequal size, while the Bonferroni method is suitable for equal as well as unequal group sizes. Scheffé's test is very conservative so as to minimize the risk of type I error. Consequently, Scheffé's is not as likely to detect true differences between groups as the other comparison tests. More comparison tests are available, but essentially they all decrease the cutoff for statistical significance as the number of group contrasts is increased. The various comparison tests are appropriate in specific circumstances, and opinions differ among statisticians about which is best.[12]

Calculations involved in ANOVA tests are complex, but can be carried out

Statistical Tests Commonly Encountered in Research

FIGURE 4.18 Between-groups variance is the difference between the means (within the brace). Within-group variance is the variability of each group, represented by arrows.

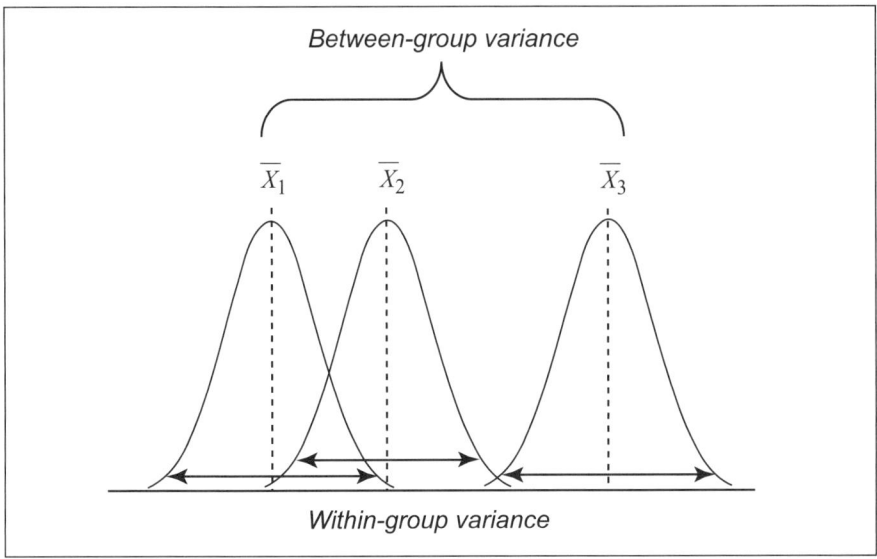

very easily on a computer that has the appropriate software. As an example, another group will be added to the hypothetical data presented in Table 4.8. A group that received physical therapy (PT) will be added to the study in addition to the chiropractic and standard medical care groups. The PT care group also has eight subjects, with the mean ROM gain being 6.38 degrees and variance being 11.13. The study's data were entered into Microsoft Excel, and the ANOVA test was carried out. The results of this analysis are shown in Table 4.11. Notice that the means of the medical and PT care groups are not very different from each other (6.75 versus 6.38), but the mean of the chiropractic care group is 13.63, which, on first glance, appears to be appreciably different from the others. An ANOVA table, like what is commonly seen in journal articles, is located below the summary information in Table 4.11. The sum of squares, mean squares, and degrees of freedom are used in the F-test. When the value of F is compared with the critical value of F, it is obvious that the group means are different overall, thus explaining the very small P value ($P < 0.001$).

TABLE 4.11 Microsoft Excel table resulting from the ANOVA test carried out on the means of the chiropractic, medical, and physical therapy care groups

SUMMARY

Groups	Count	Sum	Mean	Variance
Chiropractic care	8	109	13.625	8.55357
Medical care	8	54	6.75	7.92857
PT care	8	51	6.375	11.125

ANOVA

Source of Variation	SS	df	MS	F	P value	F crit
Between groups	266.5833	2	133.2917	14.4845	0.00011	3.4668
Within groups	193.25	21	9.2024			
Total	459.8333	23				

Note: PT, physical therapy; SS, sum of squares; *df*, degrees of freedom; MS, mean squares; F crit, critical value of F.

Since the ROM means between the groups are judged to be different overall, it is appropriate to perform a multiple-comparison test to consider pairwise differences. The data were analyzed with SPSS Version 12 using Tukey's HSD (Honestly Significantly Different) test. The SPSS printout in Table 4.12 shows that when changes in ROM for chiropractic care was compared with either medical or PT care, the difference reached statistical significance, but when medical care and PT were compared with each other, the difference did not. Indeed, the resulting *P* values were 0.967.

The example test presented here is considered a *one-way* ANOVA. ANOVA techniques can also be used to test multiple factors (treatments) using the same outcome measure, such as a two-way or three-way ANOVA.

The ANOVA test assumes that the data involved are normally distributed and that subjects were randomly assigned to groups. When these assumptions are not met, a nonparametric alternative test should be used in place of ANOVA. When the data are not normal or the variances of the groups are unequal, the Kruskal-

TABLE 4.12 SPSS Version 12 table of the results of the Tukey HSD multiple-comparisons test carried out on the ROM means of the chiropractic, medical, and physical therapy care groups

(I) Type of care	(J) Type of care	Mean Difference (I – J)	Std. Error	P Value	95% Confidence Interval	
					Lower Bound	Upper Bound
Chiro	MD	6.87500*	1.51677	0.001	3.0519	10.6981
	PT	7.25000*	1.51677	0.000	3.4269	11.0731
MD	Chiro	–6.87500*	1.51677	0.001	–10.6981	-3.0519
	PT	.37500	1.51677	0.967	–3.4481	4.1981
PT	Chiro	–7.25000*	1.51677	0.000	–11.0731	-3.4269
	MD	–0.37500	1.51677	0.967	–4.1981	3.4481

Note: Chiro, chiropractic; MD, medical; PT, physical therapy.
*The mean difference is significant at the 0.05 level.

Wallis test should be used. The nonparametric alternative test that should be used when three or more paired groups are involved is the Friedman test. The appropriate comparison test to use following either of these nonparametric tests is Dunn's test, which examines post test differences between groups.

Chi-Square Test

Chi-square tests are used to test hypotheses with categorical data (i.e., nominal and ordinal). What a chi-square test does is determine whether one set of proportions is different from another by comparing frequencies of occurrence. There are two versions of the chi-square test: the *chi-square goodness of fit* and the *chi-square test of independence*.

The *chi-square goodness-of-fit test* determines whether the observed occurrence frequencies are different from what would be expected by chance (i.e., observed frequencies "fit" against the expected frequencies). The easiest way to explain this concept is to present the following example. In a random sample of 100 Americans, one would expect to find on average about 50 males and 50 females. However, if a sample of Americans found 60 males and 40 females, would that represent a statistically significant difference from what was expected? This question is best answered using the chi-square goodness-of-fit test.

The purpose of the chi-square test is to determine how a set of proportions that have been observed by the investigator compare with a set of proportions thought to be true (expected). Accordingly, the chi-square formula calculates the difference between the observed and expected frequencies, and then divides that value by the expected frequencies to produce the chi-square statistic (χ^2).

$$\chi^2 = \frac{\Sigma(O-E)^2}{E}$$

where O represents the observed frequencies and E represents the expected frequencies.

Returning to the question about whether a sample of 100 Americans with 60 males and 40 females is truly different from what would be expected, the chi-square statistic can be calculated as follows:

$$\chi^2 = \frac{(60-50)^2}{50} + \frac{(40-50)^2}{50}$$
$$= \frac{100}{50} + \frac{100}{50}$$
$$= 4.0$$

χ^2 is evaluated for statistical significance using a chi-square table, with df equal to the number of categories minus 1. If the critical value of χ^2 is exceeded, then the test result is statistically significant (just like in the t-test and F-test). In this case, the critical value is 3.84, which the calculated χ^2 exceeded, and one can say that the sample is indeed different from the population of Americans.

The *chi-square test of independence* tests to see whether the proportions or frequencies for one category differ significantly from those of another category. This test utilizes a *2 × 2 contingency table* (also known as a *cross-tabulation table*) to organize the corresponding variables (Table 4.13) As an example, in a hypothetical study where patients were administered Gonstead versus Diversified spinal manipulative technique, a researcher could measure pain as an outcome variable such that the pain is either present or absent at the end of treatment. Table 4.14 presents data for this hypothetical study in a contingency table with "Technique used" as variable 1 and "Pain after treatment" as variable 2.

TABLE 4.13 A 2 × 2 contingency table

		Variable 2		
		Yes	No	Row Total
Variable 1	Yes	a	b	$a + b$
	No	c	d	$c + d$
Column Total		$a + c$	$b + d$	$a + b + c + d$ Grand Total

TABLE 4.14 Data for hypothetical study comparing outcomes of patients who received Gonstead versus Diversified technique in a 2 × 2 contingency table

		Pain after treatment		
		Yes	No	Row Total
Technique used	Gonstead	9	21	30
	Diversified	11	29	40
Column Total		20	50	70 Grand Total

The table contains the observed values that resulted from the Gonstead versus Diversified study. It appears that Diversified patients had better outcomes than Gonstead patients, since 9 of 30 (30%) still had pain after Gonstead treatment, and 11 of 40 (27.5%) still had pain after Diversified.

In order to determine whether the difference between the outcomes is statistically significant, CHI will be calculated. The first step is to calculate the expected values for each cell using the following formula:

$$\text{Expected } (E) = \frac{\text{Row Total} \times \text{Column Total}}{\text{Grand Total}}$$

		Row Total
9 $E = 30 \times 20/70 = 8.6$	21 $E = 30 \times 50/70 = 21.4$	30
11 $E = 40 \times 20/70 = 11.4$	29 $E = 40 \times 50/70 = 28.6$	40
Column Total: 20	50	70 Grand Total

The chi-square statistic is then calculated using these expected values with the same CHI formula that was provided above:

$\frac{(9-8.6)^2}{8.6}$	$\frac{(21-21.4)^2}{21.4}$
$\frac{(11-11.4)^2}{11.5}$	$\frac{(29-28.6)^2}{28.6}$

=

0.0186	0.0168
0.0316	0.0056

The next step is to add all of the cells together, which results in $\chi^2 = 0.0726$. The method used to calculate *df* for the chi-square test of independence is as follows:

(Number of categories for variable 1) × (Number of caregories for variable 2) − 1

In this case there is only 1 *df* because there are two categories for each variable. The chi-square test of independence can be used with more than two categories for each variable, however. Finally, refer to a chi-square table and find the critical value needed to reach significance at the 0.05 level and 1 *df*, which is 3.84. As a result, the chi-square statistic definitely did not reach statistical significance in the hypothetical Gonstead versus Diversified study, and one would conclude that the outcomes were not different. In other words, the presence of pain did not depend on the technique that was used.

There are some conditions that need to be considered before the chi-square test can legitimately be utilized. First, the observations must be completely independent of each other. A good check for violations of this condition is to make sure that the total number of observed frequencies is not higher than the number of subjects included in the study. The second condition involves the avoidance of expected frequencies that are small. Typically, when any of the expected frequencies are less than 1 or are less than 5 in more than 20% of cells, the test is not considered valid. In cases where expected frequencies do not meet this condition, an alternative to the chi-square test is available, called *Fisher's exact test*. There is no lower limit on the amount of data that is required for Fisher's exact test. All that is needed is at least one data value in each row and one data value in each column. The third condition that should be met before using chi-square is the avoidance of extremely small and extremely large sample sizes. Using chi-square with extremely small sample sizes may overlook obvious false null hypotheses and extremely large sample sizes may identify trivial differences.

Contingency tables were introduced earlier in this section for use in chi-square analysis. They are applicable to several other types of analysis and will be discussed in subsequent chapters. Contingency tables are commonly seen in journal articles and are simply tables that correspond to the relationships between categorical or *binomial* (when there are exactly two mutually exclusive outcomes) variables. An example of a binomial outcome is the relationship between patients being adjusted (yes or no) and having a headache (yes or no).

Correlation

Frequently there is a relationship between two variables such that if one increases or decreases, the other one will also increase or decrease a specific amount. This phenomenon is known as *correlation* and is a measure of a mathematical relationship that may exist between values of two or more variables.[13] *Pearson product-moment correlation coefficient* (also known as Pearson's correlation coefficient) is a commonly used correlation coefficient that is symbolized by the letter r. It numerically summarizes how strongly variables are mathematically related and represents the linear relationship between the two variables. Measurement scales utilized in calculating a correlation coefficient should be at least on the interval scale, although other types of data can be handled using specialized correlation coefficients. An example of a correlation is the relationship between the number of cigarettes smoked per day and the likelihood of developing lung cancer. Essentially, the more cigarettes a specified group of people smokes, the more cases of lung cancer will occur within the members of the group.

Values of the correlation coefficient range from −1.00 to +1.00, with +1.00 representing a perfect *positive* correlation and −1.00 representing a perfect *negative* correlation. If the variables tend to go up or down together, the correlation coefficient will be positive. Conversely, if the variables tend to go up and down in opposition, the correlation coefficient will be negative. Sometimes there is no mathematical relationship between variables, resulting in a corresponding correlation coefficient value of 0.00. In effect, the closer the correlation coefficient is to +1 or −1, the more closely the two variables are related. It is tempting to assume that a cause-and-effect relationship exists in situations where two variables are strongly correlated, but this is not necessarily so. Though a relationship may be very strong between two variables, it does not mean that one actually caused a change in the other. An example is the relationship between coffee drinking and lung cancer. Studies have shown that the more coffee people drink, the more likely they are to develop lung cancer. The problem with this reasoning is that there is a tendency for heavy coffee drinkers to also be heavy smokers, and it is the smoking that is the actual cause of lung cancer. If the influence of smoking is removed from this relationship (controlled for), it becomes apparent that coffee drinking is not at all related to the incidence of lung cancer.

A closely related measure of correlation is the *coefficient of determination*, which is the square of the correlation coefficient and is symbolized as r^2. Because r is squared in the process of calculating the coefficient of determination, it can have only positive values that range from 0.0 to 1.0. The coefficient of determination, r^2, provides information about how much of the variation in one variable can be explained by the other variable. For example, if r^2 was 0.41 in the smoking and lung cancer relationship that was just mentioned, one could say that 41% of the variability in the incidence of lung cancer could be explained by the number of cigarettes smoked per day. Other factors, such as heredity, diet, and environmental exposure, may account for the remaining 59% variability in the incidence of lung cancer.

Correlation is often represented graphically via a scatterplot, which is an *x–y* graph that is composed of symbols representing specific values for the two variables (Figure 4.19). The line through the data points is called a *regression line* or *least squares line*, which is calculated by minimizing the vertical distances between the data points and the straight line that is fitted to the data (Figure 4.22 later in this section). The regression line, in a manner of speaking, represents the average trend of all the data points on the scatterplot.

Scatterplots show the *form*, *direction*, and *strength* of the relationship between variables. The form of a scatterplot is dependent on the data, which may be linear, as shown in Figure 4.19, but can also be curvilinear or nonlinear. When

FIGURE 4.19 **Scatterplot of the relationship of height and weight, which represents a strong positive correlation.**

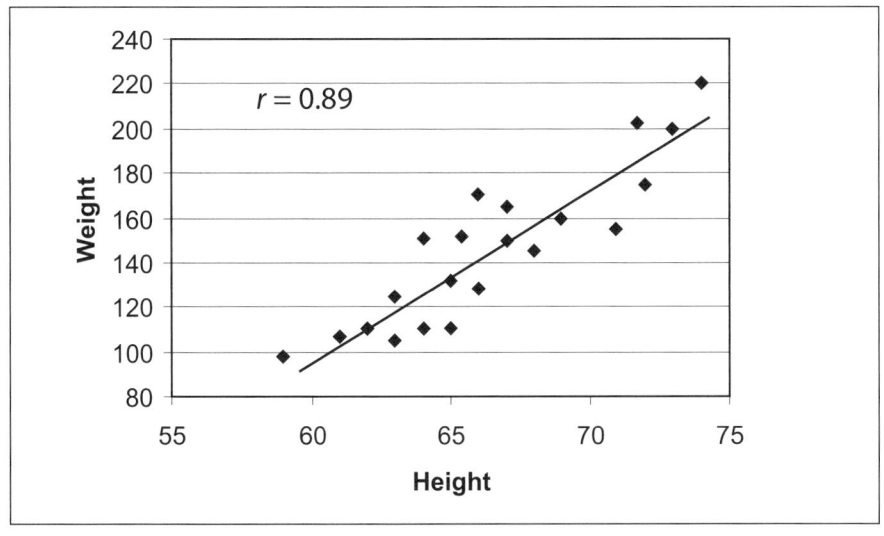

data is curvilinear, the correlation weakens after a certain point, that is, it becomes more difficult to predict how the value on the *y*-axis changes when the *x* value is changed. Thus, although Pearson's *r* is a useful measure of linear relationships, it is not appropriate when the data is nonlinear or curvilinear. An example of a curvilinear correlation is the relationship between age and strength. As people age, they get stronger to a certain point, but they eventually begin to weaken after a certain age (Figure 4.20). The correlation is said to be positive when the pattern of data in scatterplots slopes upward, and the correlation is said to be negative when the data slopes downward.

Calculation of the correlation coefficient is not affected by the specific units of measurement that are being used. Hence, calculating the value of *r* for the relationship between height and weight will be the same whether inches and pounds or centimeters and kilograms are used. Statistics software packages, including Microsoft Excel, are capable of producing scatterplots, constructing least squares lines, and calculating the value of *r* when examining relationships between variables.

Occasionally, extreme values occur that are not located close to the common grouping of data on the scatterplot (Figure 4.21). These values are termed *outliers*

FIGURE 4.20 **A curvilinear relationship between age and strength. Strength increases with age, but after a certain age it begins to diminish.**

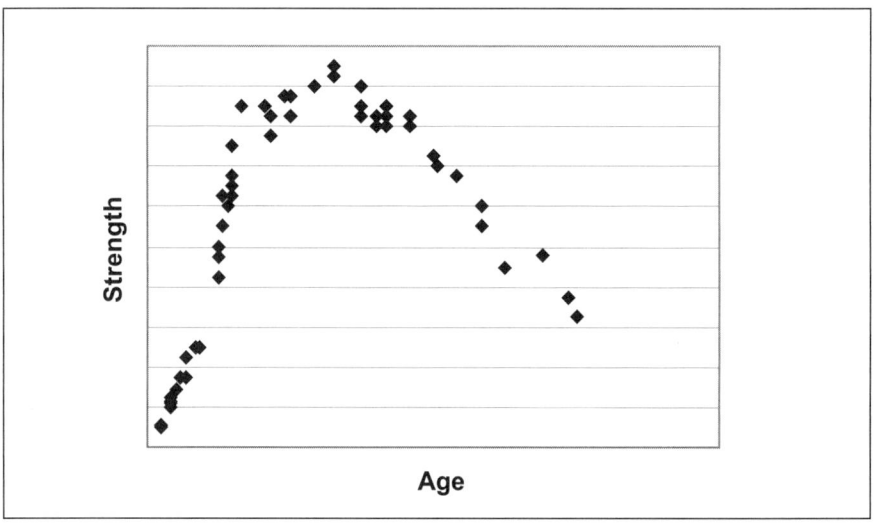

FIGURE 4.21 The data point representing a 50-inch-tall person weighing 300 pounds is an outlier. It may actually represent a short, obese person, but it was probably caused by an error.

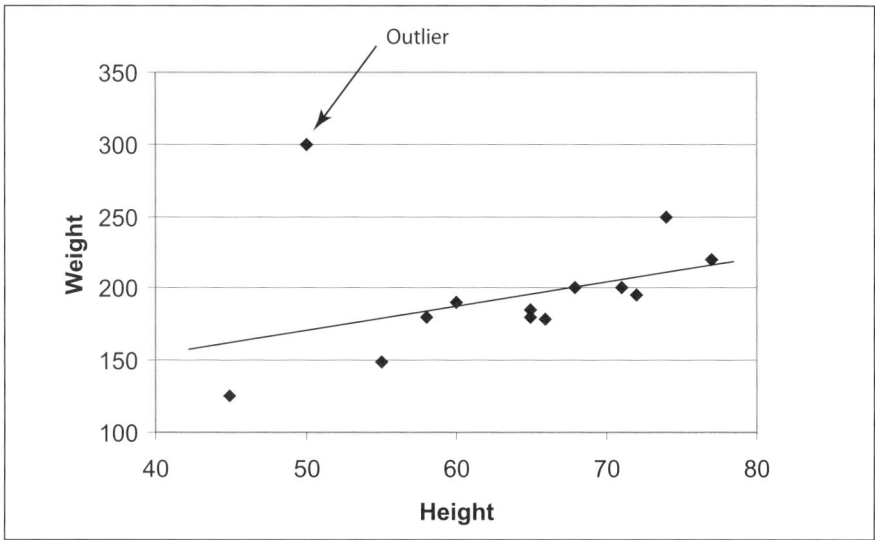

and can strongly influence the slope of the regression line as well as the value of the correlation coefficient. Outliers are clearly apparent on scatterplots as points that do not lie near the general trend of the data. They can be the result of data recording errors, values that were not sampled from the same population, an underlying subpopulation that was not normal, or legitimate extreme cases. Authors of journal articles should satisfactorily address outliers that occur in their data. Sometimes outliers are simply eliminated from the analysis because of their inordinate influence on the study's results, but this practice is inappropriate without an acceptable explanation.

Closely associated with correlation is *regression analysis*, which is the process of using the observations in a set of data to calculate the line of *best fit* passing through the data. Regression produces an equation describing the least squares line that fits the data. The equation enables one to make predictions about the direction and amount of change of the variables. The line is fitted by minimizing the sum of squared deviations (dy) of the data points from the least squares line. When the line is positioned so that the distances of all deviations are as short as possible, the line will be the best fit possible (Figure 4.22).

FIGURE 4.22 The deviations (*dy*) of the data points from the best-fit line are represented by a dashed line.

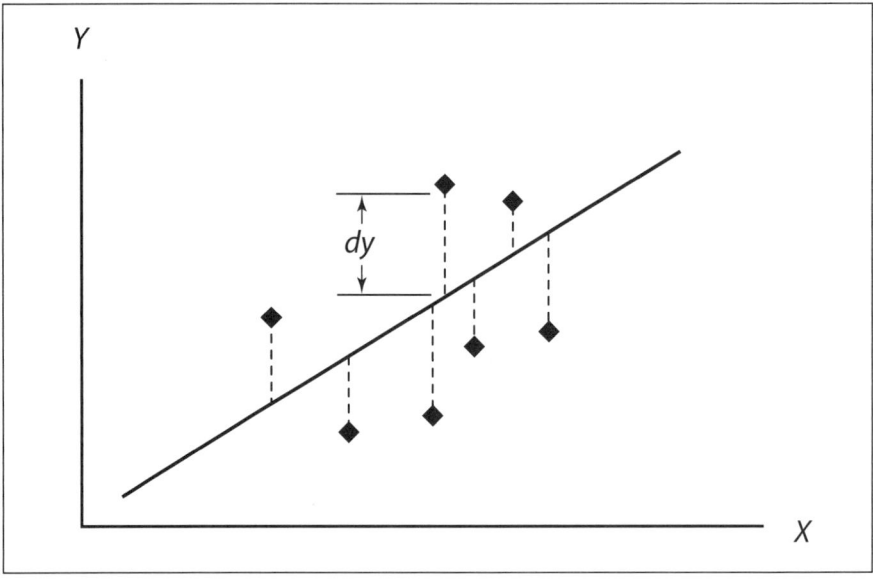

The linear regression equation is $Y = a + bX$, where a is the Y intercept, b is the slope of the line, and X is the value of the variable X. After the values for the regression equation have been calculated for correlated data, one can predict the value of an outcome variable (also known as a criterion variable) that is associated with a specified value of a predictor variable. For example, the regression equation for the height and weight data shown in Figure 4.21 is as follows: Weight = –53 + 3.7(Height). Using this equation, one could then estimate that a 66-inch tall person would probably weigh about 191.2 pounds. We have to hedge our prediction based on the strength of the correlation, because the regression equation assumes no variation in the data from which it is derived.

Thus far we have focused on the relationship between two variables, but many times outcomes are influenced by more than one factor. Consequently, several variables are often used to predict the value of an outcome variable, a process termed *multiple regression*. The equation used for multiple regression is similar to that used in simple regression, except there is more than one value for b. Thus, the form of the equation for multiple regression is $Y = a + b_1X_1 + b_2X_2 + \ldots + b_kX_k$, where X_1 is the value of the first predictor variable, X_2 is the value of the second, and X_k would continue for as many predictor variables as are being analyzed. For example, a study looking at the prognostic indicators of sciatica[14] found using multiple linear regression that driving at least 2 hours per day, carrying heavy loads at work, a high level of psychosomatic problems, and sciatica symptoms the year before study inclusion all contributed to the persistence or recurrence of sciatica.

References

1. Rosner, B. *Fundamentals of Biostatistics*. 6th ed. 2005. Belmont: Thomson Brooks/Cole.
2. Witte, R.S., and J.S. Witte. *Statistics*. 2004. Hoboken: John Wiley, 21.
3. Glaser, A.N. *High-Yield Biostatistics*. 3rd ed. 2005. Philadelphia: Lippincott Williams & Wilkins, 9.
4. Carlin, J.B., and L.W. Doyle. *2: Describing and displaying data. J Paediatr Child Health*, 2000. **36**(3): 270–4.
5. Carlin, J.B., and L.W. Doyle. *Comparison of means and proportions using confidence intervals. J Paediatr Child Health*, 2001. **37**(6):583–6.
6. Guyatt, G., et al. *Basic statistics for clinicians: 1. Hypothesis testing. CMAJ*, 1995. **152**(1):27–32.
7. Swaen, G.G., O. Teggeler, and L.G. van Amelsvoort. *False positive outcomes and design characteristics in occupational cancer epidemiology studies. Int J Epidemiol*, 2001. **30**(5):948–54.
8. Jones, T.C. *Case reports and qualitative research: Two important approaches to evaluation and communication in medical science. Braz J Infect Dis*, 2001. **5**(3):158–60.
9. Guyatt, G., et al. *Basic statistics for clinicians: 2. Interpreting study results: Confidence intervals. CMAJ*, 1995. **152**(2):169–73.
10. Trochim, W.M.K. *Research Methods: The Concise Knowledge Base*. 2nd ed. 2004. Cincinnati: Atomic Dog, 363.
11. Kuhn, D.R., et al. *Immediate changes in the quadriceps femoris angle after insertion of an orthotic device*. J Manipulative Physiol Thera, 2002. **25**(7):465–70.
12. Field, A.P. *Discovering Statistics Using SPSS for Windows: Advanced Techniques for the Beginner*. 2000. Thousand Oaks: Sage Publications, 13.
13. Guyatt, G., et al. *Basic statistics for clinicians: 4. Correlation and regression. CMAJ*, 1995. **152**(4):497–504.
14. Tubach, F., J. Beaute, and A. Leclerc. *Natural history and prognostic indicators of sciatica. J Clin Epidemiol*, 2004. **57**(2):174–9.

PART II

Research Designs Commonly Encountered in the Chiropractic Literature

CHAPTER FIVE

Experimental Designs

Part II of this book covers various types of research designs that are commonly utilized by chiropractic researchers. For two reasons, experimental designs will be covered before the other designs. The first reason is that the "classic experiment" is a randomized controlled trial (RCT), which is probably the most well-known type of research design. The second reason concerns the fact that RCTs typically have the most validity when compared with other designs, and if one understands why this is true, it becomes clear why other designs do not measure up. Before beginning the experimental design section, however, a short introduction to research methods is presented to provide a foundation for understanding some of the concepts involved in research.

Research Methods

Quantitative and Qualitative Research

Quantitative and qualitative are two broad categories of research that are classified based on the type of data involved. Generally speaking, *quantitative data* involves numbers that result from taking measurements on participants in a study, and *qualitative data* involves words from questionnaires or interviews. Quantitative research is objective, since it is based on reliable measurements, whereas qualitative research is subjective because it is derived from people providing estimations about things such as how they feel or their ability to function. Another difference between these types of research is that qualitative research is typically based on inductive reasoning, whereas quantitative research is based on deductive reasoning. *Inductive reasoning* draws on observation to create an idea or theory. *Deductive reasoning* is utilized in research to test known theories or ideas to determine whether they are true.

The involvement of researchers differs between quantitative and qualitative research. In quantitative investigations, the researcher acts as an objective observer who does not participate in or influence what is being studied. Conversely, the researcher participates in qualitative research, sometimes being immersed in it so that more can be learned about a given situation.

Quantitative research is usually esteemed more highly than qualitative because of its relationship with the scientific method. Although this may be true, qualitative research certainly has value and can provide very important information regarding many health care issues. Furthermore, the results of qualitative research can be designated with numerical values for statistical analysis. For instance, a study that found that patients had no, mild, moderate, or severe pain could code these results as 0, 1, 2, or 3, respectively. Certain statistical analyses could then be carried out on this data to provide descriptive information and to explore relationships that might exist with other variables.

Quantitative research is sometimes limited in relation to the relevance of its results to clinical practice, because the strict methods utilized in studies may not be duplicable in actual practice. Nonetheless, both quantitative and qualitative research methods are important, and both are necessary to investigate concerns of interest to the practice of evidence-based chiropractic (EBC).

Pragmatic and Explanatory Research

Pragmatic research methods are employed to determine the *effectiveness* of treatments or interventions—in other words, whether they work under real-life conditions and in terms that matter to patients. However, pragmatic studies do not provide very much information about how or why the interventions work. These types of studies are primarily designed to help make decisions about how effective new treatments are as compared with existing treatments; thus, placebos are not usually utilized.

In contrast to pragmatic research, *explanatory* research methods determine how interventions work under ideal conditions, as one would find in a controlled experiment. These studies are helpful in answering questions about the efficacy of treatments, which has to do with how and why they work. However, the strict methods involved in explanatory research are often quite different from day-to-day clinical circumstances: consequently, the results may be of limited importance to practitioners.[1] Furthermore, interventions that have demonstrated efficacy in an explanatory study may not work well in actual practice for several other reasons.[2] First, clinicians must diagnose a patient's condition correctly for the patient to even be offered the treatment. Assuming that the patient is diagnosed properly, clinicians must then provide the treatment in a correct manner (i.e., as it was done in the related study). Finally, patients must follow orders associated with the treatment protocol (e.g., keeping appointments, doing prescribed exercises, avoiding certain activities). When applying the results of explanatory research to clinical practice, quite a few factors must therefore be considered in relation to the implementation of the interventions involved.

It is important to recognize the differences between pragmatic and explanatory research, which is usually not that difficult because unique methodological issues apply to each. For example, the approach to patient selection is dissimilar between these types of research in that pragmatic studies include a wider range of patients, with exclusion from care typically only applying to patients who present with contraindications to the method of care involved in the study. On the other hand, patient selection in explanatory studies is very stringent in order to determine if the intervention is effective under ideal circumstances. Patients may be excluded from explanatory studies because of the presence of comorbid conditions, prior treatment, age, and so on. The disadvantage of this procedure is that many times it is unknown whether the intervention will then work for patients outside the study.

The distinction between pragmatic and explanatory research is not always clear-cut, often making it difficult to identify which type is involved. A given study may include components of each of these types of research, such as a study that has stringent selection criteria yet does not utilize a placebo control group.

Descriptive, Relational, and Causal Research

There are three fundamental types of research that are designed to either describe certain aspects of health-related situations, examine relationships that may exist between two or more variables, or determine whether one or more explanatory (independent) variables produces a change in one or more outcome (dependent) variables. These research types are referred to as *descriptive*, *relational*, and *causal*, respectively. They build on each other, to the extent that relational studies contain descriptive information, and causal studies include both descriptive and relational information.

We have already considered descriptive statistics, which is what is involved in descriptive designs. Thus, *descriptive research* simply looks at various aspects of the participants in a study and then numerically describes the resulting data. An example would be a study that surveys lower back pain patients in relation to their functional status and then reports the findings of the survey. There is no intervention involved in the study, only a description of what is found. This type of research is also called *observational*.

The underlying mechanism of *relational research* was covered in Chapter 4, where correlation and regression was presented. These analytic tools are used to examine relationships that may exist between two or more variables. An example of relational research would be an expanded study of the lower back pain patients just mentioned, to see if there was a relationship between participants' functional status and their employment status. A researcher would be interested in determining whether worse functional status is actually correlated with worse employment status and, if so, in generating an equation that would predict a person's potential for employment based on his or her functional status.

Causal research attempts to provide evidence that an intervention causes or somehow affects one or more outcome variables. Causal research is experimental research, which is the most demanding type of research to carry out, involving very specific methodologies. An example of causal research would be a study where a sample of lower back pain patients is randomly assigned (randomized) to receive either manipulation (the treatment group) or a simulated manipulation (the control group). Measurements would be taken on participants at the beginning and end of the study, looking for a difference between the groups' outcomes. If the manipulation group fared better, with statistically significant differences between groups, then one could say there was a causal relationship between manipulation and a better outcome.

Experimental and Quasi-experimental Research

The main difference between experimental and quasi-experimental research designs is whether random assignment (randomization) of study participants to groups was involved. If a study utilizes randomization, then it is considered experimental; otherwise, it is quasi-experimental. Experimental studies are unsurpassed as the preferred way to demonstrate cause-and-effect relationships. Quasi-experimental studies, on the other hand, provide much less evidence of cause-and-effect relationships. Nonexperiments provide practically no evidence of causality, given that they do not even compare groups like quasi-experimental studies do. Nonexperiments merely entail one group that is observed before and after the application of an intervention. Thus, the major advantage that experimental research designs have over quasi-experimental and nonexperimental research is that experimental research permits a stronger claim of causal inference.

A method of notation that can be helpful in understanding research designs uses the letter R to stand for random assignment, O for observation or measure, X for treatment/intervention, and N for nonequivalent groups. Each group is assigned one line in this method, so that the number of lines represents the number of groups involved in the study, and time progresses from left to right (Figure 5.1).[3]

FIGURE 5.1 **Notation method for the depiction of research designs. Three common designs are shown.**

The classic experiment involving randomization and two groups	R O X O R O O
Quasi-experiment with two groups but no randomization	N O X O N O O
Nonexperiment with only one group	O X O

R - Randomization
N - Nonequivalent groups (no randomization)
X - Treatment
O - Observation

Populations and Samples

One usually thinks of a population as being the total number of people within a given geographic area, like the population of Hawaii, for instance. In research, however, a *population* refers to the units from which a sample is drawn, which may include people but can also consist of events or observations. It would be nice to be able to include each and every unit when investigating the attributes of a population, but that is usually not possible because of the quantities involved. As an alternative, a smaller number of units is selected to represent the entire population. This smaller number of units is termed a sample and is defined as a subset of observations from a population.[4] The objective of taking samples is to be able to make inferences about what is happening in a population based on what is observed in a sample. To make these types of inferences, a sample must be representative of the population from which it was derived. This is accomplished by means of random selection of the sample units, a process by which each unit of the population has an equal chance of being selected (Figure 5.2).

The target population to be used in a study should be defined prior to selecting a sample. Examples of populations are migraine headache patients presenting to an HMO in the past year and lower back patients presenting to a chiropractic

FIGURE 5.2 A sample taken from a population. Can inferences about what is happening in the population be made based on what is observed in the sample?

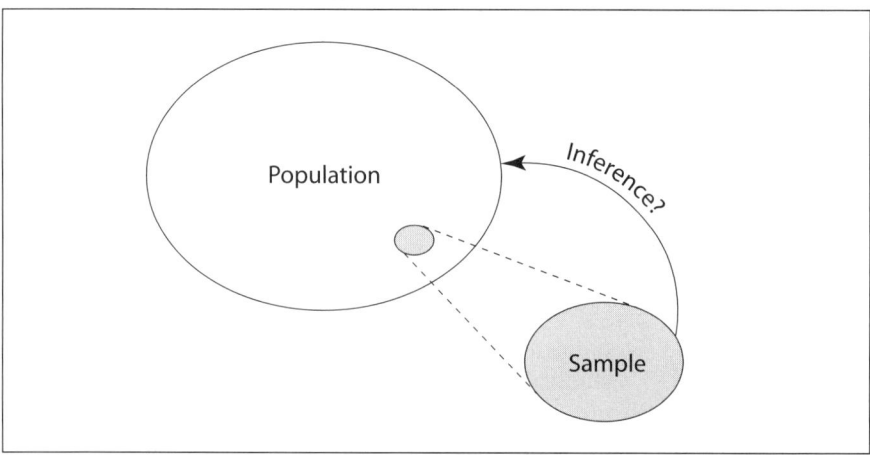

practice in the next six months. Sometimes sampling is carried out by sequentially taking every tenth patient, or some other specified number from the population. However, random number tables or computer-generated random numbers are preferred methods. When a random sample is derived from a population, any parameters that are estimated based on that sample are said to be unbiased estimates.

Random sampling is rarely employed with clinical trials; rather, patients are obtained for these studies using methods such as taking sequentially presenting patients and recruiting through advertisements. These methods are sometimes referred to as *convenience sampling* because patients are selected at the convenience of the researcher. Patients are included in a clinical trial only if they meet specific criteria, such as the severity of the condition, their history, age, gender, and so forth. Thus, one must examine the characteristics of a study's population before applying its results to a specific patient. Clinical trials utilize randomization, which is different from random sampling in that randomization denotes how patients are assigned to groups.

Journal articles that report the findings of clinical trials often include information about how the number of subjects that were included in the sample was decided. The determination of the needed sample size is an important part of a study's protocol for ethical as well as economic reasons:[5] ethically, because no more subjects should be inconvenienced or put at risk than what is actually necessary to find a treatment effect, and economically, because of the resources that are required to include unnecessary subjects. Another reason to predetermine sample size is that samples that are too small reduce the power of a study such that the study is not able to recognize a treatment effect when it is present. Conversely, samples that are excessively large will point to statistically significant differences between groups even when the difference is very small. There is a method to sample size determination that takes into account the estimated variance of the sample, the size of the clinically important treatment effect that is being sought after, and the acceptable amount of possible error.

Group Clinical Trial Designs

The RCT is regarded as the ultimate experimental research design in health care and is what comes to mind for many people when thinking of research in general. The rationale for using RCTs is to minimize a variety of biases that might occur during an experiment that could alter the study's final results. Without the use of randomization and a control group for comparison, researchers could not really be confident that the treatment or intervention actually caused the observed improvements in the patients.

The basic design of an RCT consists of a sample of patients selected from a target population that is representative of typical patients with the condition under study (Figure 5.3). This sample is then divided at random into two groups, one of which receives the genuine treatment or intervention (the intervention group) and another that receives a placebo or sham treatment (the control group). It is important to understand that RCTs typically take a long time to enroll patients; therefore, as each patient is enrolled, he or she is randomly assigned to a treatment group. There are also RCT designs that involve more than two groups.

A *placebo* is an inert substance or treatment that is used as a comparison to the active substance or treatment in an RCT. Placebos are used extensively in

FIGURE 5.3 **Flowchart of a simple randomized controlled trial.**

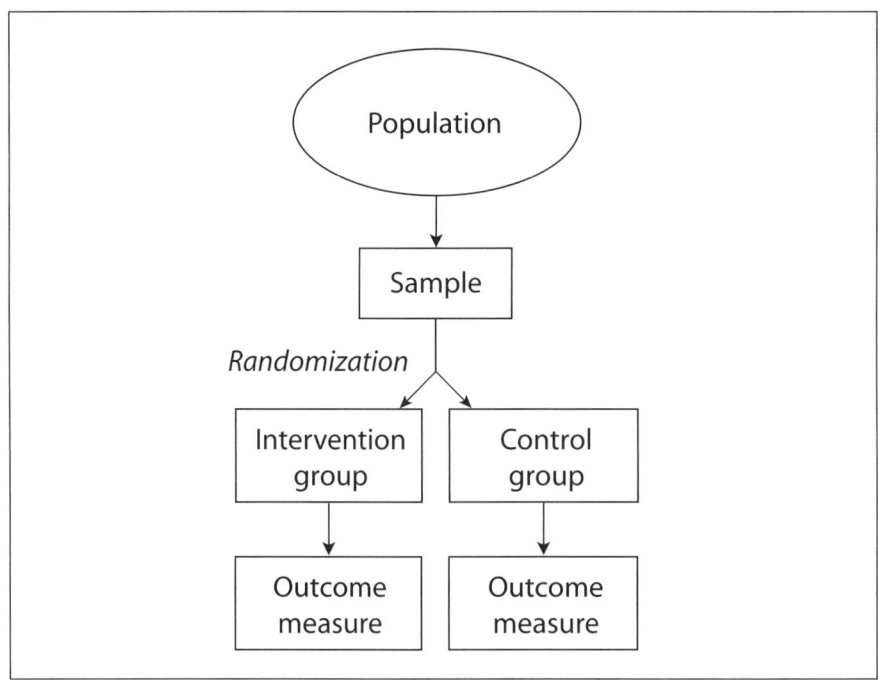

pharmaceutical trials to establish whether an active drug is more effective than a placebo. The outcomes of drug and placebo groups are compared at the end of a study to determine if the drug resulted in a statistically significant treatment effect. A *treatment effect* is the result that a treatment or intervention has on outcomes that are attributable specifically to the effect of the intervention. The treatment effect is estimated in the analysis of a study using the difference between the mean outcomes observed in a treatment group and a control group. A *sham treatment* is another type of placebo involving the application of a nontherapeutic intervention. It is delivered in such a way that it simulates the real treatment so well that the patients have a difficult time telling the difference between the two. As is discussed later, it is difficult to produce a sham chiropractic manipulation that is not easily recognized as such by patients.

The use of a placebo control group in RCTs provides an essential point of reference needed to determine the efficacy and rate of adverse effects of active treatments.[6] In addition to just looking at the improvements that the patients experienced, other factors must be considered. There are essentially three reasons why patients experience improvement with any given therapy. The first is natural history, because most acute and some chronic conditions resolve on their own. In this same category, and closely related, is the phenomenon of *regression to the mean*, in which extreme symptoms that some patients have at the beginning of a study tend to return toward a more normal state with the passage of time. The second is the specific effects of treatment involved. The third is nonspecific effects of treatment that are in some way related to the treatment, but are actually due to factors other than the treatment's active components. Nonspecific effects of treatment are often called placebo effects (Figure 5.4).

Placebo or sham treatments produce a *placebo effect*, which refers to the proportion of patients who tend to improve when they receive supposedly useless substances or interventions. The placebo effect is substantial for a variety of complaints, especially in relation to pain syndromes. The placebo effect has even been reported to influence serious illnesses. It has been observed that approximately one-third of patients who are given placebos notice improvement of their condition. The underlying mechanisms involved in the placebo effect remain a mystery, although it is thought to be triggered by the patient's belief in the treatment and his or her expectation of feeling better. The enthusiasm of the practitioner providing the treatment can help boost a patient's expectations. This assumption is based on the observation that when the placebo (pill or treatment)

Chapter 5 Experimental Designs

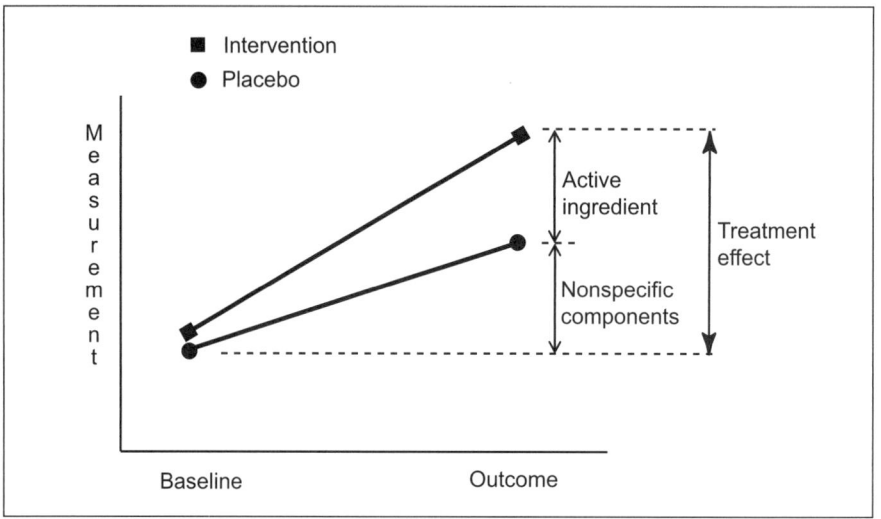

FIGURE 5.4 Nonspecific components of treatment must be removed from the treatment effect to determine the amount of active ingredient.

looks genuine, the person receiving it is more likely to believe that it will work and will therefore experience correspondingly a more potent placebo effect. Additionally, the more trust patients have in their doctor, the more likely they are to believe that a placebo will work.

Both the placebo and treatment groups typically show improvement at the conclusion of a study, but it is the difference between the groups at that point in time that matters. If it can be shown that the mean outcome of the treatment group is statistically significantly better than the mean of the control group receiving a placebo, then the treatment can be considered effective.

Randomization

The primary purpose of randomization is to attempt to make the experimental groups *equivalent* with regard to prognostic factors that may confound the measure that is being investigated. For instance, in a study looking at the effect of chiropractic manipulation on radicular leg pain, the mean pain levels at the beginning of the study should be approximately the same in the treatment group as they are in the control group. The equivalence of groups after random assignment is sometimes called *probabilistic equivalence* because there is a chance that there will be a difference between groups in spite of randomization. Moreover, chance is the only reason that groups sometimes differ after random assignment since each person has an equal likelihood of being selected for inclusion in either group.[3] If the randomization process is carried out properly, the risk of introducing biases into studies is minimized.

Randomization can be accomplished in a number of different ways. The most straightforward is to determine the assignment of each pair of study participants by a simple coin toss. Another uncomplicated method is to draw slips of paper that are labeled "placebo" or "treatment" from a hat or bin. A more sophisticated approach, and what is currently employed most commonly, is to utilize a randomization list that is generated from a random number table or from random numbers generated by a computer. Other methods include block randomization (blocking) and stratified randomization, both of which can help prevent unequal treatment group sizes.[7] Blocking involves separating subjects into homogeneous subgroups based on factors such as age or disease severity. Blocking enhances the comparison of groups during data analysis because the subgroups are more similar to each other than the intact groups. Stratified randomization separates intact groups into subgroups based on prognostic factors, such as patients with and without a history of spine trauma in a chronic lower back pain study.

The assignment of patients during randomization is often concealed from those doing the assigning to avoid the temptation of allotting patients with certain characteristics to groups where they can receive special treatment. Preferential assignment defeats the purpose of randomization and is especially harmful to a study's validity. A randomization scheme that utilizes sealed envelopes that are given to the participating clinicians as they choose which therapy to offer patients is a widely used option for concealment. Another solution is distance randomization, which turns the assignment decision over to another investigator, often at a separate facility.

The importance of concealed assignment is greater than one might think. In a review article, Kunz and Oxman[8] compared adequate versus inadequate concealment of random assignment. They found that when studies failed to adequately conceal random assignment, the apparent effects of the treatment were altered, either in support of or against the treatment. The magnitude of these distortions was as large as or larger than the size of the effects that were being investigated. Furthermore, a meta-analysis of RCTs revealed that the findings of included studies yielded larger estimates of treatment effects, which were exaggerated by 41% for inadequately concealed trials (i.e., those which did not report on the concealment approach) and by 30% for unclearly concealed trials (i.e., those which incompletely reported on concealment).[9]

Bias in Research

When *bias* is mentioned in the research setting, it refers to systematic errors introduced into a study that are attributable to problems with selection, assignment of participants to groups, or problems with the measurements involved in the study. Numerous types of biases need to be considered while reviewing articles because their presence can render a given study invalid, although no study is perfect and at least some bias will be present in all studies.

Before describing some of the more common biases, you should be aware that, in general, people react differently when participating in experiments. This was discovered in the 1930s in a study done at the Hawthorne Plant of the Western Electric Company in Chicago, Illinois. What the researchers discovered is that work productivity increased under a variety of conditions, even those that would normally be expected to reduce productivity (e.g., when rest periods were eliminated). The conclusion of the study was that the workers' behavior was not so much influenced by the interventions that were introduced as by the attention they received from the researchers. Accordingly, this phenomenon is known as the *Hawthorne effect*, and it is a factor in virtually every study involving humans.[10]

The first bias to consider is *sampling bias*, where study participants are selected in such a way that each person from the source population does not have an equal chance of being selected. The process of random selection is supposed to take care of this problem, but sometimes it is not successful. The classic example of sampling bias occurred during the campaign for president of the United States in 1936. A very large poll had predicted that President Franklin D. Roosevelt, a Democrat, would lose to Alfred Landon, a Republican. The poll was done by mailing postcard ballots to more than 10 million people, with over 2 million of them being returned. Based on the results of that poll, it was predicted in *The Literary Digest*, a popular magazine of the day, that Landon would defeat Roosevelt by a big margin. The opposite happened, however, and Roosevelt won in a landslide. The problem was that the names and addresses for the postcards were obtained from automobile registration lists and telephone books. At that time, however, many low-income residents of this country did not own automobiles or telephones. As a result, wealthy Republicans were grossly overrepresented and Democrats were grossly underrepresented in the final count.

Sampling bias is at times called *selection bias*, since it refers to a problem with the way participants are selected for a study. A better use of the term *selection bias*, especially when dealing with experimental design, has to do with systematic differences that occur between the groups being compared in a study with regard to prognosis or response to treatment. Random assignment to groups with adequate concealment about which group the participants were allocated to is the best safeguard against this form of selection bias. Random assignment does not actually remove selection bias; rather, it distributes the bias evenly between the treatment and control groups, which in effect cancels it out.

The second bias occurs when the examining or treating doctors involved in a study influence the results in accordance with their expectations or desires for a particular outcome. This phenomenon has been termed *experimenter bias* or *researcher bias* and works similar to the way that patients' beliefs influence their perceptions about the care they receive. Researchers may conduct themselves in a manner that influences study participants so much that the results of the study are changed one way or the other.

It has already been mentioned that random assignment is a powerful protection against biases in a study. Another solution is the *blinding*, or *masking*, of study participants as to which group they are in so they will not know whether they are receiving the treatment or a placebo. This type of blinding is used in a *single-blind* study. Preferably, neither the patient nor the researcher knows whether the treatment or placebo is involved, which is termed *double blinding*. *Triple blinding* is even possible, in which neither the subject, the person providing the treatment, nor the evaluator knows the group assignment of any of the subjects.

Treatment outcomes should always be measured by someone who is blind to the subjects' group assignment to avoid bias. Blinding of the treatment providers as well as the patients is also desirable, especially in explanatory studies. If treatment providers or patients are aware of their group assignment, it will be difficult to determine whether the derived benefits were from the direct effect of the treatment or from some other variable. Researchers often survey the participants at the

Chapter 5 Experimental Designs

conclusion of a study to determine if they were able to discern whether they were in the treatment or sham group, a tactic that helps evaluate the effectiveness of the blinding.

Greenhalgh[11] describes several other biases, which are listed in Figure 5.5 alongside the stages where they may occur in an RCT.

Extraneous and Confounding Variables

Experiments are carried out in a very controlled environment in which the researchers are able to manipulate the explanatory variables and then observe what happens to the outcome variables. The researchers expect to be able to say that the study's outcome is attributable to the treatment rather than to something outside the environment of the experiment. The extent to which the conclusions of such an experiment represent real occurrences is a reflection of the study's validity, in this case its internal validity. In other words, *internal validity* is the

FIGURE 5.5 **Potential sources of bias in randomized controlled trials.**

Selection bias: Unsuccessful randomization may result in nonequivalent groups.

Performance bias: Care is provided to patients inconsistently. Especially detrimental when groups are managed differently.

Exclusion bias: Dropouts are systematically different than subjects that remain in the study.

Detection bias: Patients are evaluated differently regarding the outcome measures.

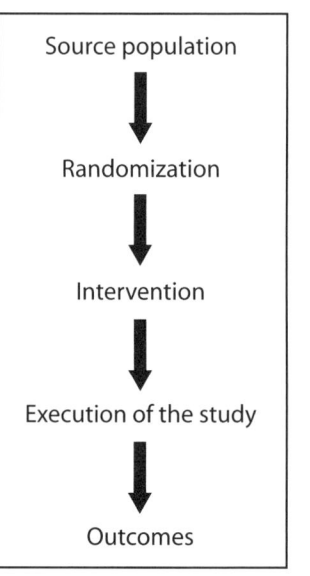

capacity of an experiment to show that the explanatory variables actually caused the changes that were observed in the outcome variables.

Sometimes uncontrolled factors have an influence on the relationship between the variables in an experiment. These *extraneous variables* affect the outcome of an experiment, even though they are not the variables that are actually being studied. They produce error in an experiment and, as a result, are undesirable. One of the most important objectives in designing experiments is to minimize or control the influence of extraneous variables. A *confounding variable* is a type of extraneous variable that introduces *systematic error* into a study because it affects the levels of the explanatory variables differently. For instance, a confounding variable might have an effect on the treatment group, but not the control group. This makes it extremely difficult to interpret the study's outcome. Extraneous variables add error variance to studies, but it is distributed uniformly between the groups when random assignment is utilized. Thus, random assignment does not actually reduce the amount of error that occurs when extraneous variables are present, but it does reduce its influence on the study's final results.

As an example of a study containing a confounding variable, consider a study investigating a new weight-loss program that involved one group receiving the new weight-loss program and another group receiving a sham program that was designed to maintain the subjects' usual nutrient intake. All subjects continued their regimen for six weeks and were weighed daily. For weigh-ins, subjects receiving the intervention reported to an office that was accessible only after walking nearly one-half mile and climbing four flights of stairs, whereas the control subjects reported to an office that was accessible in a matter of a few steps. The results of the study pointed to a favorable outcome in favor of the weight-loss group, but because of the confounding variable of exercise (walking and climbing stairs) that affected the treatment group but not the control group, one cannot be confident in its findings.

Confounding occurs primarily in quasi-experimental designs because random assignment is not utilized. Because study participants are assigned to groups in these types of studies, the individual differences of subjects have the potential to act as confounding variables. An example would be a lower back pain study in which the assignment of patients to receive active versus sham treatment was unbalanced because the researchers allocated patients based on the complexity of the case (e.g., chronicity or the presence of leg pain). Whether the procedure was intentional or unintentional, randomization would have been the best solution to prevent this type of confounding.

A number of other factors threaten the internal validity of studies. Some of the more common *threats to internal validity* are as follows:

- *History*: Participants are exposed to some historical event during the research project that affects the results but was not intended to be associated with the explanatory variable. An example would be a statewide fitness campaign that coincided with a lower back pain study and encouraged participants to do exercises that were not part of the experiment. The exercises would likely have an effect on the outcome of the study, producing an inaccurate conclusion.

- *Reliability of measures*: Unreliable measures can invalidate a study and can be caused by such things as faulty equipment, inconsistent provision of instructions to study participants, unreliable training of examiners, examiners becoming tired or bored after doing repeated examinations, or the improvement of examiners at doing the test procedures due to practice.

- *Mortality*: Participants commonly drop out of studies for a variety of reasons, which creates a problem, especially when the dropouts are somehow different from those that remain. Perhaps they were not improving, or perhaps they improved so much that they did not think they needed further care. Whatever the reasons why people drop out of studies, there will subsequently be a chance that the groups will no longer be equivalent.

- *Maturation*: Participants change during a study for reasons that are not related to the explanatory variables involved. The maturation threat is different from history in that the changes that take place due to maturation are not related to an event but to the passage of time. A simple example would be a study looking at the strength of children, where the children would be expected to get stronger as time goes by, regardless of their exposure to the study's explanatory variables.

- *Regression to the mean*: This was previously mentioned as one of the three reasons participants improve with treatment. It is also a threat to internal validity because it is difficult to determine whether changes that occurred in a study's outcomes were caused by the explanatory variables or by extreme values at the beginning of a study that migrated toward the mean because those participants' symptoms returned to a more normal state with the passage of time. This threat is particularly evident when patients are selected for inclusion to the study because they have high values at the time of screening, while patients with low values are screened out. High initial patient scores are much more likely to move toward normality than to go even higher.

Generalizability of Research Findings

Assuming that an experiment is methodologically sound and has acceptable internal validity, another concern is whether the study has external validity. *External validity* is the degree to which the results of a study are applicable to other populations and other settings, and when implemented under different circumstances. However, since experiments involve samples from populations, the first concern regarding external validity is whether the study is applicable to the source population. *Generalizability* is another term frequently used to describe the concept of external validity (Figure 5.6). Any time you are contemplating applying the results of a given study to the management of one of your patients, you should ask whether its results are generalizable to that case. Does your patient or your practice differ from those enrolled in the trial in question regarding things such as

FIGURE 5.6 Internal validity has to be with cause and effect, whereas external validity has to do with the applicability of a study to other populations, other settings, and other situations.

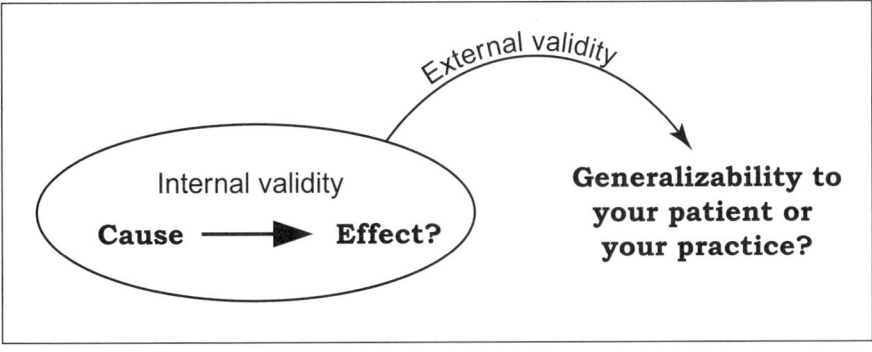

age, gender, and severity of the condition? The answers to these questions determine whether you will be able to utilize the study. For instance, can the results of a study of spinal manipulation for adult asthmatics be generalized to a pediatric patient with asthma?

The decision as to whether the external validity of any given study is adequate is a matter of judgment and depends on the clinical situation. When making decisions about external validity, one should consider things such as the traits of the study participants, the outcomes that were studied, the type of treatment that was utilized, and the setting in which the study was carried out. An example of problematic settings was evident in a lower back pain study done by Meade and associates[12] in which office-based chiropractic manipulation was compared with hospital-based physical therapy. Chiropractic care was found to be superior, but since the settings were so different (private offices versus outpatient departments at hospitals), one must wonder how much of the study's effect was attributable to the location rather than the intervention. Because of the impact these factors have on external validity, journal articles that report the results of clinical trials should provide enough information about these factors so that readers are able to make informed decisions about generalizability.

Design Options

The design of the classic experiment was presented in Figure 5.1. This design is also called the *pretest-posttest randomized experimental design*[3] and is the most commonly used design in research for several reasons. First, the design involves randomization to treatment and control groups, which drastically reduces the potential for biases. Second, the subjects in each group are evaluated before and after the introduction of the intervention. This strategy permits the statistical comparison of group means in such a way that any pretreatment differences that may have existed between the groups can be taken into account. Randomization is intended to render groups equivalent, but by chance, the groups will rarely be exactly equal. The analysis of covariance (ANCOVA) test is often utilized to analyze the data associated with this design because it factors in the pretreatment differences between groups as a covariate (Figure 5.7). Articles that report the results of ANCOVA will often use terminology such as "the effects of pretreatment differences were adjusted for during analysis." Other variables, such as differences in age or condition severity, can also be adjusted for using ANCOVA,

FIGURE 5.7 Pretreatment differences between groups can be adjusted for during the analysis using ANCOVA.

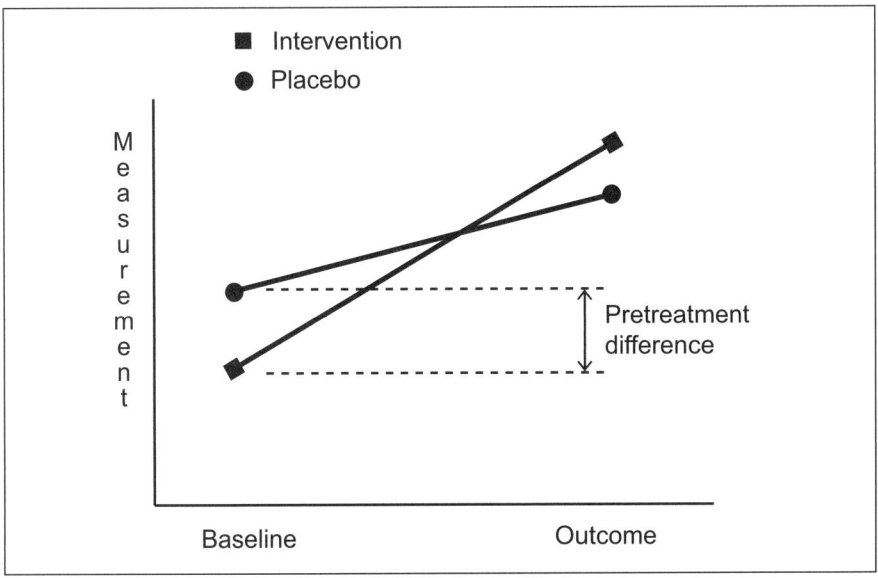

which statistically removes the effect of these covariates from the analysis. Another reason the classic experiment design is so popular is that it includes both a treatment group and a control group, which allows comparison between groups such that the active ingredient of the treatment effect can be discerned from non-specific components (Figure 5.4).

Sometimes the outcome of a treatment is not compared with a control group; rather, an alternate form of treatment is used for comparison. Typically this design involves evaluating a new therapy in comparison with an established therapy. This design, called the *two-group pretest-posttest design*, is helpful to demonstrate differences between treatments, but is not capable of establishing whether the new treatment works better than no intervention. The notation for this design is as follows:

$$R \quad O \quad X_1 \quad O$$
$$R \quad O \quad X_2 \quad O$$

The *posttest-only randomized controlled trial* is another design that is sometimes used when the sample size is large.[13] No pretest is utilized in this design, which does not allow a comparison of groups after randomization to make sure that the process was successful. This is a weaker design because of the uncertainty about the success of randomization. Larger samples are much more likely to produce equivalent groups, which will reduce the concern about randomization problems, but samples tend to be relatively small in chiropractic research. Accordingly, the posttest-only randomized controlled trial is rarely utilized within this profession. The notation for this design is as follows:

$$R \quad X \quad O$$
$$R \quad \quad O$$

Frequently, several explanatory variables are involved in a research project. For example, a study comparing the Diversified versus Gonstead spinal manipulation techniques in which patients have their spinal listings detected either by palpation or by x-ray analysis would have four different explanatory variables, two of which relate to the technique used and the other two to the spinal listings detection method. This type of design is called a *factorial design* because the independent variables are categorized as being either *factors*, which are the major independent variables (technique used and spinal listings method), or *levels*, which are the subgroups (Diversified and Gonstead along with palpation and x-ray analysis) (Figure 5.8). Factorial designs are used when two or more independent variables are involved and the investigators want to determine if any interaction exists between them. Four groups result from this design, with group 1 receiving Diversified technique and palpation as the method of analysis; group 2, Gonstead and palpation; group 3, Diversified and x-ray; and group 4, Gonstead and x-ray. Factorial designs can include more factors and levels than just two each, as was illustrated here. The notation for a two-factor by two-level (2×2) design is as follows:

$$R \quad O \quad X_{11} \quad O$$
$$R \quad O \quad X_{12} \quad O$$
$$R \quad O \quad X_{21} \quad O$$
$$R \quad O \quad X_{22} \quad O$$

Design Options

FIGURE 5.8 Major factors and levels of the explanatory variables involved in a factorial design.

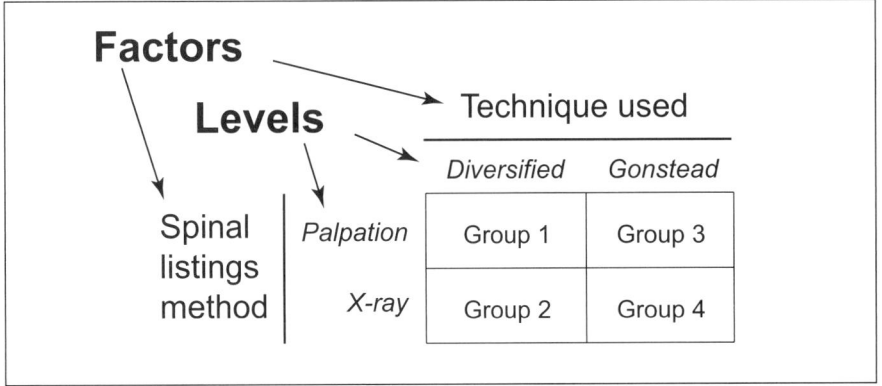

Crossover designs involve providing the treatment to one group while the other group receives a placebo or alternate treatment, and then switching assignments at some fixed point in time without the knowledge of the subjects or those administering the treatment. Thus, the members of each group receive the active treatment as well as the placebo or alternate treatment in rotation (Figure 5.9). Use of this design allows each subject to act as his or her own control, which can substantially reduce the size of the sample that is needed.[14] The notation for the crossover design with randomization is as follows:

| R | O | X_1 | O | Optional | O | X_2 | O |
| R | O | X_2 | O | washout period | O | X_1 | O |

Crossover designs have several limitations that must be taken into consideration to ensure study validity. *Carry-over effects* occur when the therapeutic effects of the first intervention continue during administration of the second intervention. Accordingly, a washout period of time is often employed to allow the effects of the first treatment to disappear before starting the second. Crossover designs are not appropriate for investigating acute conditions or those that are responsive to treatment, but they are appropriate for stable conditions such as chronic lower back pain and other conditions where outcomes revert to baseline after treatment is stopped. *High dropout rates* are caused by the fact that patients must submit to two or more periods of treatment. Recall that one of the benefits

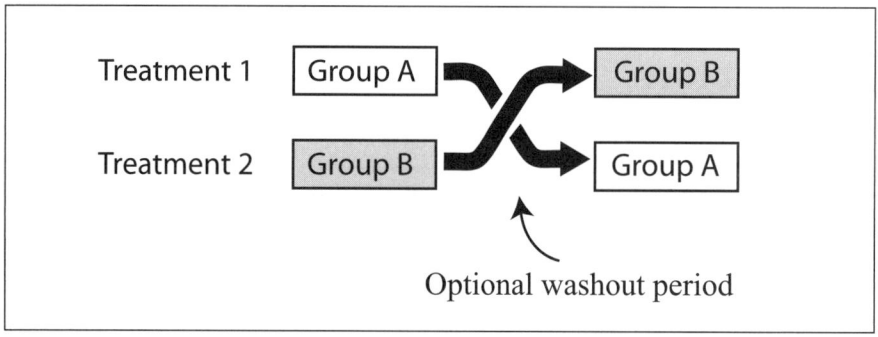

FIGURE 5.9 Crossover design.

of this design is that the sample size can be smaller; thus, when patients do drop out, the effect is more harmful to the data analysis than with other designs because the data derived from each patient contributes so much to the total. Another limitation is *treatment sequencing*, where patients have the potential to respond differently when treatment 1 is given before treatment 2 than if the order had been reversed. An example would be a study in which lower back pain patients received manipulation first, followed by stretching exercises during the second phase. The results could be quite different if the stretching were provided first because the patients might be preconditioned by the stretching to receive a better effect from the manipulation.

Quasi-experimental designs look very similar to the randomized designs just covered, minus the random assignment of subjects to treatment groups. Because of this deficiency, it is much more difficult to make claims about causality based on quasi-experimental evidence. There are quite a few varieties of quasi-experimental designs; in fact, Cook and Campbell[15] describe 11 different versions. Refer to the Cook and Campbell text for more information on this subject. Threats to internal validity can be substantially reduced when the proper quasi-experimental design is utilized. Furthermore, it is possible for a first-rate quasi-experiment to outdo a less robust RCT and generate stronger evidence. Rosner[16] went so far as to say that "a well-crafted cohort study or case series may be of greater informative value than a flawed or corrupted RCT."

RCTs have been considered by some as the only type of evidence that should be utilized in evidence-based practice, whereas Busse and colleagues[17,18] referred to quasi-experimental designs as being reasonable alternatives in many cases. These authors suggested that RCTs and quasi-experimental studies have complementary roles in research, such as when conducting RCTs would be unethical or impractical. High-quality quasi-experimental studies may be more appropriate under these circumstances.

Nonexperimental designs not only do not utilize randomization, but also do not include a comparison group. Consequently, it is not possible to credit any of the effects that are observed to the intervention that is under investigation. Several nonexperimental designs are discussed in Chapters 7 and 8. Briefly, nonexperimental designs include surveys and observational research, which describe certain characteristics of patients who have been exposed to some type of intervention or their natural setting, and case studies and case series, where the care of one or more patients is described. Even though these designs are low on the evidentiary scale and cannot support cause-and-effect relationships, they are still quite valuable because they describe unfamiliar occurrences and provide data that often leads to more complex studies. Pretreatment measures are sometimes taken in nonexperiments, in particular in case studies, but many times only one measure is involved. The outcome measure in the following nonexperiment could follow any type of intervention, or merely the observation of some variable in its natural setting:

$$X \quad O$$

Chiropractic Interventions and Experimental Methods

Experimental methods work quite well when investigating pharmacological interventions because it is reasonably straightforward to create one pill that contains an active ingredient and another identical-looking pill that is a placebo containing inert ingredients.[19] Chiropractic interventions, on the other hand, are not especially amenable to experimental methods.[20] Placebo or sham chiropractic manipulations are either so invasive that they introduce forces into the tissues that may become therapeutic or are so dissimilar from chiropractic manipulation that both the treating DCs as well as the patients are fully aware that they are involved in the placebo group. Patients may not receive a placebo effect, which is primarily based on patient expectations, if they think they are not actually being treated.

Otherwise stated, they will not improve to the extent that someone receiving a realistic placebo would. RCTs that investigate chiropractic interventions will consequently have limited validity in relation to the difficulties associated with implementing convincing placebos. Budgell[21] cautioned that one should not assume that the placebo procedures used in chiropractic clinical trials that involve physical contact or positioning of patients will not have an effect on symptoms.

A second reason chiropractic interventions are not amenable to experimental methods is related to the fact that blinding is very difficult to achieve in chiropractic research,[22] probably because patients have expectations about the treatment they will receive that are not met with most types of sham manipulations. An example of a sham manipulation designed for a study investigating chronic otitis media in children[23] "consisted of manual static and motion palpation and light touch of specific spinal segments so that the placebo treatment was identical to the active treatment except for the low-amplitude, high-velocity thrust." Another example of an attempt at devising a chiropractic placebo (simulated treatment) is seen in a childhood asthma study.[24]

> For simulated treatment, the subject lay prone while soft-tissue massage and gentle palpation were applied to the spine, paraspinal muscles, and shoulders. A distraction maneuver was performed by turning the subject's head from one side to the other while alternately palpating the ankles and feet. The subject was positioned on one side, a nondirectional push, or impulse, was applied to the gluteal region, and the procedure was repeated with the subject positioned on the other side; then the subject was placed in the prone position, and a similar impulse was applied bilaterally to the scapulae. The subject was then placed supine, with the head rotated slightly to each side, and an impulse applied to the external occipital protuberance. Low-amplitude, low-velocity impulses were applied in all these non-therapeutic contacts, with adequate joint slack so that no joint opening or cavitation occurred.

The simulated chiropractic care that was employed in this study involved considerable incursion into both the soft tissues as well as the bony structures. Just because a cavitation was not produced certainly does not exclude the possibility of a therapeutic effect. In fact, Mein and associates[22] pointed out that the simulated treatment in this study was strikingly similar to a traditional general osteopathic treatment. Furthermore, there was no attempt to blind the treating DCs in either of these studies, which introduces researcher (treater) bias and detracts from a study's validity. Treater bias will almost always be problematical in manipulation studies, except possibly trials involving instrument adjusting.[25]

The fact that chiropractic interventions are difficult to study does not excuse the profession from conducting trials that utilize experimental methods. However, the previously mentioned limitations should be considered by researchers and rectified in future trials when possible. These limitations should also be taken into account when comparing the results of manipulation trials, which may be unconvincing, with those of other therapies that are better suited to experimental methods.

Ethics in Biomedical Research

The current state of affairs regarding biomedical ethics is best appreciated within a historical context. Prior to World War II, biomedical research was unregulated; as a result, there was widespread abuse in this area, producing unnecessary harm to research participants. No doubt the most notorious example of unethical biomedical research is that of the Nazis, who carried out gruesome experiments on inmates of concentration camps. These "studies" included cases in which people were forced to swallow or were injected with deadly substances, immersed in ice water, and subjected to deadly surgeries. Also around this era, many experiments were carried out on prisoners, orphans, or mentally ill residents of state institutions, often without the subjects' knowledge. The Tuskegee Syphilis Study was a prime example, in which 400 African Americans with syphilis were observed from the 1930s until 1972 in an attempt to determine what the natural history of untreated syphilis would be. Study participants were denied appropriate medical care and deceptively subjected to invasive diagnostic tests (e.g., lumbar puncture) under the pretext that the procedures were therapeutic.

These examples of abuse to participants in research, and many others, led to the development of regulations designed to bring ethical standards to the conduct of clinical trials. The first set of rules to be developed in this area was called the Nuremberg Code because it was developed as a result of the Nuremberg military tribunals, which tried the Nazi doctors involved in abusive human experiments.

The 1947 tribunals denounced their experiments as "crimes against humanity." In response, the judges wrote a statement about permissible medical experiments, which was later called the Nuremberg Code.

The Nuremberg Code contained several unresolved issues that rendered it incomplete. First, it did not have any legal authority, thus making it unenforceable. Second, it only dealt with research on healthy participants. Third, it left the control of research entirely up to scientists, without governmental controls. In an effort to remedy these deficiencies, the World Medical Association developed the Declaration of Helsinki in 1964. The purpose of the Helsinki Document was to guide medical researchers concerning the proper ethics involved in human-subject research. A major focus of this document was to require medical researchers to clearly define the protocol of the procedures involved in human-subject experiments and submit it to a specially appointed independent ethical review committee for approval. Consequently, institutions that permit human-subject research now have institutional review boards (IRBs) to oversee the ethics of studies performed within their sphere of influence. Many biomedical journals now require a statement of IRB approval regarding the ethics of studies that deal with human subjects. Anyone contemplating such research is advised to seek appropriate approval before commencement of the study to ensure the protection of participants and the publication of the results when completed.

Another watershed event in development of ethics in human-subject research occurred when the National Commission for the Protection of Human Subjects of Biomedical and Behavioral Research issued the Belmont Report in 1979. In response to the Belmont Report, regulations were developed by the U.S. government to control the performance of federally funded research. At the heart of the Belmont Report were three underlying principles of research ethics: autonomy, beneficence, and justice. *Autonomy* has to do with the ethical principle of respect for persons. In research ethics, it is applicable in two areas: (1) An autonomous person's opinions and choices ought to be considered and his or her actions should not be obstructed, and (2) additional protections should be provided to persons with diminished autonomy. *Beneficence* provides that efforts to secure the well-being of research subjects must be enacted in a study's protocol. Under this principle, researchers are obligated to follow two rules: (1) Do not harm subjects, and (2) maximize possible benefits while minimizing possible harms. *Justice* concerns the distribution of the benefits of research and who should bear its burdens and risks. In other words, one group or particular groups should not be expected to unduly bear the burdens of research risks and one group or particular groups should not be denied the benefits of research.

The principle of *informed consent* is one of the cornerstones of ethical research. The Nuremberg Code indicated that "the voluntary consent of the human subject is absolutely essential," and the Belmont Report emphasized the idea of showing respect for research participants. Respect, in this case, requires that research subjects be given the opportunity to choose what will or will not happen to them. Accordingly, informed consent is one of the most valuable ways to ensure respect for persons involved in research.

Some readers may be contemplating or actually conducting research within their practices, ranging in complexity from case studies to some type of clinical trial. However, the issue of ethics must be considered prior to beginning such a project in order to avoid consequent problems. Foremost among these problems is the fact that research conducted without input and supervision from a legitimate ethics review board may place study participants at unacceptable risk. Furthermore, because of this omission, there is a great likelihood that the findings of such research will never be published in a reputable journal. Anyone considering engaging in practice-based research is urged to seek approval from a research ethics committee by contacting the research department at a health-related college or university. Several commercial enterprises also offer this service.

When conducting research with human subjects, several ethical issues need to be addressed so as to avoid violating research ethics and to have a reasonably good chance of getting the project approved by an ethics review board. The most important of these issues, and one that all the other issues stem from, is ensuring the safety of the participants. Second, the researcher is obligated to obtain a signed informed consent from every participant. Third, the researcher must indicate how privacy and confidentiality matters will be handled. Fourth, the researcher must spell out how adverse events will be taken care of. Finally, when one intervention is compared with another in a study, the researcher should at the outset be uncertain as to which one is superior.

It is important to note that ethics pertain to all clinical research, not just experimental designs. However, the subject is covered at this point in the book because it is the introductory chapter to the book's second part.

Appraisal Tactics

There are no rigid rules that can be applied to evaluating research; indeed, there are quite a few different methods and checklists available that reflect variable opinions as to how appraisal should be done.[26] Nevertheless, there are similarities among these methods that are directed toward the same objective, which is to assist readers of research in determining to what extent a study is valid and whether its findings are applicable to a given clinical situation. Regardless of which method or checklist is utilized, the end result is very similar. Suggestions on how to appraise the various study designs covered in this book are presented at the end of each of the applicable chapters. The material presented has been gleaned from other checklists and commentaries in an attempt to provide appraisal tools that are specific to the appraisal of chiropractic-related research.

The assessment of any form of clinical evidence first requires familiarity with the methods that were associated with the specific design being evaluated. This material was presented previously in this chapter and is presented in each of the subsequent chapters that deal with the various research designs. Once familiar with the correct methods, one can examine the components of the methods utilized in a given study and judge their degree of compliance with correct procedures. Although not required, appraisal checklists are commonly employed as aids during this process.

Three issues that should be considered when reviewing any journal article:[27,28]

1. *Are the results of the study valid?* This issue has to do with whether the methodology employed in the study was carried out correctly, whether the statements made by the authors were logical and supported by the findings of the study, and whether confounding factors were present.
2. *What are the results of the study?* If a treatment effect was demonstrated, is it large enough to be considered clinically significant.
3. *Will the results of the study help my patients?* Are the study's findings applicable to your practice or to one of your patients?

Each of these three issues comprises several steps that ultimately come together to generate an appraisal checklist. Please refer to Appendix 2 for a *gen-*

eral checklist for the appraisal of journal articles, which can be copied or used as a template to create your own checklist.

After appraising a study's evidence, you will have to make a decision about whether to apply its findings to your practice. Some studies may be assessed as being so flawed that they should be considered worthless, whereas others may appear unimpeachable and, subject to clinical applicability, should readily be utilized. However, as was mentioned in Chapter 1, rating the validity of evidence is rarely black and white; consequently, some portions of an article may be deemed acceptable, whereas others are totally disregarded. This process of appraising and determining the applicability of research evidence boils down to a judgment call on your part, but the tools of appraisal can be very helpful in making the right decision.

Appraising Randomized Controlled Trials

As was presented in this chapter, very specific protocols are utilized in carrying out RCTs; accordingly, their appraisal is essentially a matter of determining whether each of the necessary steps was actually completed and, if so, whether they were implemented properly. Things that should be considered when appraising RCTs are listed here, along with explication when necessary. These items are also included in the *checklist for the appraisal of therapy articles* that can be found in Appendix 3.

- *Was a clear and logical study question presented?* RCTs should clearly state a question that takes into account the population that is being studied, the intervention that is to be utilized, and what outcomes are being measured.

- *Was random assignment to treatment and control groups carried out correctly?* Randomization methods that were utilized in the study should be described and should appear to be likely to produce equivalent groups. If done by coin toss, sealed envelopes, random numbers table, or by computer, then randomization was probably appropriate. If it looks as if the sequence of assignment to groups could be guessed by either participants or study personnel, it is probably inappropriate. Methods used to balance the randomization, such as stratification or blocking, should be described and justified.

- *Was randomization successful?* Were the groups well balanced after randomization, especially regarding the severity of the outcomes under investigation? The groups should also be equivalent with respect to medical histories and demographic information. Any differences noted between groups at the beginning of the trial should be considered as possible confounders.

- *Was the study population adequately described?* Participants that are selected for a study should be appropriate to the type of information being sought. The population should adequately reflect such characteristics as the condition under study, a particular age group, or the general population. The makeup of the study population is also a major factor regarding the applicability of the findings to clinical practice. Essentially, study participants should be similar enough to your patient population or to the patient in question to be able to generalize the study's findings.

- *Were the study's inclusion and exclusion criteria described and were they reasonable?* Patient selection in some studies is so restrictive that the results of the study may not be applicable to your patient or practice. For instance, many studies that have dealt with whiplash have excluded patients with grade III injuries (those having neurologic signs),[29] even though these types of patients are commonly seen by chiropractors. One would have to be cautious about extrapolating findings from a study that did not include patients similar to the one in question.

- *Were study personnel as well as participants blinded as to group assignment?* Although blinding is difficult with chiropractic interventions, the researchers should make an effort and describe their methodology. Determine what efforts were made by the researchers to achieve blinding and consider how much it matters in that particular case. Consider, however, that Schulz and coworkers[9] estimated an exaggeration of treatment effect by 17% in studies that were not double blinded. Frequently, researchers evaluate how successful blinding was after the study has concluded by asking both clinicians and patients to what group they thought the patient was assigned. If too many patients or clinicians are able to guess the assignment correctly, then blinding was not really effective. Moreover, Kunz and Oxman[8] indicate that the correctness of a study's blinding procedures may be a more sensitive means of appraising bias than checklists that are used to evaluate their quality.

- *Was the sample size large enough to find a treatment effect if one was present?* Higher-quality articles provide calculations of the number of participants needed in the study in order to have enough power to discern a treatment effect when one is actually present. Small samples increase the risk of a type II error; accordingly, it is important for researchers to make sure they have included enough participants in the study. Unfortunately, this calculation is reported less than 25% of the time in chiropractic journals[30] and less than 20% in the spine surgical literature.[31]

- *Were the groups treated equally, excluding the intervention, throughout the study?* Were treatments and examinations carried out at the same time intervals? Did it appear that study participants received the same amount of attention from the clinical personnel? If differences in the way participants were handled are discovered, consider the possibility that performance bias may have altered the results.

- *Were all of the study participants accounted for at the end of the study?* The number of participants completing a study should equal the number starting the study, minus dropouts and those eliminated for some reason. When some participants are lost to follow-up, their outcomes should still be analyzed according to the groups to which they were originally assigned. This practice is called an *intention-to-treat analysis* because patients who are randomly assigned to a group are analyzed together, even if they failed to complete the study or receive the treatment. Be aware that Kruse and colleagues[32] reviewed 100 articles in which authors claimed to have performed an intention-to-treat analysis and found that 47% of the time they had not.

- *Are the results of the study statistically significant?* How large a treatment effect was reported? Were the appropriate statistical tests utilized and were statistics calculated correctly? It is not that uncommon for authors to choose an incorrect statistical test to analyze the data in a study.

- *Are the results of the study clinically significant?* Although statistical significance is almost always addressed, clinical significance is not. Researchers will often define what differences would be considered clinically important at the outset of a study. If the minimum differences to attain clinical importance are not met, the results would not be considered important to clinicians, even if statistical significance was attained.

- *Were the outcomes that were measured clinically important?* Outcomes that are clinically important are those that are of interest to patients. Essentially, patients want to feel less pain and function better. In contrast, they are not nearly so concerned about improvements such as their orthopedic tests or palpation tenderness.

- *Who sponsored or funded the research?* Approximately 70% of the funding for clinical drug trials is from commercial sources,[33] and consequential biased findings are often reported.[34] Chiropractic research is not immune to this type of bias, although different commercial interests are involved. For instance, a study that was sponsored by or authored by someone closely connected with a chiropractic technique that is commercially promoted to the profession may have a tendency to be biased. The same could be said about research sponsored by vendors of nutritional supplements or therapeutic or diagnostic devices.

- *Were the conclusions appropriate?* All conclusions that are presented in articles should be consistent with and supported by the studies' findings. Be cautious about authors who put a spin on their findings in an attempt to support their point of view.

These questions can be applied to the appraisal of quasi-experimental studies as well, excluding the questions that deal with randomization. However, one should keep in mind when appraising quasi-experimental studies that although their external validity may sometimes be better than RCTs, their internal validity is always uncertain. Because of the high potential for confounding and bias associated with inadequate internal validity, it is difficult to use nonrandomized studies to demonstrate cause-and-effect relationships.

References

1. Roland, M., and D.J. Torgerson. *Understanding controlled trials: What are pragmatic trials? BMJ*, 1998. **316**(7127):285.
2. Haynes, B. *Can it work? Does it work? Is it worth it? BMJ*, 1999. **319**(7211):652–3.

3. Trochim, W.M.K. *Research Methods: The Concise Knowledge Base*. 2004. Cincinnati: Atomic Dog.
4. Witte, R.S., and J.S. Witte. *Statistics*. 6th ed. 2001. Fort Worth: Harcourt College Publishers.
5. Macfarlane, T.V. Sample size determination for research projects. *J Orthod*, 2003. **30**(2):99–100.
6. Preston, R.A., et al. Placebo-associated blood pressure response and adverse effects in the treatment of hypertension: Observations from a Department of Veterans Affairs Cooperative Study. *Arch Intern Med*, 2000. **160**(10):1449–54.
7. Roberts, C., and D. Torgerson. Understanding controlled trials: Randomisation methods in controlled trials. *BMJ*, 1998. **317** (?):1301–10.
8. Kunz, R., and A.D. Oxman. The unpredictability paradox: Review of empirical comparisons of randomised and non-randomised clinical trials. *BMJ*, 1998. **317**(7167):1185–90.
9. Schulz, K.F., et al. Empirical evidence of bias. Dimensions of methodological quality associated with estimates of treatment effects in controlled trials. *JAMA*, 1995. **273**(5):408–12.
10. Shi, L. *Health Services Research Methods*. 1997. Albany: Delmar Publishers.
11. Greenhalgh, T. How to read a paper: Assessing the methodological quality of published papers. *BMJ*, 1997. **315**(7103):305–8.
12. Meade, T.W., et al. Randomised comparison of chiropractic and hospital outpatient management for low back pain: Results from extended follow up. *BMJ*, 1995. **311**(7001):349–51.
13. Portney, L.G., and M.P. Watkins. *Foundations of Clinical Research: Applications to Practice*. 2nd ed. 2000. Upper Saddle River, NJ: Prentice Hall.
14. Louis, T.A., et al. Crossover and self-controlled designs in clinical research. *N Engl J Med*, 1984. **310**(1):24–31.
15. Cook, T.D., and D.T. Campbell. *Quasi-experimentation: Design and Analysis Issues for Field Settings*. 1979. Chicago: Rand McNally College Publishing.
16. Rosner, A. Fables or foibles: Inherent problems with RCTs. *J Manipulative Physiol Ther*, 2003. **26**(7):460–7.
17. Busse, J., et al. User's guide to the chiropractic literature-IA: How to use an article about therapy. *J Manipulative Physiol Ther*, 2003. **26**(5):330–7.
18. Busse, J., et al. User's guide to the chiropractic literature-IB: How to use an article about therapy. *J Manipulative Physiol Ther*, 2003. **26**(8):525–32.
19. Liebert, M.A. The efficacy paradox in randomized controlled trials of CAM and elsewhere: Beware of the placebo trap. *J Altern Complement Med*, 2001. **7**(3):213–8.
20. Hawk, C., et al. A randomized trial investigating a chiropractic manual placebo: A novel design using standardized forces in the delivery of active and control treatments. *J Altern Complement Med*, 2005. **11**(1):109–17.
21. Budgell, B.S. The placebo, the sensory trick and chiropractic. *Chiropractic Journal of Australia*, 2004. **34**(2):58–62.
22. Mein, E.A., et al. Manual medicine diversity: Research pitfalls and the emerging medical paradigm. *J Am Osteopath Assoc*, 2001. **101**(8):441–4.
23. Sawyer, C., et al. *A feasibility study of chiropractic spinal manipulation versus sham

spinal manipulation for chronic otitis media with effusion in children. J Manipulative Physiol Ther, 1999. **22**(5):292–8.
24. Balon, J., et al. *A comparison of active and simulated chiropractic manipulation as adjunctive treatment for childhood asthma. N Engl J Med*, 1998. **339**(15):1013–20.
25. Hawk, C., et al. *Preliminary study of the effects of a placebo chiropractic treatment with sham adjustments. J Manipulative Physiol Ther*, 1999. **22**(7):436–43.
26. Lohr, K.N. *Rating the strength of scientific evidence: Relevance for quality improvement programs. Int J Qual Health Care*, 2004. **16**(1):9–18.
27. Guyatt, G.H., D.L. Sackett, and D.J. Cook. *Users' guides to the medical literature. II. How to use an article about therapy or prevention. A. Are the results of the study valid? Evidence-Based Medicine Working Group. JAMA*, 1993. **270**(21):2598–601.
28. Guyatt, G.H., D.L. Sackett, and D.J. Cook. *Users' guides to the medical literature. II. How to use an article about therapy or prevention. B. What were the results and will they help me in caring for my patients? Evidence-Based Medicine Working Group. JAMA*, 1994. **271**(1):59–63.
29. Spitzer, W.O., et al. *Scientific monograph of the Quebec Task Force on Whiplash-Associated Disorders: Redefining "whiplash" and its management. Spine*, 1995. **20**(8 suppl):1S–73S.
30. Long, C.R., T.G. Nick, and C. Kao. *Original research published in the chiropractic literature: Evaluation of the research report. J Manipulative Physiol Ther*, 2004. **27**(4):223–8.
31. Bailey, C.S., C.G. Fisher, and M.F. Dvorak. *Type II error in the spine surgical literature. Spine*, 2004. **29**(10):1146–9.
32. Kruse, R.L., et al. *Intention-to-treat analysis: Who is in? Who is out? J Fam Pract*, 2002. **51**(11):969–71.
33. Bodenheimer, T. *Uneasy alliance—clinical investigators and the pharmaceutical industry. N Engl J Med*, 2000. **342**(20):1539–44.
34. Djulbegovic, B., et al. *The uncertainty principle and industry-sponsored research. Lancet*, 2000. **356**(9230):635–8.

CHAPTER SIX

Literature Review Designs

Literature review may be defined as a systematic, explicit, and reproducible way of identifying, evaluating, and interpreting all of the research findings and scholarly work available on a particular topic.[1] Literature reviews comprise a particular type of research design that is considered to be descriptive or observational because it primarily involves the observation of other authors' work. Reviews can target research findings that deal with a particular condition, a type of treatment, a diagnostic method, or other technology. Three different types of literature reviews may be encountered: narrative reviews, systematic reviews, and meta-analyses (Table 6.1). Each of the three review types presents the collective findings of research on a given topic, but they are distinct regarding the methodologies employed in their production.

Narrative reviews are characterized by the fact that they do not follow strict systematic methods to locate and synthesize the findings of the articles that are involved. Narrative reviews are often selective regarding the articles that are included, which has a tendency to introduce bias because authors may choose to incorporate articles that support their hypothesis and exclude those that do not. Furthermore, this type of review does not utilize rigorous methods to appraise the included articles, which can lead to a distortion of the results.

Systematic reviews, on the other hand, employ very strict, well-defined methods of locating, appraising, and synthesizing all of the research that is available on a given topic. A systematic review is actually an efficient scientific

TABLE 6.1 The three types of literature review designs

Narrative review	• Selective review of the literature that broadly covers a specific topic
	• Does not follow strict systematic methods to locate and synthesize articles
Systematic review	• Utilizes exacting search strategies to make certain that the maximum extent of relevant research has been considered
	• Original articles are methodologically appraised and synthesized
Meta-analysis	• Quantitatively combines the results of studies that are the result of a systematic literature review
	• Capable of performing a statistical analysis of the pooled results of relevant studies

technique.[2] Appraisal instruments are utilized to assist in the evaluation of the articles included in systematic reviews to ensure impartiality. The ultimate goal of a systematic review is to determine the estimated comparative effectiveness and safety of a treatment. Cook and colleagues[3] provided an excellent definition of a systematic review: "the application of scientific strategies that limit bias to the systematic assembly, critical appraisal, and synthesis of all relevant studies on a specific topic."

A *meta-analysis* is essentially a systematic review that incorporates an additional step that combines the quantitative data from the included articles using specific methodological and statistical procedures. A definition of a meta-analysis is as follows: "a systematic review that employs statistical methods to combine and summarize the results of several studies."[3] Because of the rigorous methods involved, readers of systematic reviews and meta-analyses ought to be able to reproduce the study's quantitative section and come up with similar results.[4]

Other terms are sometimes used to identify narrative reviews, including *overviews*, *clinical reviews*, *unsystematic reviews*, and *updates*, to name a few. This type of review typically covers a topic broadly, whereas the subject matter of systematic reviews and meta-analyses is more focused.[5] A systematic review may also be referred to as a *qualitative systematic review* since the findings of the included studies are synthesized to produce a conclusion that represents the middle ground of their results, rather than statistical combining of the data. In contrast, meta-analyses (also known as *quantitative systematic reviews*) do use statistical methods to combine the results of the studies that are included in a systematic review. Both quantitative and nonquantitative reviews extensively examine all relevant literature on a given topic in an effort to synthesize the collective information and draw a conclusion about what was included. Moreover, new hypotheses that were not presented in the individual studies of reviews can be tested in meta-analyses.[4]

Reviews can be located quickly when searching PubMed by clicking on the Limits tab and selecting "Review" or "Meta-analysis" from the Publication Types drop-down menu. The "Review" option retrieves both narrative and systematic reviews, while leaving out other types of studies. The "Meta-analysis" option only retrieves review articles that have combined the quantitative data of the included studies. These search-limiting strategies can be quite valuable when one wants to narrow down a search yet still be able to find information that represents the comprehensive literature on a specific topic.

Narrative Reviews

Narrative reviews have a number of similarities with systematic reviews, but are lower in the hierarchy of evidence because they do not employ many of the safeguards needed to control against bias. Specifically, they typically do not employ systematic methods in their development and preparation; for that reason, they should not be used as evidence to draw conclusions about the effectiveness of treatments. Narrative reviews often mix the authors' opinions with evidence; hence, they are prone to present a biased viewpoint. Montori and associates[6] defined them as "summaries of research that lack an explicit description of a systematic approach." On the other hand, they are often quite valuable in evidence-based chiropractic (EBC) because they summarize in general what is contained in the literature and provide a viable source for relevant background information. Like any form of research, narrative reviews vary in their quality and must accordingly be appraised to ascertain their degree of validity.

Narrative reviews are often written by authors who are considered to be experts in a given field. These types of reviews are comparatively easy to carry out and compose. As such, many review authors are inclined to write them. Practitioners are likely to prefer reading them over more complex designs, because they present the views of an expert on a given topic concisely and in a manner that can be read and comprehended quickly without having a lot of background knowledge. However, narrative reviews have the potential to contain numerous problems, and because they are unmethodical, it may be impossible to replicate their results.

When writing narrative reviews, authors often have their own opinions on the topic; accordingly, they may try to find studies to support their viewpoint when conducting the literature search. After the articles are selected, narrative review authors are often inclined to take a subjective and disorganized approach when analyzing the information. A common method is to simply add up the number of studies in favor of one side of an issue or the other and then espouse the view presented by the side that is in the majority. Unfortunately, this system may overlook things in the individual studies such as the research design that was utilized, the effect size, and the sample size; thus, it is clearly inadequate.

These casual methods often introduce a variety of biases that render the review's findings unreliable. For instance, *selection bias* (also known as *reference bias*) occurs when an author chooses articles during the search that support his or her conclusions, to the exclusion of articles with opposing views. To evaluate the extent of this problem, Schmidt and Gotzsche[7] considered 70 narrative review articles and found them to be severely biased. They indicated that the citations that were utilized in these reviews clearly favored the viewpoints presented by the authors. This type of search process does not present an accurate portrayal of the literature, and the resulting review may lead undiscerning readers astray. This is unfortunate, because clinicians often look to these types of reviews to acquire guidance from the experts and to obtain evidence for their practices. At any rate, review readers must keep these weaknesses in mind and attempt to identify potential biases.

Systematic Reviews

Systematic reviews are distinct from narrative reviews primarily in relation to the degree to which procedural quality is assured (Table 6.2). These distinctions should be taken into consideration when deciding whether a systematic or narrative review is most appropriate. A number of attributes distinguish systematic reviews from other reviews: (1) They deal with specific clinical questions, (2) an all-inclusive search of the literature is involved, (3) the criteria used to identify relevant articles are explicit, (4) the validity of the studies that are included is evaluated, (5) dissimilarities between the results of the studies are investigated, and (6) the results of the included studies are qualitatively or quantitatively syn-

TABLE 6.2 Differences between narrative and systematic reviews

Feature	Narrative Review	Systematic Review
Topic	Typically broad-scoped	Focused research question
Data sources and search strategy	The search strategy and databases that were used may not be provided	The search strategy is explicit and comprehensive, with a list of all databases that were utilized
Authorship	A recognized expert or experts on the topic	A team of experts having methodologic and clinical expertise
Article selection criteria	Typically not specified	Consistently applied inclusion and exclusion criteria
Searching	May be extensive, intended to locate literature on the topic area in question	Extensive, intended to locate all primary studies on a particular research question
Appraisal of included articles	Indefinite; may be variable	Critical appraisal is meticulous, typically involving the use of data extraction forms
Synthesis	A qualitative summary is usually provided	A qualitative summary is provided (quantitative when the data can be pooled)
Inferences	Sometimes evidence-based	Usually evidence-based

Source: Adapted from Cook, D.J., C.D. Mulrow, and R.B. Haynes. Systematic reviews: Synthesis of best evidence for clinical decisions. *Ann Intern Med,* 1997. **126**(5):376–80.

thesized.[8] Additionally, Montori and associates[6] reported that systematic reviews included twice as many citations as narrative reviews that were published in the same journals, which is the product of the rigorous search methods involved in systematic reviews. One of the most important outcomes of these methodical procedures is the curtailment of potential biases. The specific scientific strategies

Chapter 6 Literature Review Designs

that are employed in the assembly, critical appraisal, and synthesis of the studies included in the review considerably limit the influence of biases.[9]

Systematic reviews are initiated in response to clinical questions for which several primary studies exist, yet uncertainty about the topic remains. They can be very helpful when looking for evidence to answer clinical questions that deal with treatments or diagnostic tests. Ideally, they provide unbiased conclusions that are based on all of the collective literature that is available. Nevertheless, the negative effects attributable to authors' opinions are not entirely avoided by the thoroughness of systematic reviews, and the potential for selection bias is still of concern, although its impact is certainly reduced. Hence, their conclusions should not be accepted without first critically appraising the entire review. Also, since a systematic review is only designed to answer a specific patient care question, the information provided may be too narrow to completely answer a given EBC question.

When carrying out systematic reviews, the quality of the studies being evaluated is the primary determinant for inclusion of articles. Generally speaking, only randomized controlled trials (RCTs) are included in systematic reviews, while articles using other types of study designs are categorically eliminated. RCTs are considered to be the only design that adequately controls for confounding variables and biases; accordingly, they are more likely to provide reliable information than other sources of evidence.[10] When these confounding variables and biases are not controlled, there is a higher potential for studies to overestimate the treatment effects. This notion was disputed by Concato and colleagues,[11] however, who compared nearly 100 studies that included both RCTs and observational studies and found that the average results of the observational studies were very similar to those of the RCTs.

By design, systematic reviews cover a focused topic. As such, clinical questions that are not targeted specifically toward that particular topic may go unanswered or at least partially unanswered. An example would be a systematic review that dealt with the management of patients with whiplash injuries. The review would be expected to cover optimal therapies, but may provide no information about which patients should be x-rayed, receive MRI, or undergo electrodiagnostic tests. Also, combinations of therapies or co-management scenarios most likely would not be addressed. Narrative reviews that address most or all of those questions are probably available. However, their conclusions may differ as a result of the inherent weaknesses found in narrative reviews. Consequently, they need to be appraised for quality in order to decide which conclusions are acceptable to incorporate as evidence.

Conducting and writing a systematic review is a multistep process that is somewhat variable, but typically is as follows:

1. A clear therapeutic question must be created that incorporates the intervention to be studied and the pertinent outcomes, and also describes the patient population.
2. A comprehensive literature search is executed that includes all published, as well as unpublished, literature on the topic. Indeed, 77.7% of authors of systematic reviews thought that unpublished material should definitely or probably be included in the review process.[12] Search terms are targeted to the intervention, the outcome, and the appropriate patients. To reduce the potential for bias, all of the literature on the topic must be searched, including indexed journal articles, conference proceedings, and even unpublished reports. Ideally, non-English sources are included.
3. Studies that were located during the literature search are selected for inclusion in the review corresponding to the components of the question presented in step 1.
4. Each included study is appraised for quality, and its findings are recorded. In better systematic reviews, more than one independent reviewer is involved in the appraisal process.
5. The findings that were noted in step 4 are then synthesized to generate an overall conclusion about the effectiveness of the intervention.
6. The review's conclusion is discussed and placed in perspective regarding the influence of bias and the relevance of the findings to clinical practice.

The stages involved in performing a systematic review are presented in Figure 6.1 and are based on recommendations from the Centre for Reviews and Dissemination.[13]

The strategy used in searching the electronic databases should be fully described so that the process could be replicated by another researcher if desired. The description of the search strategy should include the following components: the name of database that was searched, the date the search was performed, the time frame encompassed, a full list of the search terms that were utilized, and identification of the languages that were used in the search. When

FIGURE 6.1 Stages and phases involved in a systematic review.

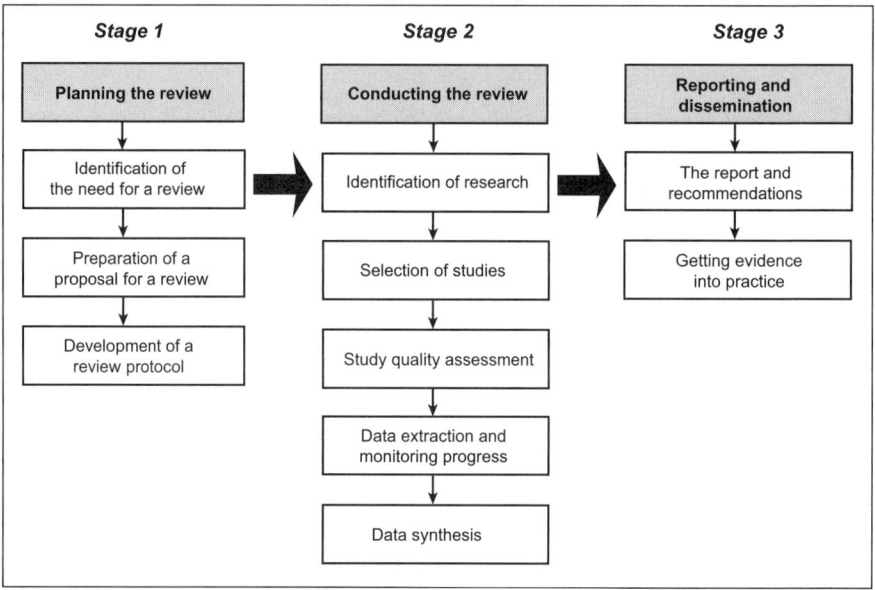

other sources of information are searched (e.g., conference proceedings, unpublished studies, or hand-searching of journals), the involved methodology should be fully described.

It was previously mentioned that the appraisal of articles should utilize more than one independent reviewer. Particularly important is the decision to accept or reject articles after applying the specified inclusion/exclusion criteria. There is no universally accepted methodology that can be applied when determining the quality of a given study.[14] Thus, the process is, to a certain extent, a judgment call, and reviewers sometimes disagree. They can often resolve these conflicts, but this is not possible when only one reviewer is involved.

Rather than rejecting articles altogether, sometimes statistical methods are used to weight studies according to their assessed validity so that the more valid studies have more influence on the review's final result. Weighting of studies is usually based on their methodological quality, the precision of their results based on the width of the associated confidence interval, and their degree of external validity. The weighting of articles is carried out by the reviewers and, because it is a somewhat subjective process, may result in discrepancies.

A limitation that may affect both narrative and systematic reviews is *publication bias*, the phenomenon whereby studies with statistically significant results are more likely to get published than those with nonsignificant results. Publication bias is often attributable to the author or funding source not considering the results of a "failed study" worthwhile to submit to a journal, or to journals being hesitant to publish studies that fail to show positive results. Articles that are not present in the literature will not be found in a search; thus, they will not become part of a review. Reviews that are affected by this bias are prone to give an overoptimistic view of the effectiveness of a given therapy. The chance of this bias occurring is why a thorough search in a systematic review should include sources other than journals. Publication bias *in situ* is an analogous type of bias, in which some of the results from a study are published, while other parts are suppressed.[15] There are several methods currently in use that attempt to detect and rectify publication bias, but their dependability has been questioned.[16] Therefore, when evaluating any kind of review article, keep in mind that the results may be subject to publication bias, which, when present, it is difficult to detect.

Meta-analyses

A *meta-analysis* is a type of systematic review that statistically combines the results from a number of studies in order to generate a single estimate of the effect of a treatment. The unit of analysis in meta-analyses is the findings of the original studies that are included, whereas clinical studies examine individual patients. The procedures involved in meta-analyses have been in use and presented in the literature since the 1950s, though the actual term was not used until 1976.[4] The key objective of a meta-analysis is to provide an estimate of the "average" treatment effect that exists among the studies included in the review.[17] Studies with exceptionally high or low results are offset by the studies in the middle, which in effect moderate the extremes. This averaging process can be very useful to practitioners because the results represent a reasonable approximation of the true value of the treatment effect size.

Considering what was just presented about averaging the results of studies in a meta-analysis, one should bear in mind that the process does not simply involve calculating an arithmetic average. If this were done, the results would often be misleading because studies with small samples are more prone to chance variations than are larger studies. Consequently, they should be given less weight so they will have less of an influence on the final estimate of treatment effect. Thus, meta-analyses typically employ methods that calculate a weighted average, whereby larger studies have more of an influence on the final estimate than smaller studies.

Meta-analyses have the ability to increase the power of individual studies by combining their data, which essentially increases the sample size. As was noted in Chapter 5, studies presented in the chiropractic and spine surgical literature frequently include too few subjects to detect true differences between the groups. As a result, there is a higher potential for type II error to occur in the articles that are read by chiropractors. This deficiency is somewhat ameliorated when studies are combined in meta-analyses.

Meta-analyses provide detailed information about how the included studies were selected, how the information was extracted, and how the findings were combined. These procedures permit readers to objectively appraise the methods and even allow others to replicate the research, if desired. Meta-analyses should have specific inclusion criteria in order to focus the topic on one area. If the inclusion criteria are too broad and too many studies are included, problems may arise when trying to compare dissimilar studies. For instance, if a meta-analysis were to incorporate studies that investigated manipulation for lower back pain, and the inclusion criteria allowed some studies involving patients with acute injuries and others involving chronic cases, there would likely be problems.

A meta-analysis involves the pooling of data from two or more studies; however since no two studies will have exactly the same findings, disparities will surely exist. Sometimes these disparities are small and sometimes they are large, depending on factors such as the quality of the studies, differences in study methodologies, different populations, and so forth. When conducting meta-analyses, often numeric scores are calculated to reflect the quality of the individual studies, and then a corresponding weight is assigned prior to statistical analysis.

The terms *homogeneity* and *heterogeneity* are sometimes used to describe the degree to which studies included in meta-analyses are comparable. *Homogeneity* refers to similarities among included studies that render them amenable to comparison, whereas *heterogeneity* refers to dissimilarities among studies that hamper or even prevent realistic comparison. As you would expect, homogeneity is preferred in meta-analyses. When planning reviews, most authors try to establish inclusion criteria to generate a relatively homogeneous set of studies. In practice, however, systematic reviews frequently exhibit substantial heterogeneity. Statistical tests are available to determine the amount of heterogeneity present in a meta-analysis, but their use is complex; consequently, they are underutilized.[18] Essentially, these statistical tests assess whether the observed differences in the studies' results are real or due to chance using a chi-square test.

There are a number of factors that contribute to heterogeneity in meta-analyses that should be considered. First, there may be heterogeneity in the makeup of the study samples due to differing inclusion and exclusion criteria; differences in the patients' baseline health status; patient population differences caused by disparate geographical locations; the use of matched controls versus those selected independently; comparison groups that receive either no treatment, placebo, or a standard treatment; or differences in the treatment, such as the method of delivery or frequency of care that was provided. Second, there may be heterogeneity in relation to the study design, such as differing patient dropout rates or the way in which dropouts were managed in the statistical analysis, or the length of time allowed for patient follow-up. Third, heterogeneity may occur with regard to the handling of patients' comorbid conditions, the handling of complications, the degree of freedom that practitioners had in controlling patient care, or the outcome measure that was employed. A fourth type of heterogeneity is sometimes referred to as *statistical heterogeneity*, which occurs when the observed treatment effects of the included studies are more dissimilar than what would be expected by chance.[19]

With all of the looming heterogeneities that are possible in meta-analyses, there is a fair likelihood that authors will combine data that is too dissimilar and, as a consequence, draw erroneous conclusions. Moreover, inconsistency among the results of studies in a meta-analysis reduces the confidence that one may have about any associated treatment recommendations.[20] A meta-analysis may actually be worthless if the included studies are too dissimilar from a clinical perspective.[19] For instance, it makes no sense to combine studies in a meta-analysis that involve treatments that utilize different types of comparison groups. Similarly, it is not appropriate to combine studies that utilize outcomes that are too dissimilar.

Nevertheless, a small amount of heterogeneity is acceptable and may actually serve to demonstrate that the results of a given treatment are consistent across a variety of conditions, which reinforces confidence in the treatment. If the variation between the results of studies is sizeable, however, it may be deceptive for authors to provide a value representing the overall treatment effect.

Mulrow[21] notes that the mixture of multiple reviewed studies in a systematic review offers an interpretive perspective that cannot be provided by any one study. This new perspective is attributable to the fact that studies integrated in systematic reviews, even though they deal with similar questions, often use different eligibility criteria, different definitions of disease, different methods of measuring or defining exposure, variations of a treatment, and different study designs. In effect, the results of all studies in a review would not be expected to be exactly the same. However, it is suspicious and degrades the findings of a review when some studies demonstrate a positive effect while others do not show any benefit at all, or possibly even a harmful effect.

As was stated previously, one of the major benefits of meta-analyses is their capacity to reduce the influence of studies with extremely high or low results through averaging. However, they cannot magically neutralize problems that may exist in the included studies, and their final value is constrained by the quality of the articles that make up the meta-analysis. Flaws that were present in the original studies may even be reinforced or amplified in the process of conducting a meta-analysis. This is why it is important for authors to critically appraise the articles before statistically combining them. An example meta-analysis was conducted by Assendelft and associates,[22] which investigated manipulation for the treatment of lower back pain. Comparison treatments were classified into seven categories, and pain and function was classified as either acute or chronic. The authors then analyzed this heterogeneous data using regression models to adjust for differences between the studies. They went on to report that the primary limitation of their review was the uneven quantity and quality of the original studies, and that this problem was common to many other systematic reviews.

The sizes of the treatment effects of studies in meta-analyses are typically displayed in a characteristic graph, commonly called a *forest plot* (Figure 6.2).[23] Each study is represented by a black square, which corresponds to a point estimate of the study's effect size, and a horizontal line extending to either side of the box, which corresponds to the 95% confidence interval of the effect size. The true value of the treatment effect would be present within this confidence interval 95% of the time if the study were repeated again and again. A vertical line bisects the graph and corresponds to zero or no treatment effect. If the 95% confidence inter-

FIGURE 6.2 **Graph of treatment effects for studies A through D. Zero represents no effect, positive values favor the treatment, and negative values favor the control or comparison. Studies B and D would be considered statistically significant in this case because their confidence intervals do not cross the bisecting line.**

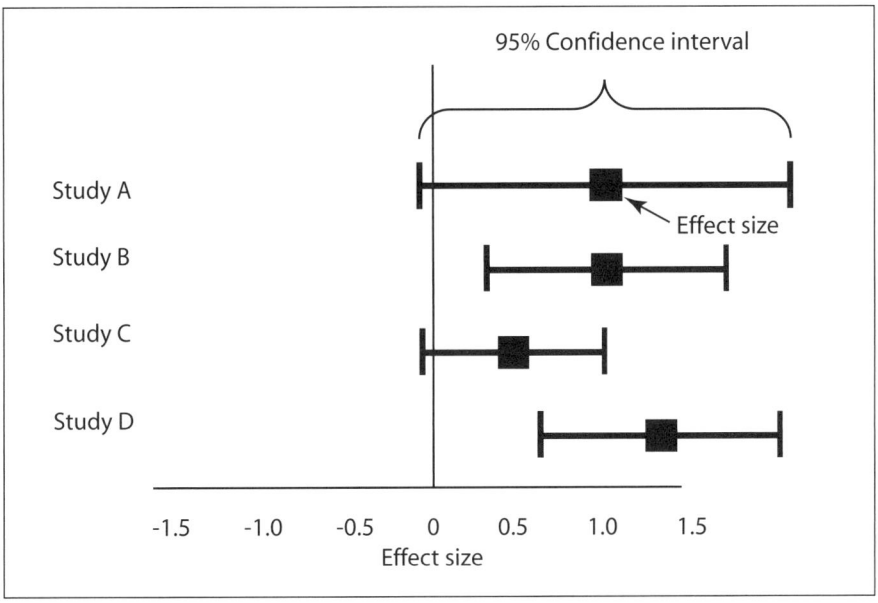

val of a study crosses over the vertical line and includes zero, then the difference between the treatment and control groups is not statistically significant. Sometimes the sizes of the black squares vary in these graphs to portray the weights of the various studies. Also, a diamond with a confidence interval line is sometimes placed at the bottom of the graph to represent the overall estimate calculated from the meta-analysis.

Effect size is essentially the difference between the means of the treatment and control groups in a study. However, when effect sizes from different studies are combined in a meta-analysis, often the units of measurement that were used are not comparable. To resolve this problem, the effect sizes are standardized to produce the *standardized mean difference*, which can be found by dividing the effect size by the pooled standard deviation. This form of standard deviation has been adjusted for the differences in the sizes of the groups. After this correction, the effect size then represents the standardized difference between group means and provides the relative magnitude of the experimental treatment.[24] It can be calculated by several different methods, but a common and simple approach is to find Cohen's *d* using data presented in the published studies. Cohen's *d* is calculated on continuous data by dividing the difference between the means of the two groups by their pooled standard deviation. The same concept is used when more than three groups are involved in a study. With two groups, the formula is as follows:

$$d = \frac{\overline{X}_t - \overline{X}_c}{S_{pooled}}$$

where

d = Cohen's *d* (the effect size)
$\overline{X}_t$ = the mean of the treatment group
$\overline{X}_c$ = the mean of the control group
S_{pooled} = the pooled standard deviation

If the outcome measure is dichotomous, such as the presence of pain versus no pain, or disability versus no disability, then an odds ratio or relative risk must be used instead of Cohen's *d*. An *odds ratio* can be calculated by comparing the odds of an outcome being present in patients who received treatment with the odds of the same outcome being present after a control intervention. For example, in a study involving manipulation for the treatment of lower back pain, the odds of patients in the treatment group having back pain versus no back pain can be compared with the odds of having back pain in the control group. Consider a hypothetical study involving 25 patients in each group. At the study's conclusion, 5 of the treatment group were still experiencing pain, while 10 of the control group still had pain. The odds of having pain in the treatment group would be 5:20 (0.25), whereas it would be 10:15 (0.66) in the control group. The odds ratio is then calculated by dividing 0.25 by 0.66, which equals 0.38; consequently, the odds of having back pain after manipulation would be less than after the control intervention. An odds ratio of 1.0 represents the case where there is no treatment effect and corresponds to an effect size of zero, as shown in Figure 6.2.

The *relative risk* (also known as *risk ratio*) can be determined by comparing the risk of having the outcome of interest in the treatment group with that of the control group. For example, in a manipulation study involving 25 lower back pain patients in each group, if pain was present in 5 of 25 patients in the treatment group and 10 of 25 in the control group, the relative risk would be $5 \div 25 = 0.2$, compared with $10 \div 25 = 0.4$. Thus, the relative risk would be $0.2 \div 0.4 = 0.5$, and one could say that there would be less risk of having pain after manipulation versus the control intervention.

Meta-analyses are generally considered most valid when the included studies are RCTs, although Egger and associates[25] reported that about half of the meta-analyses they looked at were derived from observational studies. These included mainly cohort and case-control studies that dealt with interventions or etiological associations. Because these studies frequently involve large numbers of subjects, it is not that difficult for the associated meta-analyses to produce results that seem plausible but are actually false. This misinterpretation of the findings of observational studies is because they are much more susceptible to the effects of biases and confounding factors than are RCTs. Thus, when observational studies are included in a meta-analysis, estimates of the true treatment effect reflect this unreliability and are not dependable. Accordingly, it is generally unsuitable to statistically combine the results of observational studies.[26] On the other hand, when RCTs are the focus of a meta-analysis, it is assumed that each study offers an unbiased estimate of the treatment effect and that any variability among the various studies is attributable to random variation. As a result, the calculated treatment effect provides an unbiased estimate of the true treatment effect. This whole matter is controversial, however, since Concato and associates[11] reported that well-designed observational studies, compared with RCTs, produce similar results in a review when dealing with the same topic.

It is unlikely that a given treatment effect from a meta-analysis would be the same across different patient subgroups that may be present in the included studies. Subgroups are based on various patient characteristics, such as disease severity, age, gender, patient history, and so on. For instance, young patients may have an entirely different response to a treatment than the elderly. Likewise, lower back pain patients with concomitant leg pain would be expected to respond to treatment differently than patients without complications. Because of the potential for practitioners to derive erroneous conclusions from meta-analyses that are composed of dissimilar patient strata, *subgroup analysis* is frequently carried out to determine whether certain outcomes or findings vary between patient groups. This procedure helps readers to distinguish the effects of a treatment specific to the strata involved, although the power of the results will decline as a result. An example of a subgroup analysis would be a comparison of studies in which blinding was adequate versus those with inadequate blinding. As one might expect, the results from the subgroups may be quite different. The main problem with subgroup analyses is that the original patient samples are split up; consequently, the results of the associated meta-analyses will be less likely to reach statistical significance.

Meta-regression is a statistical procedure that is sometimes used to adjust for differences between studies in meta-analyses. It is actually an extension of subgroup analyses in which diverse characteristics of the studies are investigated simultaneously. However, meta-regression is seldom possible because it requires that at least 10 trials be included in a meta-analysis. Meta-regression is very similar to simple regression, which was discussed in Chapter 4. The predictor variables are the characteristics of the studies that are being investigated, and the outcome variable is the overall estimate of treatment effect. Thus, the outcome variable (overall effect) is predicted based on the values of one or more of the predictor variables.

A s*ensitivity analysis* is similar to a subgroup analysis, but it considers nonpatient characteristics such as treatment variations, study methodology, the statistical analysis that was employed, and so forth. Sensitivity analyses are typically used to determine the extent that heterogeneity contributed to the results of a meta-analysis. If the results of a meta-analysis are weak, a sensitivity analysis could possibly demonstrate statistically significant treatment effects when different methods are used.[27]

Antman and colleagues[28,29] described an interesting technique called *cumulative meta-analysis*, which involves carrying out repeated meta-analyses as new RCTs are published and incorporating the latest data in the overall estimate of effect size. This method has the potential to reveal the ultimate effect of a therapy as soon as a new study sways the cumulative results toward statistical significance. By retrospectively analyzing RCTs, a cumulative meta-analysis can also identify the specific point in time when a given treatment effect first reached a level of statistical significance. Antman and associates were able to show that traditional reviews failed to mention important advances in treatment that were identified by a cumulative meta-analysis. The primary advantage of this procedure is that clinicians do not have to wait for a full-scale systematic review to be conducted in order to discover the ultimate results of a therapy. Furthermore, researchers can recognize whether more studies are needed to establish the effectiveness of a therapy or how likely additional studies would be to change the results of the cumulative evidence. When a significant treatment effect becomes obvious through cumulative meta-analysis, additional studies would probably be unnecessary.

Comparison of Literature Review Designs

At times it may be difficult to determine whether a given review is systematic or narrative because there are no strict rules that can be applied to the construction of either type. Moreover, some narrative reviews are carried out in a strict manner, looking much like systematic reviews. Likewise, some systematic reviews may be carried out carelessly and look like the narrative variety. McAlister and coworkers[30] examined the quality of review articles published in six popular general medical journals and found that only a minority of them indicated that their authors had employed rigorous methods to identify, evaluate, and synthesize articles. McAlister and associates thought these deficiencies probably weakened the validity of the conclusions that were presented in the reviews.

Narrative reviews, in particular, have several drawbacks, which are usually overcome by systematic reviews or meta-analyses. Narrative reviews are naturally prone to bias because they are largely subjective in relation to their unmethodical approach. Without the use of systematic methods, authors of reviews are often in conflict with regard to basic issues, such as what to do with quantitative evidence that is discovered or which types of studies to include. Narrative reviews typically cover a broader topic than systematic reviews, which are usually more focused. Consequently, narrative reviews tend to provide a general viewpoint on a topic that is more likely to be derived from a biased review of the evidence. Additionally, the process of deciding which studies to include in a narrative review may be discriminatory and inclined to support the beliefs of the authors. Studies that are in agreement with their beliefs may be more likely to be cited, while conflicting studies are ignored.

Another problem with narrative reviews concerns their approach to drawing conclusions from the studies that are integrated. It is usually unclear as to how the conclusions follow from the data that were examined. A common practice is to count the number of studies that support one side of a topic and then make a comparison with the number in support of the opposite side. The opinion with the highest number of supporting articles wins, which is reflected in the review's conclusion. What this practice does not take into consideration, however, are differences between the included studies concerning the magnitude of the treatment effect, the sample size, and the research design that was utilized. These variables are taken into consideration in systematic reviews and meta-analyses. Because of these limitations, it is not uncommon for a mixture of narrative reviews on a given topic to draw conflicting conclusions.

Systematic reviews and meta-analyses, on the other hand, are much more objective and can help resolve conflict when other sources of evidence are in disagreement. Nevertheless, the findings of any type of literature review can be contradictory as a result of disagreement between the findings of the reviews or because of divergent interpretations and inferences made by the authors.[31] Moreover, one review may conclude that a particular intervention is beneficial, whereas another may suggest that there is no benefit or that it is possibly even harmful. These differences become especially important when they are used to make decisions about health care. When disparity exists among reviews, it may be explained by examining the search criteria and methods that were utilized in the studies to see if they were actually carried out differently.

Treatment recommendations are frequently offered in the Discussion sections of review articles, as well as in original articles and practice guidelines. However, the validity of these recommendations is variable and depends, to a large extent, on the rigor of the studies from which they were derived.[32] As might be expected, comprehensive systematic reviews involve the highest rigor, making them the most valid and hierarchically higher than the other sources of treatment recommendations. The next step down in this hierarchy is high-quality evidence-based practice guidelines, followed by less rigorous systematic reviews. The lowest level of rigor and the weakest validity for treatment recommendations occurs when the evidence is derived from narrative reviews.

Systematic reviews and meta-analyses are not faultless, however, and when several are done on the same topic, they sometimes reach contradictory conclusions.[33] To address some of the problems inherent in these types of reviews, more and more biomedical journals are requiring authors to conform to the QUOROM

(Quality of Reporting of Meta-analyses) Statement.[34] This statement provides guidance to authors, directing them through each of the steps involved in the preparation of a review, which ensures uniformity and accurate reporting. The QUOROM Statement consists of a checklist and flow diagram that can be used by review authors to ensure the appropriateness of searches, article selection, validity assessment, data abstraction, study characteristics, data synthesis, and trial flow. The QUOROM Statement is rapidly being adopted by many journals, which is expected to improve the quality of and to bring uniformity to forthcoming reviews. Table 6.3 contrasts the relative potentials of well conducted versus poorly conducted meta-analyses. Table 6.4 contrasts the advantages and disadvantages of narrative versus systematic reviews.

Although systematic reviews and meta-analyses in general provide more reliable evidence that is hierarchically higher than narrative reviews, they appear to be read much less frequently. Loke and Derry[35] found that in the first week after publication of articles in the electronic version of the *British Medical Journal*, there was an average of 4,148 web hits per article for narrative reviews and only 1,168 hits per article for primary research papers or systematic reviews. The authors thought that the readability of articles was the problem and that steps should be taken by authors and journal editors to simplify articles and make them more attractive to readers. At the time of this writing, journals have not changed in response to this admonition.

TABLE 6.3 **Comparison of the potentials of well-conducted versus poorly conducted meta-analyses**

Well-Conducted	Poorly Conducted
• Provide a more objective appraisal of the evidence than narrative reviews	• May be biased due to exclusion of relevant studies
• Provide a more precise estimate of a treatment effect	• May be biased due to inclusion of poor-quality studies
• May explain heterogeneity between the results of individual studies	

Source: Adapted from Egger, M., G.D. Smith, and A.N. Phillips. Metanalysis: Principles and prodcures. *BMJ*, 1997. **315**(7121):1553–7.

TABLE 6.4 Advantages and disadvantages of narrative versus systematic reviews

	Advantages	Disadvantages
Narrative reviews	• Present a general overview covering a specific topic that provides primary information or an update, or both • Fairly easy for novice authors to prepare	• May not provide the best available answers to focused questions • Findings are less reliable
Systematic reviews	• Present a comprehensive review of the literature based on all available research with regard to a focused research question • Provide an estimate of the "true" answer to the research question	• Specialized expertise of reviewers is required • Involve a formal research protocol • Findings are only relevant to a single question

Structure of a Review Article

Review articles are written in a format that conforms to the typical anatomy of a scholarly article (introduced in Chapter 2): Abstract, Introduction, Methods, Results, Discussion, and References. This is because literature reviews are actually a category of research, which derive their conclusions from original sources of information. The general contents of the sections of a review article are presented here.

The *Introduction* section of a literature review should present the background and context of the problem that inspired the authors to carry out the study in the first place. The topic under investigation should be clearly defined, along with an explanation about how it applies to clinical practice. Additionally, novel terms should be defined in this section.

The importance and need for the review should be established early on by showing that there are gaps in the literature on the topic, as well as the extent of its negative impact on society. The significance of the problem should be explained in enough detail to justify the need for the review. This is typically accomplished by describing how prevalent the problem is and how much it costs society in terms of human suffering as well as monetarily. It is also helpful when a review conveys how likely it is that patients with the condition will present to chiropractic offices. A description of the course of the disease, existing outcomes and treatment options, and a synopsis of existing research are other factors that are commonly included in the introduction.

Systematic reviews should be founded on well-constructed questions[36] that not only provide direction to the review but also assist readers in determining its applicability to their individual clinical circumstances. Questions that lack focus may result in the authors making wrong decisions about which studies to include and how they should be summarized. Well-constructed questions should help to establish the review's inclusion criteria, which may involve such things as the characteristics of the population of interest, exposures, features of the control, outcomes that were utilized, and study design. Furthermore, review authors should specify which types of studies would be considered appropriate in answering the questions. As with any useful clinical question, the outcomes should be relevant to the patients under study.

The *Methods* section should describe the search process and all strategies that were involved, including a list of the databases and other sources of evidence that were used. The search terms that are used and limits on years or languages should be mentioned. Specific search criteria are required so as to limit the number of retrieved references to a manageable quantity, thus making the review doable. It is not feasible for review authors to include all articles that are even peripherally related to the topic under investigation. On the other hand, the boundaries of the search must not be so restrictive that relevant studies are overlooked.

Information should be provided that specifies how the studies were appraised for validity and what criteria were used to include or exclude them from the review. Reviews should utilize primary sources of information as the basis for establishing the level of evidence. Secondary information sources, such as unsystematic reviews or textbooks that simply cite an original source, must be avoided. In addition to information about how the validity of articles was determined, there should also be a description of the procedures used to ascertain the relevance of primary studies, how the data were extracted and synthesized, and how heterogeneity was handled. One of the primary reasons for including so much detail in this section is to enable others to replicate the study's results if the search were carried out again.

Rating instruments are typically used to measure the validity of included studies, although the reliability of these instruments varies dramatically. A study that used 25 different rating instruments to assess the quality of 17 trials found that some studies determined to be of high quality using one instrument were considered to be of low quality using another instrument.[37]

The *Results* section presents the outcome of the search process, including the number of articles that were retrieved from the search as well as how many of the articles were excluded from the review and which of the inclusion criteria they failed to meet. Readers should look for evidence of selective referencing, which is the tendency for authors to include only information that supports their point of view. The characteristics of the various studies should be described and contrasted in this section. Tables are often presented, which provide the reader with an overall perspective of the research that was assembled. A review article's Results section may sometimes be very short, with much of the detail about the articles that were retrieved being provided in the Discussion section.

The *Discussion* section should cover a number of subtopics that relate to the main focus of the review. Various aspects of the condition under consideration are typically included, such as details about its etiology and pathophysiology, and information concerning its diagnosis and treatment, as well as what kind of prognosis can be expected. The Discussion section is where the findings of all of the articles that were included in the review are synthesized to generate an integrated conclusion. This conclusion provides a new perspective on the topic that is typically more reliable than any of the individual articles making up the review. It is important that the study question be answered in this section in such a way that it accurately corresponds to what was asked in the introduction. At this point, review authors may have a tendency to unfairly emphasize research that agrees with their viewpoint and underrate that which does not.

The quality of the articles that were included in the review should be critically evaluated and the results presented in this section. Tables and figures (such as Figure 6.2) are typically used to illustrate the spectrum of studies and highlight key points. When the results of the review are controversial, an impartial review will call attention to the full range of the disparity and discuss discrepancies, as well as any unresolved questions. Limitations that might influence the validity of the review's conclusions, as well as conflicts of interest, should be acknowledged.

The structure of the Discussion section of review articles may acceptably vary from review to review, depending on the topic under study. For instance, the Discussion section of a literature review that focuses on therapy issues will be different from one that involves diagnostic tests. When available, reviews often provide information on cost-effectiveness analyses that is useful when comparing the costs and benefits to health of alternative interventions. This information is also valuable to those who make decisions about the implementation of health care services.

There may or may not be a separate section entitled *Conclusions*; often it is incorporated within the Discussion section. The conclusion is the bottom-line of a literature review and should be in agreement with the evidence that was included in the review. It should not merely repeat the contents of the entire article; instead, it should call attention to exactly what new information readers can gain from the review. Conclusions are generated in somewhat of a subjective manner, however, and authors have the leeway to defend articles that support their viewpoint or to challenge those that do not. Much of this subjectivity is controlled for by utilizing systematic methods, but it may still exist in the best of literature reviews.

The *References* section should be comprehensive, with all of the articles that were included in the review appropriately referenced. References should be derived almost entirely from peer-reviewed journals, although conference proceedings, textbooks, and government documents are sometimes included. Articles from evidence sources that are not peer-reviewed are generally not trustworthy and should rarely be referenced in a good review article. Sometimes unpublished information may be included in a review; nevertheless, because such material has not been subjected to peer review, its validity is undeterminable. Some journal articles include exhaustive reference lists, which may be appropriate in some instances. However, there should be no padding, and, other than the articles that specifically relate to the direct focus of the review, only enough articles to make a point should be cited. Depending on which style a journal subscribes to, the formatting used in References sections is variable. The Declaration of Vancouver "Uniform Requirements for Manuscripts Submitted to Biomedical Journals" is a style that is commonly encountered in the biomedical literature; it can be freely accessed on the Internet at http://www.icmje.org/.

Appraisal Tactics

Even though the process of conducting systematic reviews and meta-analyses follows an explicit set of criteria, the finished products still require critical appraisal to verify if they actually met the accepted standards for carrying out a review. Furthermore, after establishing their level of validity, one still needs to determine whether the information provided will be helpful in practice.[38] When looking for evidence, one should strive to locate reviews that are as up to date as possible. Recent reviews are typically more helpful than earlier works because the latter may not include recent advances in the field. When newer research findings are not included in a review, the article's information may no longer be valid.[39] Keep in mind, however, that the process involved in researching, writing, and publishing a review may take a year or more; thus, even the latest review may be behind the most current research.

Literature reviews should incorporate a comprehensive search that examines more than just MEDLINE, especially when exploring chiropractic-related topics.[40] Conversely, a search that only involves databases that are specific to chiropractic or manipulation and excludes MEDLINE is likely to miss important references.[41] Therefore, reviews that search multiple databases are preferred, and single-database searches would be considered methodologically flawed. The search strategy should be clearly described, and the criteria used for study inclusion should be mentioned. If the reasons for selecting and including studies in the review are missing or incomplete, the review may not be valid.

In addition to electronic database searches, hand-searching of individual journals and the Reference sections of the articles included in a review should be carried out.[42] Databases do not include all studies, or it may be difficult to locate studies due to vague or misleading search terms that the database used to index articles. Items such as conference abstracts and articles published in journal supplements are not typically included in databases, yet they may contain information pertinent to the review. Also, RCTs can be missed during an electronic search, even though a MEDLINE record actually exists, because the publication type terms "randomized controlled trial" or "controlled clinical trial" are missing.[42]

Checklists are invaluable aids in the appraisal of review articles;[43] therefore an appraised checklist for *literature review articles* is included in Appendix 4 of this book that is generic to all types of review articles. Specific checklists have been generated by other authors to address the different types of review articles (i.e., narrative, systematic, and meta-analysis).[44]

To assist with the appraisal of review articles in general, the following are some questions that one should ask when reading review articles:[30,45-47]

- *Was a clear study question asked?* It is particularly important for systematic reviews to have a definite purpose, but this question also applies to narrative reviews. When the article's purpose is clearly stated at the outset, it lets the reader know that the study was well planned. Without a clear study question, a review will lack direction and produce lackluster conclusions.

- *Was the study question focused on a specific clinical issue?* Not only must a review's study question be clear, but to help practitioners make clinical decisions, it also must be focused on a specific clinical issue that is relevant to patient care. Review articles that are too broad may incorporate information on the etiology, diagnosis, prognosis, treatment, and prevention of a given condition. This sort of information may be of interest to practitioners seeking background information on a topic. However, these types of reviews do not typically provide reliable information that can answer evidence-based clinical questions.

- *Were the inclusion/exclusion criteria that were used to select articles provided and were they appropriate?* It is important that authors list the criteria that were used to select articles for inclusion in the review. If they are listed, readers can be more confident that the authors did not unfairly cite studies that support their own position. Selection criteria may address the type of study, the methods employed, the population that was studied, the intervention used, or the outcomes. The more explicit the selection criteria are, the more focused the review will be. Clinicians should also make certain that the selection criteria match up with the clinical question that initially prompted the search for the review article.

- *Was an adequate literature search conducted?* The search terms employed should be capable of locating the full extent of available research relating to the study question. Appropriate databases should be selected that are likely to cover the review topic effectively. The time period that the search involved should also be clearly stated.

In assessing the adequacy of the literature search, one should judge whether an adequate attempt was made to obtain all relevant studies. Review authors should examine the References sections of the included articles to see if they can locate other articles that may have been missed during the search, and this process should be described in the Methods section. Some experts advocate personally contacting researchers who are actively investigating the topic for supplementary information.[45] Essentially, the methods of the literature search should be described in enough detail so that another person could duplicate the results. After evaluating the search methods, one should consider what the likelihood was that relevant studies were missed during the search.

- *Was the validity of the studies included in the review assessed?* Poorer-quality reviews may incorporate articles without subjecting them to systematic appraisal, even though it is quite common for flawed studies to appear in the literature. Therefore, to generate a high-quality review, the methodology of articles included in a review must be carefully assessed in a systematic way and the authors should clearly describe the appraisal criteria that were used. Narrative reviews do not typically utilize these kinds of strict appraisal methods, which weakens not only their validity but also their usefulness in solving clinical problems. Some of the attributes of studies that should be assessed by reviewers are the methods of randomization, the extent that blinding was utilized, and whether the allocation to groups was concealed.

- *Were the studies appraised in a dependable manner?* Ideally, the articles will be reviewed by more than one reviewer, using a reliable appraisal instrument that is likely to produce consistent results. The likelihood that the assessment findings of a given study are correct is strengthened when several reviewers agree regarding its validity. Sometimes the actual appraisal instrument that was used by the reviewers is included in an appendix, which allows readers to evaluate the study's methodology more closely.

- *Were the included studies randomized trials?* The strength of a literature review is considerably enhanced when it deals with randomized controlled trials. Reviews that include observational studies are useful to understand the current status of a given topic, but provide little evidence to support treatment. However, when observational research is all that is

available, it qualifies as being the best evidence and would be valuable to assist with patient care.
- *Were the results of the included studies similar?* Frequently, some of the studies in a review show a significant beneficial effect while others show little positive effect, or possibly even a negative effect. One would not expect the treatment effects to be identical for all of the included studies, although one should be concerned when these discrepancies are large. The authors should discuss this lack of consistency between studies and suggest possible reasons why it occurred. Sources of heterogeneity of studies may include clinical factors (e.g., dissimilar participants, interventions, or outcomes), methodological factors (e.g., sample size or method of randomization), or simply results that are contradictory by chance. Subgroup analysis or meta-regression may be used to determine the degree to which the characteristics of the studies affected the treatment effect sizes. However, make sure that sufficient numbers of studies are involved in the review to allow the use of these techniques.
- *Do the results of the synthesis logically flow from the studies that were included?* The synthesis and resulting conclusions should accurately represent the collective information contained in the articles that were obtained in the literature search. The potential for bias in this part of the review is noteworthy, since authors have a certain amount of latitude in the way they interpret and judge the articles. If the conclusions are not supported by the literature that was reviewed, then the validity of the entire article is in doubt.

    Some reviews merely summarize the results of the incorporated studies by comparing the number with positive findings to the number with negative findings. The main problem with this method is that large studies are weighted equally with small studies, even though the larger studies should have proportionally more influence on the review's overall results. Also, when the total numbers of positive and negative studies are simply added and compared, the relative validity of the studies may not be taken into consideration.
- *If the review dealt with therapy, was an estimate of treatment effect provided?* In meta-analyses, the results of each study are generally summarized in a figure that presents the effect size of each study. Often, a meta-analysis provides an overall (pooled) estimate of effect size. The

precision of the treatment effects reported in the studies included in a review can be evaluated by observing the size of the associated confidence intervals. Wide confidence intervals degrade the precision of the treatment effect estimates. Heterogeneity of the studies may prohibit the use of quantitative summaries. However, in these cases, weighting of studies by validity or sample size or both may still be possible.

- *Do the results of the review help with the care of patients?* A useful review should provide information that permits readers to determine the applicability of its findings to clinical practice. Ideally, the populations included in the review should be representative of the specific patient under care in order to successfully make use of the results. Among the benefits of a literature review is the fact that a wide range of patients is typically included by combining the results from diverse populations involved in the individual studies. One must still be careful in this area, especially if the patient is very young, very old, very ill, and so on. Additionally, the outcomes that are covered in a review should be clinically important in order to be of assistance with the care of patients.

    Problems may arise when attempting to apply the results of a review to patient care if the intervention involved in the review differs somewhat from the intervention that is intended for the patient. For instance, there may be a problem if a literature review shows that mobilization is effective in the treatment of low back pain, yet a practitioner applies the results of that review to support the use of manipulation.

- *Were directions for future research offered?* After assessing the sum of all research on a topic, review authors are in an especially good position to determine what specific types of studies should be carried out in the future. The inclusion of suggestions for future research is a sign of a high-quality review. When they are missing, the review's quality is undermined.

References

1. Fink, A. *Conducting Research Literature Reviews: From Paper to the Internet.* 1998. Thousand Oaks: Sage Publications.
2. Mulrow, C.D. *Rationale for systematic reviews. BMJ*, 1994. **309**(6954):597–9.
3. Cook, D.J., D.L. Sackett, and W.O. Spitzer. *Methodologic guidelines for systematic reviews of randomized control trials in health care from the Potsdam Consultation on Meta-Analysis. J Clin Epidemiol*, 1995. **48**(1):167–71.

References

4. Egger, M., and G.D. Smith. *Meta-analysis: Potentials and promise.* BMJ, 1997. **315**(7119):1371–4.
5. Siwek, J., et al. *How to write an evidence-based clinical review article.* Am Fam Physician, 2002. **65**(2):251–8.
6. Montori, V.M., et al. *Systematic reviews: A cross-sectional study of location and citation counts.* BMC Med, 2003. **1**(1):2.
7. Schmidt, L.M., and P.C. Gotzsche. *Of mites and men: Reference bias in narrative review articles: a systematic review.* J Fam Pract, 2005. **54**(4):334–8.
8. Montori, V.M., M.F. Swiontkowski, and D.J. Cook. *Methodologic issues in systematic reviews and meta-analyses.* Clin Orthop Relat Res, 2003. Aug. (413):43–54.
9. Cook, D.J., C.D. Mulrow, and R.B. Haynes. *Systematic reviews: Synthesis of best evidence for clinical decisions.* Ann Intern Med, 1997. **126**(5):376–80.
10. Kunz, R., G. Vist, and A.D. Oxman. *Randomisation to protect against selection bias in healthcare trials.* The Cochrane Database of Methodology Reviews, 2002. Issue 4. Article No. MR000012. DOI: 10.1002/14651858.MR000012.
11. Concato, J., N. Shah, and R.I. Horwitz. *Randomized, controlled trials, observational studies, and the hierarchy of research designs.* N Engl J Med, 2000. **342**(25):1887–92.
12. Cook, D.J., et al. *Should unpublished data be included in meta-analyses? Current convictions and controversies.* JAMA, 1993. **269**(21):2749–53.
13. Centre for Reviews and Dissemination. *CRD Report 4. Undertaking Systematic Reviews of Research on Effectiveness: CRD's Guidance for Carrying Out or Commissioning Reviews.* 2nd ed. 2001. York, England: NHS Centre for Reviews and Dissemination, University of York.
14. Greenhalgh, T. *How to read a paper: Papers that summarise other papers (systematic reviews and meta-analyses).* BMJ, 1997. **315**(7109):672–5.
15. Phillips, C.V., *Publication bias in situ.* BMC Med Res Methodol, 2004. **4**(1):20.
16. Terrin, N., et al. *Adjusting for publication bias in the presence of heterogeneity.* Stat Med, 2003. **22**(13):2113–26.
17. Davey Smith, G., M. Egger, and A.N. Phillips. *Meta-analysis. Beyond the grand mean?* BMJ, 1997. **315**(7122):1610–4.
18. Dinnes, J., et al. *A methodological review of how heterogeneity has been examined in systematic reviews of diagnostic test accuracy.* Health Technol Assess, 2005. **9**(12):1–113.
19. Deeks, J., J. Higgins, and D.G. Altman. *Analysing and presenting results.* In *Cochrane Handbook for Systematic Reviews of Interventions 4.2.4*, J.P.T. Higgins and S. Green, eds. 2005. Chichester, UK: John Wiley & Sons, 246.
20. Higgins, J.P.T., et al. *Measuring inconsistency in meta-analyses.* BMJ, 2003. **327**(7414):557–60.
21. Mulrow, C.D. *Systematic reviews: Rationale for systematic reviews.* BMJ, 1994. **309**(6954):597–99.
22. Assendelft, W.J.J., et al. *Spinal manipulative therapy for low back pain: A meta-analysis of effectiveness relative to other therapies.* Ann Intern Med, 2003. **138**(11):871–81.
23. Lewis, S., and M. Clarke. *Forest plots: Trying to see the wood and the trees.* BMJ, 2001. **322**(7300):1479–80.
24. Thalheimer, W., and S. Cook. *How to calculate effect sizes from published research articles: A simplified methodology.* 2002. http://work-learning.com/effect_sizes.htm.

Chapter 6 Literature Review Designs

25. Egger, M., M. Schneider, and G. Davey Smith. *Spurious precision? Meta-analysis of observational studies. BMJ*, 1998. **316**(7125):140–4.
26. Smith, G.D., and M. Egger. *Meta-analyses of observational data should be done with due care. BMJ*, 1999. **318**(7175):56.
27. Zed, P., et al. *Systematic reviews in emergency medicine: Part II. Critical appraisal of review quality, data synthesis and result interpretation. Can J Emerg Med*, 2003. **5**(6):406–11.
28. Antman, E.M., et al. *A comparison of results of meta-analyses of randomized control trials and recommendations of clinical experts. Treatments for myocardial infarction. JAMA*, 1992. **268**(2):240–8.
29. Lau, J., et al. *Cumulative meta-analysis of therapeutic trials for myocardial infarction. N Engl J Med*, 1992. **327**(4):248–54.
30. McAlister, F.A., et al. *The medical review article revisited: Has the science improved? Ann Intern Med*, 1999. **131**(12):947–51.
31. Jadad, A.R., D.J. Cook, and G.P. Browman. *A guide to interpreting discordant systematic reviews. CMAJ*, 1997. **156**(10):1411–16.
32. Guyatt, G.H., et al. *Users' guides to the medical literature: XVI. How to use a treatment recommendation. Evidence-Based Medicine Working Group and the Cochrane Applicability Methods Working Group. JAMA*, 1999. **281**(19):1836–43.
33. Egger, M., G.D. Smith, and A.N. Phillips. *Meta-analysis: Principles and procedures. BMJ*, 1997. **315**(7121):1533–7.
34. Moher, D., et al. *Improving the quality of reports of meta-analyses of randomised controlled trials: The QUOROM statement. Quality of Reporting of Meta-analyses. Lancet*, 1999. **354**(9193):1896–900.
35. Loke, Y.K., and S. Derry. *Does anybody read "evidence-based" articles? BMC Med* Res *Methodol*, 2003. **31**(3):14.
36. Counsell, C. *Formulating questions and locating primary studies for inclusion in systematic reviews. Ann Intern Med*, 1997. **127**(5):380–7.
37. Juni, P., et al. *The hazards of scoring the quality of clinical trials for meta-analysis. JAMA*, 1999. **282**(11):1054–60.
38. Hunt, D.L., and K.A. McKibbon. *Locating and appraising systematic reviews. Ann Intern Med*, 1997. **126**(7):532–8.
39. Shaughnessy, A.F., and D.C. Slawson. *Getting the most from review articles: A guide for readers and writers. Am Fam Physician*, 1997. **55**(6):2155–60.
40. Aker, P.D., et al. *Searching chiropractic literature: A comparison of three computerized databases. J Manipulative Physiol Ther*, 1996. **19**(8):518–24.
41. Murphy, L.S., et al. *Spinal palpation: The challenges of information retrieval using available databases. J Manipulative Physiol Ther*, 2003. **26**(6):374–82.
42. Hopewell, S., et al. *A comparison of handsearching versus MEDLINE searching to identify reports of randomized controlled trials. Stat Med*, 2002. **21**(11):1625–34.
43. Oxman, A.D. *Checklists for review articles. BMJ*, 1994. **309**(6955):648–51.
44. Scottish Intercollegiate Guidelines Network. *Methodology checklist 1: Systematic reviews and meta-analyses*. In *SIGN 50: A Guideline Developers' Handbook*. 2004. Edinburgh, UK: Scottish Intercollegiate Guidelines Network.

45. Oxman, A.D., D.J. Cook, and G.H. Guyatt. *Users' guides to the medical literature. VI. How to use an overview. Evidence-Based Medicine Working Group. JAMA*, 1994. **272**(17):1367–71.
46. Zed, P., et al. *Systematic reviews in emergency medicine: Part I. Background and general principles for locating and critically appraising reviews. Can J Emerg Med*, 2003. **5**(6):331–5.
47. Hunt, D.L., and R.B. Haynes. *How to read a systematic review. Indian J Pediatr*, 2000. **67**(1):63–6.

CHAPTER

SEVEN

Case Designs

Reports that cover the management of a single patient or a series of patients who have a similar condition, exposure, or outcome are considered case designs. There are three different varieties of case designs: case reports, case series, and single-subject time series. A *case report* is simply an article that describes and discusses the clinical management of one or a few patients, which may include components such as complaints, examination findings, diagnosis, treatment, and outcome. *Case series* incorporate some of the same elements as case reports, but they involve more than just a few patients. The *single-subject time series* is a variation of the case report that tracks a patient's condition using multiple sequential assessments while a treatment is applied and withdrawn.

Case Reports

The "Instructions for Authors" of the *Journal of Manipulative and Physiological Therapeutics*[1] describes case reports as "accounts of the diagnosis and treatment of unusual, difficult, or otherwise interesting cases that may have independent educational value or may contribute to better standardization of care for a particular health problem when correlated with similar reports of others." Case reports are vital to the advancement of knowledge about patient care because they report new or unusual aspects of chiropractic practice that are of interest to and highly relevant to practitioners. Almost any type of patient or method of patient management that has not yet been presented in the literature would be worth reporting in a case report.[2] They are considered to be descriptive studies because they do not report on any experimental data (i.e., they are not controlled, there is no random assignment to groups, and they are usually retrospective). Because of this, case reports cannot be used to establish cause-and-effect relationships. On the other hand, they are educational to practitioners and often inspire important questions that may lead to future research.

Case reports can be an excellent vehicle for practitioners to learn how to recognize new or rare conditions, as well as unusual clinical presentations of known conditions.[3] The reporting of such cases may alert the chiropractic community to new problems, leading to the development of hypotheses and subsequent broader-based studies. Case reports should not be considered primarily as clinician-to-clinician communications. Actually, they may be better thought of as clinician-to-scientist communications because they provide ideas for future research.[4] There are many instances in the literature where valuable knowledge has resulted from the unusual cases that are the building blocks of case reports.[5] The information they provide should not be considered as merely anecdotal, since they present important data to other practitioners relating to patient management, as well as regarding what actually happens in clinical practice.[6]

There are basically two categories of case reports: retrospective and prospective. *Retrospective case reports* are typically the result of a practitioner who notices something unusual during the management of a patient that he or she thinks would make the case interesting to other practitioners. After beginning care or at the completion of care, the practitioner decides to write a report on the case and submit it for publication. For example, in the course of treating a patient's cervical spine injury, there may appear to be significant improvement in a coexisting visual problem, which may be a new or unusual relationship. This type of case would be a prime candidate for a case study. *Prospective case reports* are planned ahead of time by a practitioner who has an interest in a particular condition and has already researched the topic and planned the management of a related case. The next patient who presents with the condition will be a candidate for inclusion in a prospective case study. It does not necessarily have to be a previously unreported condition; rather, the case could be reported because it involves a unique treatment strategy or diagnostic procedure.

Case reports are typically brief in comparison with other types of journal articles; also, they require relatively little time to prepare. Thus, they are capable of communicating clinical observations that are newsworthy in a timely manner, which allows other practitioners to become acquainted with this new information quickly. Even though case reports contain less information and provide less evidence than other types of research,[7] they are widely read by practitioners because of their high relevance to clinical practice. Furthermore, they describe the entire decision-making process involved in the management of an individual patient, whereas reports of experimental research only describe the intervention or measurement that was involved.[8]

Huth[9] described four types of case reports:

1. The unique case, which has never before (or very rarely) been described in the literature.
2. The case with an unexpected association between two or more conditions, which may represent a newly described causal relationship.
3. The case of an unusual presentation or pattern for a previously recognized condition.
4. The case that develops unexpectedly and implies either a therapeutic or an adverse effect to an intervention.

The *unique case* variety of case report represents a distinctively different or new condition that a practitioner thinks will be of enough interest to his or her colleagues to warrant reporting in a scientific journal. An important first step for a potential author in this situation is a thorough search of the pertinent databases to find out if the condition has been previously described in the literature. If the literature search does not generate comparable cases, then the condition may indeed be new or unique. However, one must always consider that the search might have been incomplete or that the condition was previously labeled differently, which would generate an unproductive search.

Case reports that involve an *unexpected association* typically result from a patient presenting to a practitioner with two rare conditions. The association of these conditions may point to a causal relationship. An example might be a patient who presents with vertebrobasilar insufficiency and concomitant cauda equina syndrome. These are both uncommon conditions that affect the nervous system, and their presence in one patient may imply that the underlying etiological mechanisms are the same. However, one must keep in mind that the coexisting occurrence of two conditions may be merely coincidental and that the case study has no way of ruling out this possibility.

The *unusual presentation* form of case report involves a patient who presents with a condition that is not typical in some way. For instance, abdominal aortic aneurysms are not that unusual to find in adult chiropractic patients, especially in the elderly, but if the patient was 10 years old, it would be unusual and thus worthy of publication as a case report. The patient may have had an underlying disorder that led to the aneurysm, which would also be described in the report.

Cases involving an *unexpected development* in a condition can be related to either a positive or negative response to a given intervention, as long as it is atypical. An example of this type of case report, which is commonly seen in the medical literature, is cervical artery dissection and resulting stroke following cervical manipulation. Some authors have suggested that a causal relationship exists because of the regularity of this occurrence, but there are too many confounding variables in effect to make such a claim.[10] There are, however, quite a few cases of stroke that have occurred in close temporal proximity to cervical manipulation; consequently, there is high suspicion that at least a contributing relationship exists, especially when it occurs in otherwise healthy individuals very soon after the manipulation. Nonetheless, since so many cervical manipulations are provided without incident and since more than 90% of cervical arterial dissections do not appear to be related to cervical manipulation,[11] there is still uncertainty.

Case reports have many limitations, which has resulted in their being placed in a low position in the hierarchy of evidence. As a result of these limitations, they cannot be used to establish causal relationships, although they can point to future research that might be suitable to address the issue being presented. In particular, the possibility that natural progression of the condition is what actually resulted in a patient's improvement can never be fully addressed without at least the inclusion of a control group. When natural progression affects a case study, patients may indeed improve with treatment, but the outcomes might have been the same whether treatment was provided or not. In addition, it is impossible to distinguish the amount of improvement that is related to placebo effects from the treatment effects without a control group.

Another limitation is related to the fact that the case being presented may not reflect what the condition's typical response would be to a given treatment. Consider a hypothetical situation in which a condition was treated by hundreds of chiropractors across the country using manipulation, and nearly all of the involved patients failed to improve. One of these chiropractors, however, observed a near miraculous response to treatment and consequently submitted a case report for publication. That one successful case was actually atypical and does not represent the true effect of manipulative treatment for that condition. Accordingly, it is not possible to determine whether an intervention is effective based on a case report.

Another major limitation of case reports is that patient care is delivered in an environment that is not controlled, as it is in an experiment. As a result, patient care may be influenced by a number of extraneous factors, which further degrades the likelihood of determining a cause-and-effect relationship and limits the generalizability of the case to other patients. Limited generalizability not only applies to other practitioners and their patients but also to other patients of the case report's author. Indeed, even if the author of the case report applied the same case management strategies to another patient with the same condition under similar circumstances, the results might be entirely different. In spite of all these limitations, case reports still have a legitimate and important purpose in the overall scheme of research (Table 7.1).[12]

Because of their brevity as well as their subject matter, the structure of a case report deviates to some extent from that of a full research paper. When presented in journals, they typically incorporate the following sections: Abstract, Introduction, Case Description, Discussion, and References. The main difference in this format from other types of journal articles is the inclusion of a Case Description section instead of Methods and Results sections. The Case Description section is

TABLE 7.1 **The purposes and limitations of case reports**

Purposes	• Detect rare conditions
	• Educational value
	• Learn how other doctors manage certain cases
	• Generate hypotheses
Limitations	• Susceptible to many biases
	• Unable to test hypotheses
	• Does not determine the effectiveness of an intervention
	• Unable to generalize results to other patients or practices

the heart of and the longest section of a case report and is primarily what distinguishes it from the other types of articles.

The *abstract* of a case report may be either in a narrative or a structured format, depending on the journal, but the majority now require the structured variety. A case report is typically quite short (e.g., the text word limit for case reports submitted to the *Journal of Manipulative and Physiological Therapeutics* is approximately 1,500 words), but an abstract that provides a brief summary of the report is still required. The content of the abstract should acquaint the reader with the most important features of the case and why it is worth reporting.

The *Introduction* section is usually rather brief, providing background information about the condition at issue and its underlying pathology. It should clearly explain what motivated the case report (i.e., what is unique, unexpected, or unusual) and why it represents something that is worth reporting. The introduction provides a short review of the literature in enough detail so that readers will be able to recognize that the case has merit. This section should not reference every possible commentary on the subject—only that which is current and important in order to lay a foundation for the case report.

This short literature review should be expanded in the Discussion section and its information contrasted with what was presented in the rest of the case report. The introduction usually has some educational value given that the literature review presents information about the condition under investigation, such as etiology, typical patient presentation, and the value of standard treatments. If the literature review reveals an abundance of previous publications in the topic area, the case report may be superfluous and one must wonder whether another one will add any new knowledge.

The *Case Description* section, as its name implies, presents features of the case that have to do with the diagnosis, intervention, and outcome. It is equivalent to the combined Methods and Results sections found in other types of journal articles. Thus, it should describe everything that is relevant to the case in chronological order, while omitting unrelated features such as negative tests that do not directly deal with the problem. There should be enough thoroughness in the description of patient management so that, if desired, interested readers would be able to duplicate the procedures that were presented.

The features of case management that are typically included in the Case Description section include the chief complaint, medical history (including pertinent family history), diagnostic workup, diagnosis, treatment (if provided), outcome, and any follow-up actions that may have been carried out. Normal values should be provided when uncommon laboratory tests are utilized. Differential diagnoses should be discussed, along with a presentation of the rationale for ruling out other possibilities.

Case management may not involve treatment if, for instance, the patient was referred to another provider because the condition was outside the scope of chiropractic practice. However, the patient's final outcome following application of the referral intervention will often be presented. Case management should be derived from evidence-based material when possible, but because evidence is frequently lacking, case reports are often published without adequate support from research. This may be appropriate as long as the authors provide adequate information about what was done and justify why it was done.

The *Discussion* section (also known as the Comments section) should provide a rational basis for why the case is considered important and educational, as well as what makes it unique, unexpected, or unusual. Essentially, the purpose of the Discussion section is to clarify unanswered questions that remain from the Case Description section. An interpretation of the study's findings should be offered, although the authors must provide evidence supporting any statements that are made. Alternative explanations should be addressed, along with an explanation of why they were not accepted in this particular case. Limitations of either the methods that were employed or the evidence that was presented should be mentioned. Conclusions should also be substantiated by the existing evidence. The authors should identify what questions warrant further research and offer suggestions as to the appropriate types of studies that should be conducted.

This section should also discuss how this case either confirms or refutes the literature presented in the Introduction section. For example, if a case is conveying new information, one could say, "While previous studies on the topic of chiropractic and asthma did not demonstrate the effectiveness of chiropractic care, this report describes a case wherein the patient's asthma completely resolved subsequent to a brief treatment period under chiropractic care."

The format of traditional case reports has been criticized because they frequently do not produce a logical flow of information. In an attempt to remedy this shortcoming, Bayoumi and Kopplin[13] have promoted the concept of the *storied case report*, which is essentially a case report that reports on two interconnected stories: that of the patient's illness and that of the doctor's diagnosis and treatment. For the most part, this approach attempts to arrange the order in which data is presented so that it communicates these stories. They point out that the language of the storied case report should be targeted toward telling a story and should be sensitive to the patient's experiences.

The preparation of case reports, which merely involves the review of the clinical records of three or fewer patients, is not typically considered to be human-subject research and therefore does not require approval from an institutional review board (also known as human subjects review boards, ethics review boards, etc.). As discussed in Chapter 5, institutional review boards are committees that oversee research involving human subjects in a given institution. Even if their approval is not required, patient confidentiality should always be respected, and any personal information that might allow someone to identify a patient (e.g., name, social security number, date of birth, or any other identifiers) should not be used in publications or scientific presentations. Occasionally photographs or other information that potentially might identify patients are utilized in case reports. In these situations, the patients must give written consent prior to the submission of the report for publication. If you are thinking about doing a case report, and I encourage all practitioners to do just that, a cautious approach should be taken and consent should be obtained in any case where it might be possible for the patient's identity to be surmised—for instance, in a case where the patient has a rare condition and becomes identifiable because demographic information is included about the patient's city of residence, age, gender, and so forth. In light of recent HIPAA regulations, many journals are moving toward more strict consent requirements. Consequently, all subjects of case reports should consent and sign an Informed Consent form. The fact that the patient consented should be mentioned in the published article.

The case reports editor for the journal *Physical Therapy* pointed out four reasons that 90% of the case reports that were submitted to that journal were returned to the authors for revision:[8]

1. *Claims of cause-and-effect relationships between interventions and outcomes*. As mentioned previously, case reports are descriptive and do not generate experimental data; therefore, no cause-and-effect claims can be made.

2. *Lack of information about the reliability and validity of measurements.* The article should provide references to published research that shows that the outcome measurements that were used are reliable and valid so that readers can have confidence in the study's findings.
3. *Lack of detail about the examination and the intervention.* Procedures should be described in enough detail that another practitioner could reproduce them with one of his or her own patients if desired.
4. *Lack of detail about decision making.* Based on the examination findings, diagnosis, and prognosis, information should be presented about why the authors chose to use the intervention that was employed, why certain tests were carried out, and so on.

Case reports have become less and less acceptable for publication in some of the major journals.[9] In fact, a few medical journals have stopped publishing them altogether because they provide little or no reliable information on the cause or prognosis of a condition, the usefulness of diagnostic tests, or the effectiveness of interventions. As a result of these limitations, they have been portrayed as the "least publishable unit in the medical literature."[14] However, case reports that describe adverse events that are somehow related to an intervention are still likely to be reported even in these journals.[15] Case reports of adverse events are often confirmed by more rigorous research methods, although sometimes their conclusions are found to be erroneous. The true frequency of these mistakes is unknown because it has rarely been investigated,[12] but a review that looked at case reports dealing with drug side effects that were eventually confirmed determined that 35 of 47 were in fact correct.[16]

The *British Medical Journal* initiated a new type of article in 1998, dubbed the *evidence-based case report*, which was designed to demonstrate how evidence can be applied during the various phases of patient care.[15] Evidence-based case reports do not report new findings; instead, they illustrate the process involved in locating and applying evidence to a given clinical circumstance. These types of case reports are still considered useful and are likely to be published even when little or no high-quality evidence is available. This is because the information is important to readers who should be aware of gaps in the evidence. One instance of an evidence-based case report in the chiropractic literature was written by Lisi and Bhardwaj,[17] who reported on the management of a patient with postsurgical chronic cauda equina syndrome and commented on the evidence base that was available to support treating the condition using chiropractic adjustments. Evidence-based case reports are an excellent addition to the chiropractic literature, and it is hoped that more will be forthcoming.

The terms *case study* and *case report* are normally used interchangeably; however, some consider case studies to represent a specific type of nonexperimental research design, while case reports merely depict certain aspects of clinical practice.[18] Moreover, case studies describe the management of a patient or two more comprehensively than case reports. Case studies utilize various methods of observation to generate qualitative or quantitative data or both to examine and predict treatment response or the natural history of a condition.

Case Series

A *case series* report is a presentation of the management of more than a few patients who have something in common (e.g., the same diagnosis, history, or treatment). Essentially, the patients involved in a case series are provided an intervention, and then their outcomes are assessed. Sometimes case series report on adverse events that occur to individual patients, which are aggregated to find out if there are any common etiological factors. Case series have been described as "a group of patients with similar diagnoses or undergoing the same procedure that are followed over time."[19] The *Journal of Manipulative and Physiological Therapeutics* defines a case series in its "Instructions for Authors" as "a retrospective comparative assessment of the diagnosis and treatment of several cases of a similar condition, i.e., the comparative evaluation of two or more (perhaps hundreds) of case reports."[1] Case series are based on the retrospective study of patient records, typically from a single practice or institution. They can provide valuable information about case management and trends that are apparent in outcomes, and provide clues about causation.

Patients in a case series make up a group in which all have a similar diagnosis or experience the same intervention, such as a particular adjustive procedure. No comparison group is included in this type of study design, which severely limits its usefulness as a form of evidence. When there is no comparison group, it can look as if there is a relationship between an intervention and an outcome when there actually is not. Occasionally the results of case series are compared to values derived from historical controls, although this does not represent a legitimate comparison. Like case reports, case series are useful for generating hypotheses and are frequently the first studies to be carried out in the course of researching a topic. Carey and Boden[19] identified a number of characteristics that they thought case series should possess, which are as follows: a clearly defined study question, a well-described study population, a well-described intervention, the use of valid outcome measures, appropriate statistical analyses, well-described results, conclusions that are supported by the data presented, and an acknowledgment of funding sources.

All research designs can be influenced by bias, but case series are particularly susceptible. Consequently, they are more likely than other designs to have their results swayed, making them a less trustworthy form of evidence. The first bias to consider is *selection bias*, which involves the author choosing patients preferentially. As a rule, there are no criteria for patient selection in case series; accordingly, this bias will almost always be present. In the worst cases, authors may include only those patients having the best outcomes. To reduce the influence of this bias, authors commonly select consecutively presenting cases, which helps, but does not eliminate the problem. Another bias that is common in case series is *observation bias*, where the doctor's beliefs or expectations about treatment have an effect on outcomes. Because there is no blinding in case series, there is no way to control for this bias.

Like case reports, natural progression of the condition can make the results of an intervention look much better than what they really are, although this effect is somewhat lessened when a group of cases is presented. Heterogeneity of disease stages occurs when patients do not have to meet suitable inclusion/exclusion criteria, as is required in clinical trials; this also can misrepresent the findings in case series. When patients initially have extreme values and then seem to improve, it may actually be due to the phenomenon of *regression to the mean*, yet may falsely be attributed to the intervention. Regression to the mean occurs because extreme test values have a tendency to move toward the group's mean over time. Although not part of a case series study, a comparison group that does not receive the intervention can be helpful in identifying this effect. There is also the possibility that the author of a case series was just lucky and by chance had good results using a particular intervention (or observing adverse events) on a given series of patients.

Case series often compare their results with those of other case series in the Discussion section. This practice is also potentially biased since authors may select comparisons that make their results look good. Furthermore, authors may submit only those series of cases that have the best outcomes for publication. This is unfortunate because, ideally, clinicians should not only have the opportunity to read about what works in practice, but also what does not work.

Case series are sometimes very useful in highlighting a clinical condition and thus have educational value. They can also stimulate interest in further research on a given topic. Nonetheless, especially in the types of conditions managed by chiropractors, very rarely can they be used to draw conclusions about the relationships between interventions and outcomes. Only in conditions where morbidity or mortality is almost 100% and the condition is radically decreased by the intervention are case series sometimes able to support such conclusions.

Case series are similar to, but distinct from, cohort studies, which are covered in Chapter 8. Briefly, however, a cohort study identifies a group of patients with something in common and then follows them forward in time to observe any changes that may occur, whereas case series merely describe a group of patients retrospectively.

Occasionally a meta-analysis of case reports or case series or both on a given topic is generated from the literature, which can sometimes draw important new conclusions.[12] Limited statistical analyses can then be performed on the data derived from the reports. However, these conclusions sometimes turn out to be wrong after more definitive research has been carried out because of the inherent limitations of case designs. Thus, meta-analyses of case studies are best used to point out trends and patterns that may be apparent in patient care, followed by more sophisticated research that is capable of examining cause-and-effect relationships. As an example, I was involved in a literature review that looked at the relationship between chiropractic manipulation of the neck and developing internal carotid artery dissection.[20] We reviewed all studies that had reported on this relationship, but only found case reports and case series. The only form of "meta-analysis" that could be done was to add the total number of reports that were found in the articles (13 reported cases). After considering that a temporal relationship was the only implicating factor in these cases, that there was a high potential for confounding, and that no studies suitable for establishing cause-and-effect relationships had been carried out, we concluded that there was no evidence that could support a causal relationship.

Single-Subject Time Series Designs

Single-subject time series designs (SSTSDs) involve the study of a single patient in which repeated measurements are taken while an intervention is systematically applied and withdrawn. The objective of implementing a treatment-on/treatment-off regimen such as this is to observe differences in the measurements of outcomes that might occur during each phase. If there is a noticeable improvement during the time that the treatment is being applied, it may help to establish that the treatment is effective for that patient. The patient essentially acts as his or her own control as measurements are taken during the phase when no treatment is provided. There are several different types of SSTSDs, but they all essentially comprise various arrangements of observation and treatment phases. A number of different synonyms are commonly used to represent SSTSDs, including the following: single-case experimental design, time series design, small-n design, n-of-1 trial, and within-subject comparison.

Ordinarily, the initial phase of an SSTSD is the *baseline phase*, where at least three repeated measures of the outcomes of interest (dependent variables) are taken prior to beginning any treatment. The purpose of taking repeated measures is to demonstrate stability of the condition, although this may take more than three repetitions in some cases. Being a period where no treatment is administered, the baseline phase reveals the natural state of the patient's condition and becomes the standard for evaluating the effect of treatment. This phase is analogous to a control group in clinical trials, since both provide a standard with which to compare the treatment. After the baseline phase has been completed, the treatment (independent variable) is started, which begins the *intervention phase*. Outcomes are also measured at least three times during this phase, and the length of time involved should be about the same as the baseline phase. Any changes in the dependent variables that occur during this phase can be attributed to the intervention.

The use of repeated measures during treatment and nontreatment phases in SSTSDs enhances their validity and reduces the probability that the results are due to chance. To further boost validity, all measures of outcome that are used should be objective and measurable. They should be clinically relevant as well. Examples of some suitable outcome measures include range of motion examination; pain and disability questionnaires; and patient diaries that catalog such things as distance able to walk, amount of pain medication needed, frequency of pain, and so on.

SSTSDs cannot be considered merely qualitative case studies, since they purposely investigate the effect of a treatment in a quasi-experimental manner. Indeed, the independent variable or variables are manipulated (applied and then withdrawn) in SSTSDs as they are in experimental research.[21] Case studies may include some manipulation of the independent variable, but it is not done with the intention of observing changes of the dependent variable over repeated observations. Another distinction between case studies and SSTSDs is that the former are merely narrative reports of the management of patients, whereas SSTSDs are capable of producing quantitative results.

Keating and colleagues[22] pointed out that the strength of evidence for SSTSDs lies somewhere along a continuum between a well-documented case study and a randomized controlled trial (RCT). In fact, an SSTSD can be the strongest evidence available regarding individual patients and may improve confidence in therapeutic decisions.[23] SSTSDs can be very useful in clinical practice when RCTs have shown a small treatment effect for a particular condition and, as a result, the clinician has strong reservations about initiating treatment. When there is doubt, an SSTSD is undoubtedly the best way to establish whether a particular treatment is effective for an individual patient.[24]

RCTs have been criticized because they often are not relevant to individual patients, since their findings are based on the average effects found in groups of patients. Although these findings can usually be generalized to other populations, they may not apply to individual patients. In other words, just because a given treatment was shown to be effective in a group of patients does not necessarily mean that it will be of benefit to a particular patient. On the other hand, since SSTSDs involve only a single subject, they cannot be generalized to other populations, or even other individuals for that matter. The results are only representative of the subject who was involved in the study. Sometimes, however, when the findings of other published single-subject studies are similar, the results can be applied to other patients.[25]

The fundamental SSTSD is the *AB design*, where A corresponds to the baseline or observation phase and B corresponds to the intervention phase. This design is fairly weak, however, because it has very little control over threats to internal validity, and, unless the outcome changes dramatically between phases A and B, it does not support a cause-and-effect relationship between the intervention and the outcome. Consequently, the AB design by itself is not very useful in practice, and the minimum structure of an SSTSD should involve at least three consecutive phases: baseline, intervention, and follow-up (ABA). The ABA design carries the process one step further by adding another observation phase, thus having the potential to provide much stronger evidence in support of a cause-and-effect relationship (Figure 7.1). This evidence is particularly strong if the second A phase (follow-up) returns to near-baseline levels. When the distinction between phases is not impressive, additional phases can be added (e.g., ABAB) until it becomes obvious that the patient either does better while receiving the intervention or does not. Repeated pre- and posttesting helps rule out confounding variables so that the treatment effect, if there is one, can be seen more clearly. The ABA design is sometimes referred to as the *withdrawal design* because treatment is withdrawn during the final A phase.

The results of SSTSDs are normally plotted on a graph and then examined to determine if changes in the outcome measures occurred in the level, trend, and slope between the baseline and intervention phases. *Level* refers to changes in the value of the dependent variable before and after the intervention. *Trend* refers to changes in the direction of the dependent variable and can be characterized as accelerating, decelerating, stable, or variable. The *slope* of a trend refers to the rate of change of the data or the angle that is formed by the data. The graph can be visually inspected to assess patient responses over time; alternatively, the data can be analyzed using statistical methods. Both of these methods were reported to function about the same as far as their ability to determine the true treatment effects in single-subject designs.[26] However, graphs are the most popular method

FIGURE 7.1 **Single-subject time series design showing multiple observations over three phases.**

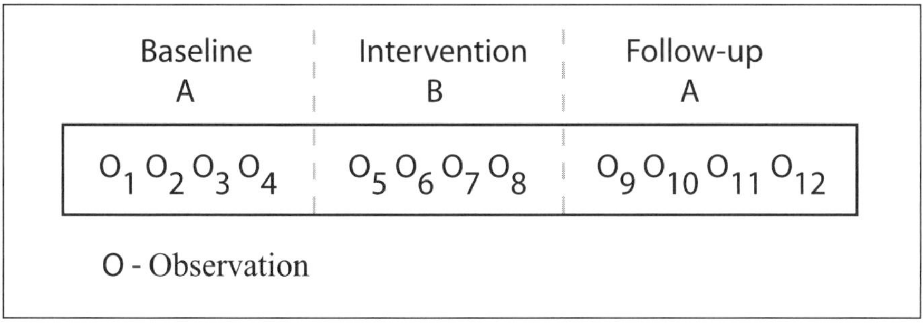

Baseline A	Intervention B	Follow-up A
$O_1\ O_2\ O_3\ O_4$	$O_5\ O_6\ O_7\ O_8$	$O_9\ O_{10}\ O_{11}\ O_{12}$

O - Observation

and have the advantage of being easily understood by both clinicians and patients. Ottenbacher[27] reported less confidence in graphed data, however, and indicated that some form of statistical analysis should be used together with visual inspection. It is helpful if the intervention under investigation has a rapid onset and offset of action in order to see clear distinctions between the phases on graphs.[28] Figure 7.2 is a graph that illustrates a hypothetical SSTSD investigating a chronic pain syndrome in a single patient.

The statistical analysis of SSTSD data is somewhat controversial, even though a number of different methods are available. The binomial test is probably the most straightforward and is commonly encountered. This test is per-

FIGURE 7.2 Simple ABA design with a minimum number of measures. Dashed lines correspond to the point of change between the observation and intervention phases.

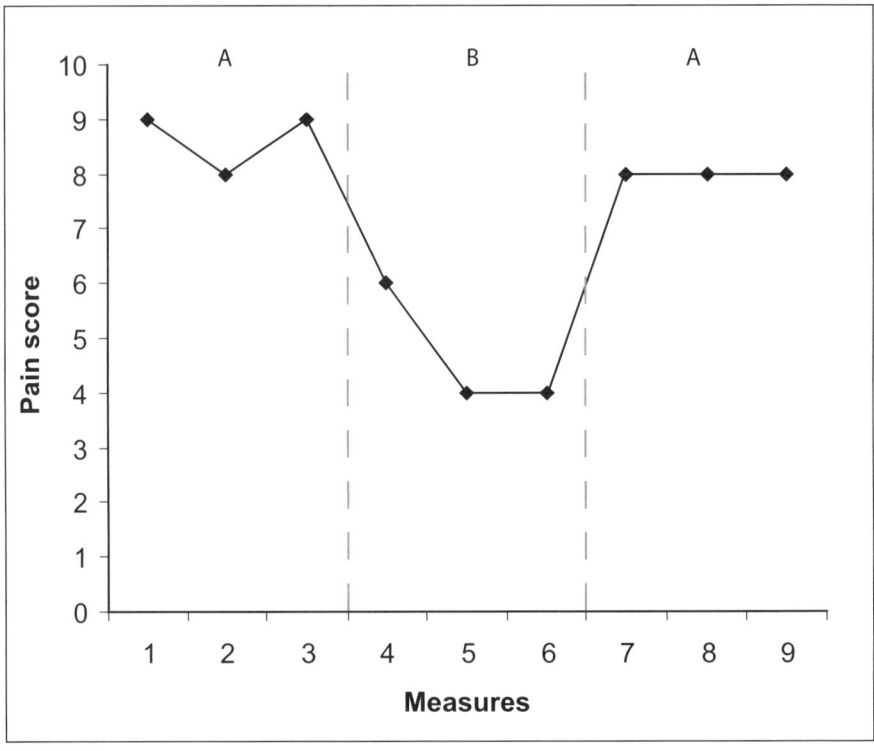

formed by calculating the probability of getting y number of successes (a positive treatment effect) by chance, given x number of events (pairs of baseline and treatment phases). Each pair of AB phases is examined to see whether the treatment was successful. Next, the number of treatment pairs and the number of successful pairs are each totaled. Finally, the probability that this number of successes could have occurred by chance is calculated. For example, in an SSTSD that utilized three treatment pairs and in which treatment was successful in each pair; the probability that the results were due to chance would be calculated as follows:

$$0.5 \times 0.5 \times 0.5 = 0.125$$

Thus, if all pairs were successful in a study, it would take at least five AB pairs to reach the 0.05 level of significance.

The statistical significance of data from SSTSDs can also be evaluated using a paired t-test or repeated-measures ANOVA test (or their nonparametric equivalents). These tests provide more power than the binomial test because they take into consideration not only the direction but also the magnitude of the treatment effect in each pair. Other methods of analysis and less common tests may also be encountered when reading research articles. Refer to the book *Foundations of Clinical Research: Applications to Practice*, by Portney and Watkins, for more information.[29]

A variation of the AB design is the ABAC design, where C represents an alternate intervention. The design involves an observation phase that is followed by an intervention phase consisting of treatment B, then a second observation phase, which is finally followed by an alternate treatment C intervention phase (Figure 7.3). Treatment C appears to be more effective than treatment B in Figure 7.3, but notice that the measure in the second observation phase did not revert to baseline values. Consequently, the added improvement seen with treatment C may have merely been due to a carry-over effect from the first phase of treatment, and the same results might have occurred if treatment B had been repeated. In cases where there is a carry-over effect after withdrawal of the treatment, a washout period is often necessary. This design, as well as the ABA design, works best with reversible conditions that return to pretreatment values when the intervention is withdrawn. Conditions for which treatments have long-lasting or irreversible effects are not suitable candidates for these designs.

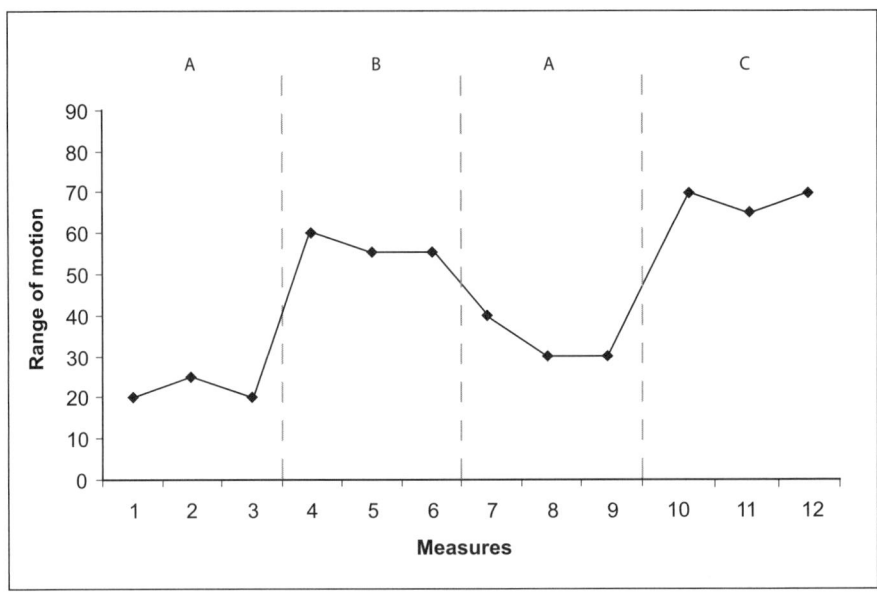

FIGURE 7.3 ABAC design showing that treatment C is apparently more effective than treatment B. Dashed lines correspond to the point of change between the observation and intervention phases.

SSTSDs are best suited for use with chronic conditions that are reasonably stable. Acute or unstable conditions are not suitable because the measures of outcome would vary considerably between phases regardless of the inclusion of an intervention phase. Even with chronic conditions, however, just because a patient responds to a particular intervention does not necessarily mean that there was a cause-and-effect relationship. The patient might have experienced a spontaneous remission or a placebo effect, or the condition may be cyclical and the patient merely presented at a time that coincidently made the treatment response look favorable. For instance, the symptoms of multiple sclerosis characteristically increase and decrease in a recurring fashion over periods of months and years. Many other conditions (such as arthritis and systemic lupus) are known to have periods of flare-up and remission, which must be considered when an SSTSD involves one of these patients (Table 7.2). In these cases, however, replication of

TABLE 7.2 Features of conditions that are suitable candidates for the SSTSD

- Condition is chronic.
- Condition is stable.
- Spontaneous remission is not likely.
- Previous treatment has had limited success.
- No concurrent treatment is involved.

---

the cycles involved in an SSTSD by adding phases and showing that the outcomes consistently improve when the treatment is applied can further support a cause-and-effect relationship. The ideal situation for demonstrating a treatment effect would be a stable baseline phase, followed by an obvious change in the level or slope of the outcome measure during the intervention phase, and then a return to the original baseline levels during the second A phase.

Just as some conditions are better candidates for conducting SSTSDs than others, some forms of treatment are better than others as well. Treatments that have a rapid onset of action when applied and a rapid termination of action when withdrawn are best suited for SSTSDs. Treatments that continue to act even after they are stopped are not as desirable because they require a washout period to allow the measures to return to a baseline state. However, this may create methodological problems if the interlude lasts longer than a few days.

Another type of AB design is the *multiple-baseline design* (also known as *replicated AB design*), which can help control for extraneous variables in SSTSDs. This design involves the use of three or more subjects who have similar complaints and are provided a similar intervention. The basic AB design is carried out on each patient, but their baselines are of differing lengths of time, and no withdrawal of treatment is involved. Differences in the measurements are then analyzed between the phases within each subject, but there is a comparison across subjects as well, which makes this analysis different from the basic AB design.[18] A cause-and-effect relationship is strengthened using this design because the likelihood that extraneous factors occurred by chance at the specific time that treatment was started on each patient would be small (Figure 7.4). What was just described could also be termed a *nonconcurrent multiple-baseline design* because patients are included in this type of study as they present for treatment, and patient care is not necessarily provided at the same time.

FIGURE 7.4 Hypothetical example of a multiple-baseline design involving three patients; each has a different-length baseline phase. Dashed lines correspond to the point of change between the observation and intervention phases.

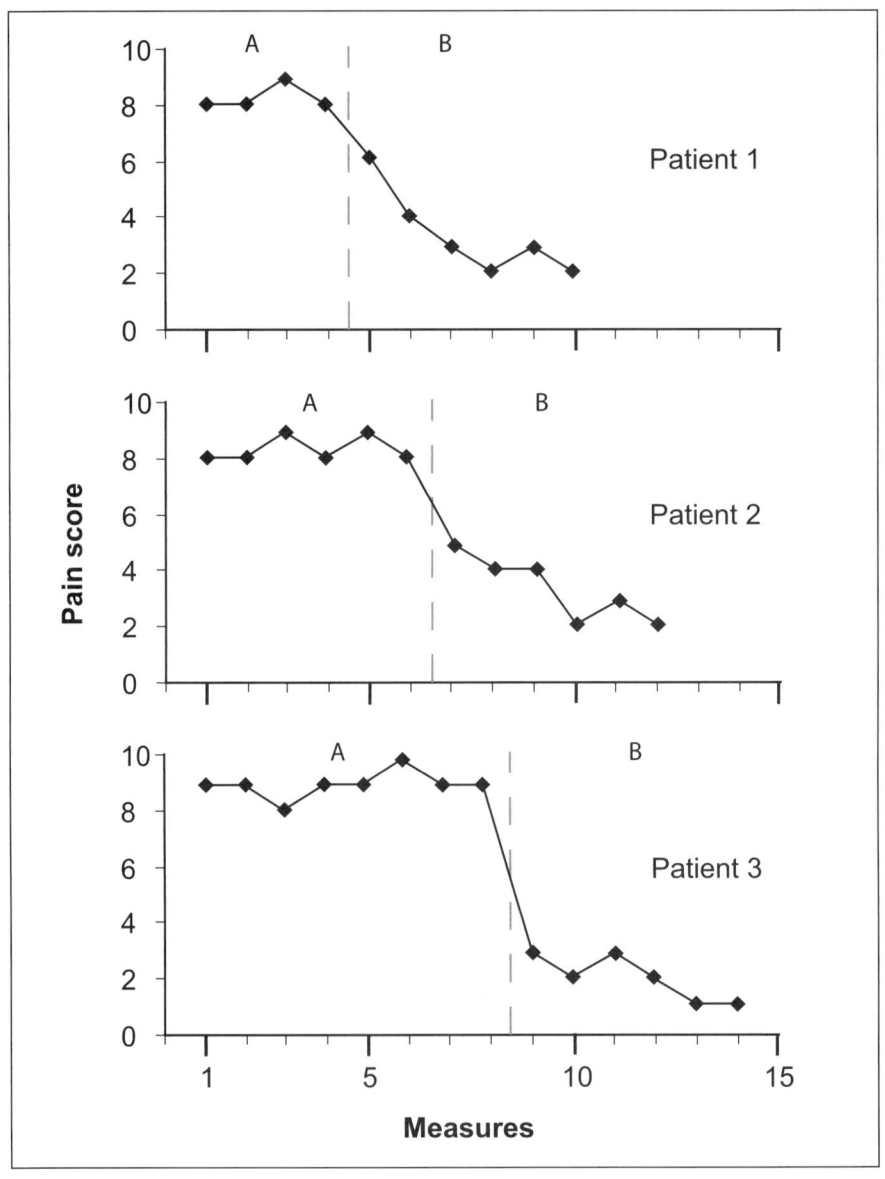

Single-Subject Time Series Designs

A variant of the multiple-baseline design is the *simultaneous replication design*,[21,30] where three or more patients are followed at the same time using an AB design as described previously. However, in this instance all patients start the study at the same time and their baseline scores are tracked concurrently. The intervention is applied to the first patient, and then in sequence across the other study participants. The first patient is started on the intervention at the outset. The intervention is initiated for each subsequent patient only after a clear treatment effect has been observed in the previous patient, until all patients have been included. This technique helps control for confounding factors, making it much less likely that the observed changes in the dependent variable were due to external events than in the typical single-patient AB design. Because the intervention is introduced to one patient and produces a change in the independent variable while the baseline measures of the other patients remain unchanged, the chance that something caused the change other than the intervention diminishes. As in the basic multiple-baseline design, this relationship is further strengthened when the dependent variable changes only after introduction of the independent variable.

Instead of using several subjects to implement the multiple-baseline design, it can also be carried out using one subject by measuring several dependent variables instead of just one. An example would be a single-subject study that measured ranges of motion, pain scores, and disability levels in a patient with chronic back pain. The multiple-baseline strategy strengthens the external validity of an SSTSD, especially when it duplicates the study's findings across three or more patients or dependent variables. Furthermore, the power (the probability of finding a treatment effect if there actually is one) of the individual AB design is extremely low, whereas it is much higher in multiple-baseline designs.[21]

Sackett and associates[31] described the n-of-1 RCT, where randomization is made possible by giving a single patient either a placebo or authentic medication, in place of just withdrawing an intervention. The authors thought that these types of trials were a very valuable aid in making treatment decisions. Randomization is achieved in n-of-1 RCTs by obtaining the assistance of a pharmacist to randomly administer a drug or placebo to the patient. Blinding can be accomplished in this design because neither the doctor nor the patient knows whether the real medication or placebo is involved. As a result, n-of-1 RCTs provide the strongest evidence for making decisions about the best treatment for a particular patient. Unfortunately, this scheme would be difficult to carry out with manipulation as the independent variable because the chiropractor would always know if a placebo (sham) therapy was being administered. The patient, too, would most likely be able to distinguish whether he or she was receiving a real treatment. Alternatively, n-of-1 studies with limited randomization and blinding are well suited for chiropractic research, and their use has been recommended.[22] An example of limited blinding in a modified chiropractic n-of-1 study was presented by Knutson,[32] who measured leg-length discrepancies and was blinded as to the status of the patient's condition on that particular visit. In a patient with scalenus anticus syndrome, he was able to show that when the patient's legs became equal following an upper cervical adjustment, skin temperature was more symmetrical in the hands. Random assignment is also possible with manipulation as the independent variable in the multiple-baseline design by randomly assigning each patient to one of the variable-length baseline periods that are available.

The SSTSD is a form of research that should commonly be carried out by chiropractors for several reasons: (1) to discover the most favorable form of treatment for a given patient, (2) to reassure both the patient and practitioner that a particular treatment is actually helpful, and (3) to contribute articles to peer-reviewed journals. This third point will add to the collective information about chiropractic care for the condition under investigation and will also help enhance the credibility of the practitioner who writes the article. Practitioners can tailor treatment specifically to the needs of an individual patient using this approach, which should facilitate providing the best care for the specific problem being addressed.

There are several patient circumstances that are good candidates for single-subject studies. The first is when a practitioner is not certain whether a planned treatment will be effective in a particular patient; possibly because the patient has already been to other practitioners and tried a variety of therapies without benefit. In a case such as this, an SSTSD would be useful to see if noticeable improvements actually occur with the current treatment. The second circumstance is when a patient has already started treatment, but it is not really apparent to either the patient or practitioner that the treatment is actually helping. The third is when the patient is undergoing another type of treatment or is self-treating, but the practitioner thinks that it may be ineffective or possibly even interfering with the patient's progress. The fourth occurs when the practitioner or patient suspects that some of the patient's symptoms may actually be caused by the treatment being provided. An example would be a chronic neck pain patient who developed headaches while under chiropractic care. The final circumstance is when there is doubt about what the ideal combination of therapies or frequency of care should be for a given patient to be optimally beneficial. There may be other circumstances that call for a single-subject study in addition to what was listed here—essentially, any time either the patient or practitioner has questions about the effectiveness of a patient's treatment.

The usual approach clinicians use to determine whether a treatment is effective in an individual patient is to observe the patient's response to care by the use of various measures of outcome. However, this environment is uncontrolled, and, as a result, many factors may mislead practitioners when this approach is used. To mention a few of these factors, the practitioner or the patient or both may be so confident about the potential of the intervention that they misinterpret the results of the care that was rendered. Natural progression of the condition may have occurred simultaneously while the patient was under care, and the patient thus would have improved whether treated or not. Also, the patient may have merely experienced a placebo effect and the treatment was actually of no value. In spite of these limitations, SSTSDs are often useful to determine the best care for an individual patient.

SSTSDs can be thought of as partnerships between the clinician and the patient; thus, the patient must be agreeable and even enthusiastic about working jointly in order to successfully carry out the study. There will likely be compliance problems if this is not the case, and the study's results will be inaccurate. Accordingly, practitioners should be fastidious about patient selection and their subsequent instruction in the protocol that will be utilized.

There are ethical considerations that affect SSTSDs as well.[29] The first has to do with denying treatment to patients during the observation phase, even if only for a limited period of time. This concern does not really apply to the type of patients and interventions found in chiropractic, but is reserved for cases where withholding treatment would actually be harmful. Chiropractic patients who would be candidates for SSTSDs have chronic conditions that are not likely to deteriorate during limited periods of time without active treatment. However, for a patient to be eligible for this type of research, the practitioner must be unsure about the effectiveness of the treatment involved. In these cases it may actually be unethical to administer an intervention on an ongoing basis without testing its effectiveness at some point. Bear in mind that the patient does not have to be completely denied any form of care during the observation phase, only the specific intervention being investigated. The patient can continue to receive other forms of treatment, as long as they were in use during the baseline phase. For instance, a patient with chronic headaches could continue to take over-the-counter pain medication while an SSTSD was conducted with manipulation as the independent variable. Another example would be a patient with a chronic shoulder problem who continues to receive ultrasound and electrical stimulation during the observation phase while being denied spinal and extremity manipulation.

The second ethical consideration that specifically applies to SSTSD studies has to do with informed consent. Patients should be fully informed about what is involved in the study in which they are about to participate, and they should consent to it in writing. They should be informed that they have the right to withdraw from the study at any time and for any reason without the loss of treatment in the future. Additionally, patient confidentiality must be respected and assured to them as part of the informed consent procedure. Many clinicians already have informed consent documents that they routinely use on all patients, but it is recommended that a tailored document be utilized with patients who are involved in SSTSDs.[33]

A third ethical consideration relative to SSTSDs has to do with the distinction between routine patient care and scientific investigation. Routine patient care may appropriately incorporate a "scientific" approach in the pursuit of the optimal treatment for a particular patient, and this includes SSTSDs. It is also acceptable to retrospectively write up the management and findings of an SSTSD case that results from such patient care and submit it to a journal for publication. On the other hand, circumstances are different when the predetermined intent of patient care includes the performance of a research project. The practitioner then becomes an investigator and, in addition to providing treatment, collects data for the research project. This practice is outside the bounds of routine patient care; hence, the patient should be informed that a new relationship exists (patient/investigator) and that he or she is the object of a scientific investigation. Two conditions point to treatment qualifying as research: (1) Data is collected with the intent to publish the findings in a journal or present them at a conference, and (2) there is intent to produce new information that goes beyond current standard care. In addition to obtaining informed consent when clinical research is carried out, even in a private practice setting, it is essential to obtain approval from a legitimate institutional review board before beginning. Colleges and universities that conduct biomedical research (including chiropractic colleges) may be able to assist practitioners in obtaining such approval if the need arises.

Chronic low back pain and neck pain are such common conditions in chiropractic practices that a special form has been provided in Figure 7.5 to serve as a

FIGURE 7.5 Single Subject Time Series Design Experiment

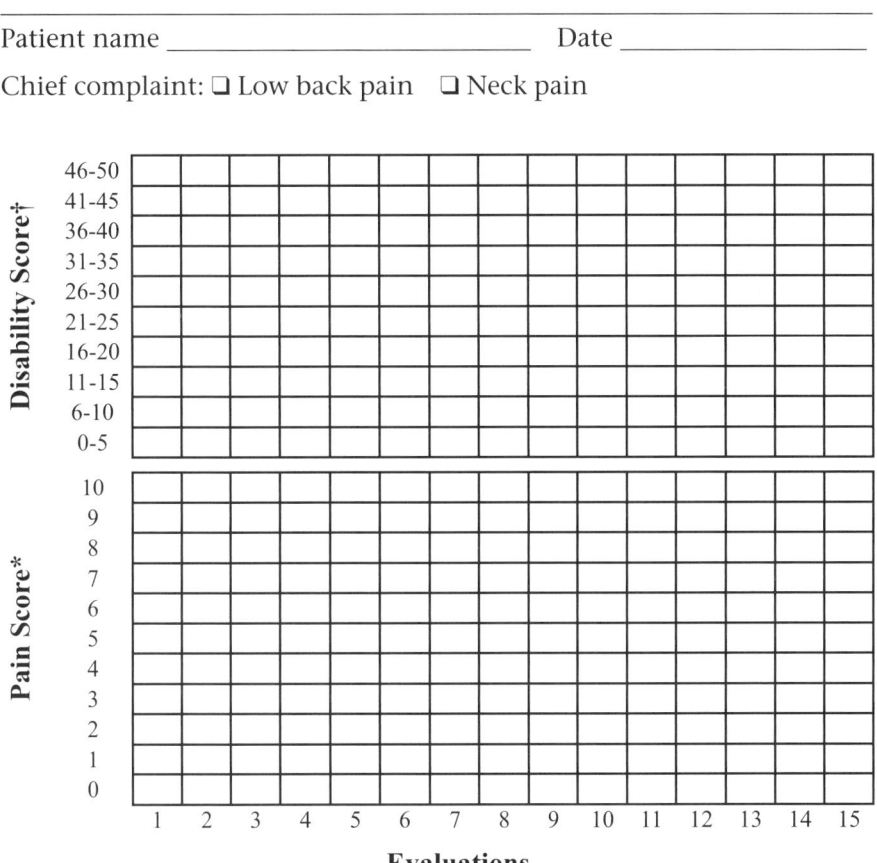

O = Observation phase
X = Intervention phase

• Numeric pain scale with 0 = no pain and 10 = worst pain imaginable
† Oswestry Low Back Pain Disability Questionnaire or Neck Pain Disability Index (raw score)

tally-sheet to assist practitioners as they follow their patients in SSTSDs. When completed, this form actually produces a graph of the case management of a patient involved in an SSTSD. The patient does not need to return to the office during phases of observation, but can take home copies of the appropriate questionnaires and complete them at scheduled times. Once completed, the forms can be returned to the office at a convenient time for evaluation. The Oswestry Low Back Pain Disability Questionnaire or the Neck Disability Index are used to evaluate the level of disability, depending on the area of involvement, and an 11-point numeric pain scale is used to assess pain. In-office measures, such as range of motion, may be utilized as well, but must be analyzed separately. Other "take-home" outcome measures can also be used in this type of study, such as the SF-36 heath survey questionnaire, condition-specific questionnaires, and measures of activity level.

Appraisal Tactics

Although a great deal of information is available on the subject of how to appraise the various types of articles that may be encountered in evidence-based practice, very little guidance exists regarding case reports and case series. This is probably because case reports are so low in the hierarchy of evidence; in addition, their findings cannot be generalized and then used as evidence in patient care. Nevertheless, they do have educational value that is of interest to clinicians and important to obtain. This makes knowledge of appraisal tactics necessary so that practitioners are able to gain as much as possible from their reading and avoid wasting time with poorly written articles.

Case reports, as with all the other types of research articles, should adhere to the general format of a scholarly publication. They typically incorporate each of the previously mentioned case report sections (i.e., Abstract, Introduction, Case Description, Discussion, and References). An immediate red flag should be raised if any of these elements are missing or incorrectly labeled; note, however, that some journals may have atypical manuscript requirements, and synonyms are sometimes used.

Case reports are often the first attempt at scholarly writing for many authors. As a result, the potential for methodological and grammatical errors is higher than with other types of articles. Most of the time, the report will have gone through the peer-review process prior to publication, which should catch most, but not all, of these flaws. Nonetheless, readers should be especially vigilant when appraising these articles; thus, a *checklist for the appraisal of case reports* is provided in Appendix 5. Some specific questions should be asked in the course of reviewing case studies, as follows:

- *Does the Abstract provide an accurate description of the case and its implications?* This issue is often taken for granted by readers; indeed, the abstract is often the only part of an article that is actually read. However, abstracts may not correctly represent the material presented in the body of an article. A study that sampled 88 articles from five major general medical journals and then compared data presented in the body of the paper with the accompanying abstracts found that from 18% to 68% of the abstracts contained inconsistencies.[34] With this in mind, realize the limitations of abstracts and use them primarily as screening tools to help locate interesting articles that will later be read in their entirety.

- *Is the case really unique or uncommon?* It may be appropriate to replicate the same topic in several case reports, but there comes a point at which further publications of this type would be uninteresting and any new studies should be carried out using more sophisticated study designs. This does not hold true to the same extent regarding case reports of harm, since it is important to observe patterns of problems that may develop as a result of a particular form of treatment. As was previously mentioned, however, case reports and series cannot determine cause-and-effect relationships, although they can be used to identify patterns and suggest appropriate future research.[35]

- *Was the literature review adequate?* Case reports are not required to incorporate comprehensive reviews of the literature, but they should at least point out the most current relevant research on the topic and indicate how it relates to the current case. The references should come from valid information sources—peer-reviewed journals, for the most part.

- *Was a rationale for reporting the case presented that effectively highlights its importance?* Why was the report written in the first place? Was it needed, or is the information already well known among practitioners? Authors should present a convincing argument that justifies the writing of the case report. Readers may not want to continue with the rest of the article if this argument is weak.

- *Was the case adequately described in the Case Description section?* The case should be described clearly and concisely, yet comprehensively enough to cover all relevant information. The patient's health history, examination, diagnosis, treatment, and final outcome should be fully presented, omitting irrelevant findings. Descriptions of treatment should be thorough, providing information about things such as the type of manipulation that was utilized, areas treated, and details about physiotherapy and rehabilitation interventions, as well as the frequency and duration of care. Another practitioner should be able to reproduce the study in one of his or her own patients based on the description that was provided.

- *Was the study population described adequately?* In case series, there should be an explicit definition of what constitutes a case. Selection criteria may be based on such things as a specified diagnosis; examination, laboratory, or radiographic findings; or condition severity. For instance, in a series of patients with radicular leg pain, the case definition would probably mention a positive straight leg raise test and/or MRI evidence of disc herniation as inclusion criteria.

- *Were the outcome measures suitable for the given clinical circumstances?* Outcome measures utilized in case studies do not always have to be validated by research, but they should certainly be quantifiable. Vague descriptions of treatment outcomes, such as "the patient's cervical spine felt significantly better" or "there was less lumbar muscle spasm," are inadequate. When novel diagnostic or assessment strategies are utilized, they should be fully described.[36] The results of less common clinical or laboratory tests should be presented together with normal values. If an attempt to draw inferences is to be made from the results of single-case experiments, as in the case of meta-analyses of SSTSDs, then it is important for the outcome measures to be valid and reliable.[21]

- *Did the author present convincing evidence in support of the diagnosis that was presented?* Readers should not be required to make assumptions based on conjecture; rather, evidence derived from the case results and the literature review should be presented in a logical manner that supports the diagnosis. Differential diagnoses that were considered and why they were eliminated should also be mentioned.

- *Did the author point out the study's limitations and suggest alternate explanations?* All types of research, case reports in particular, have limitations, and these should be plainly identified. For instance, other possible explanations for the findings of the case should be mentioned, such as natural progression of the condition, extraneous factors, and placebo effects.

In addition, basic limitations inherent to case reports should be pointed out, such as the lack of a control group and limited generalizability.

- *Were suggestions for future research offered?* One of the fundamental reasons for writing case reports is to highlight new or unique cases and to pave the way for more definitive studies; thus, authors should suggest the most appropriate methods to research the topic in the future.

- *Were suggestions provided to assist other practitioners in the management of similar cases?* To a large extent, the educational value of case reports lies in their ability to be of assistance to practitioners who may encounter patients with similar conditions. As such, authors should offer suitable advice that is based on the literature review as well as the results of the case.

- *Was enough evidence presented to support the author's conclusions?* Conclusions should logically follow from the case description. As with reports of any type of research, no unsupported statements should be offered. In particular, the author should not make groundless assertions about the effectiveness of the intervention that was involved or suggest that other practitioners will obtain similar results.

References

1. Instructions for authors. *J Manipulative Physiol*, 2005.
2. Rothstein, J.M. *Case reports: Still a priority. Phys Ther*, 2002. **82**(11):1062–3.
3. Hoffman, J.R. *Rethinking case reports. West J Med*, 1999. **170**(5):253–4.
4. Haynes, B. *Advances in evidence-based information resources for clinical practice.* In *AMPA Annual Meeting.* 2001. New York City: American Medical Publishers Association.
5. Martyn, C. *Case reports, case series and systematic reviews. QJM*, 2002. **95**(4):197–8.
6. Green, B.N., C.D. Johnson, and A. Adams. *Writing narrative literature reviews for peer-reviewed journals: Secrets of the trade. J Sports Chiropr Rehabil*, 2001. **15**(1).
7. Sackett, D.L., et al. *Evidence-Based Medicine: How to Practice and Teach EBM.* 2nd ed. 2000. Edinburgh: Churchill Livingstone.
8. McEwen, I.R. *Case reports: Slices of real life to complement evidence. Phys Ther*, 2004. **84**(2):126–7.
9. Huth, E.J. *Writing and Publishing in Medicine.* 3rd ed. 1999. Baltimore: Williams & Wilkins.
10. Chestnut, J.L. *The stroke issue: Paucity of valid data, plethora of unsubstantiated conjecture. J Manipulative Physiol Ther*, 2004. **27**(5):368–72.
11. Haneline, M., and G. Lewkovich. *An analysis of the etiology of cervical artery dissections: 1994–2003. J Manipulative Physiol Ther*, 2005. **28**(8):617–22.

12. Vandenbroucke, J.P. *In defense of case reports and case reries. Ann Intern Med*, 2001. **134**(4):330–4.
13. Bayoumi, A.M., and P.A. Kopplin. *The storied case report. CMAJ*, 2004. **171**(6):569–70.
14. Grimes, D.A., and K.F. Schulz. *Descriptive studies: What they can and cannot do. Lancet*, 2002. **359**(9301):145–9.
15. Godlee, F. *Applying research evidence to individual patients. Evidence based case reports will help. BMJ*, 1998. **316**(7145):1621–2.
16. Venning, G.R. *Validity of anecdotal reports of suspected adverse drug reactions: the problem of false alarms. Br Med J (Clin Res Ed)*, 1982. **284**(6311):249–52.
17. Lisi, A.J., and M.K. Bhardwaj. *Chiropractic high-velocity low-amplitude spinal manipulation in the treatment of case of postsurgical chronic cauda equina syndrome. J Manipulative Physiol Ther*, 2004. **27**(9):574–8.
18. Backman, C.L., and S.R. Harris. *Case studies, single-subject research, and N of 1 randomized trials: Comparisons and contrasts. Am J Phys Med Rehabil*, 1999. **78**(2):170–6.
19. Carey, T.S., and S.D. Boden. *A critical guide to case series reports. Spine*, 2003. **28**(15):1631–4.
20. Haneline, M.T., A.C. Croft, and B.M. Frishberg. *Association of internal carotid artery dissection and chiropractic manipulation. Neurologist*, 2003. **9**(1):35–44.
21. Onghena, P., and E.S. Edgington. *Customization of pain treatments: Single-case design and analysis. Clin J Pain*, 2005. **21**(1):56–68; discussion 69–72.
22. Keating, J.C., Jr., et al. *Toward an experimental chiropractic: Time-series designs. J Manipulative Physiol Ther*, 1985. **8**(4):229–38.
23. Johannessen, T., and D. Fosstvedt. *Statistical power in single subject trials. Fam Pract*, 1991. **8**(4):384–7.
24. Jull, A., and D. Bennett. *Do n-of-1 trials really tailor treatment? Lancet*, 2005. **365**(9476):1992–4.
25. Johannessen, T., D. Fosstvedt, and H. Petersen. *Statistical aspects of controlled single subject trials. Fam Pract*, 1990. **7**(4):325–8.
26. Bobrovitz, C.D., and K.J. Ottenbacher. *Comparison of visual inspection and statistical analysis of single-subject data in rehabilitation research. Am J Phys Med Rehabil*, 1998. **77**(2):94–102.
27. Ottenbacher, K.J. *Reliability and accuracy of visually analyzing graphed data from single-subject designs. Am J Occup Ther*, 1986. **40**(7):464–9.
28. Johnston, B.C., and E. Mills. *n-of-1 randomized controlled rrials: An opportunity for complementary and alternative medicine evaluation. J Altern Complement Med*, 2004. **10**(6):979–84.
29. Portney, L.G., and M.P. Watkins. *Foundations of Clinical Researc : Applications to Practice*. 2nd ed. 2000. Upper Saddle River: Prentice Hall.
30. Gemmell, H., and B. Jacobson. *Appropriateness of the replicated AB design in chiropractic field research. Chiro J Aust*, 1991. **21**(2):42–6.
31. Sackett, D.L., et al. *Clinical Epidemiology: A Basic Science for Clinical Medicine*. 2nd ed. 1991. Boston: Little, Brown & Company.
32. Knutson, G.A. *Thermal asymmetry of the upper extremity in scalenus anticus syndrome, leg-length inequality and response to chiropractic adjustment. J Manipulative Physiol Ther*, 1997. **20**(7):476–81.

33. Guyatt, G., et al. *Users' Guides to the Medical Literature: A Manual for Evidence-Based Clinical Practice*. 2002. Chicago: AMA Press.
34. Pitkin, R.M., M.A. Branagan, and L.F. Burmeister. *Accuracy of data in abstracts of published research articles. JAMA*, 1999. **281**(12):1110–1.
35. Levine, M., et al. *Users' guides to the medical literature. IV. How to use an article about harm. Evidence-Based Medicine Working Group. JAMA*, 1994. **271**(20):1615–9.
36. Green, B.N., C.D. Johnson, and W.F. Updyke. *Reading and evaluating case reports: Deciding what to use in practice-part 2. J Amer Chiropr Assoc*, 2002. **39**(5):38–41.

CHAPTER EIGHT

Epidemiology

Epidemiology is a branch of science that investigates the frequency and distribution of diseases in a defined population in an attempt to determine their causes, to discover ways to alleviate them, and to prevent their reoccurrence. Epidemiologic studies observe people in their natural setting over a period of time, at one point in time, or retrospectively in order to describe specific traits that may be present among members of a population. Some epidemiologic studies compare outcomes in groups of subjects who either have or have not been exposed to some *risk factor* (also known as *predictor variable*) specifically to see if the exposed group developed a higher incidence of disease. In a case such as this, it would be unethical for researchers to ask a group of patients to do or take something that was known to be harmful (e.g., to smoke a pack of cigarettes each day or expose themselves to known carcinogenic substances). Thus, even these types of studies are usually observational. Data is typically collected for epidemiologic studies by such means as surveys and reports from health care personnel and health departments, and the unit of analysis is the group or population involved rather than the individuals.[1] The resulting data is analyzed using a variety of statistical techniques to discover patterns and correlations that may exist.

Probably the easiest way to understand the concept of epidemiology is to consider the early work of Dr. John Snow,[2] who is widely recognized as the father of epidemiology. Snow lived in London, England, during an extensive cholera epidemic that killed thousands of people. Up until that point, no one understood what caused cholera, although some thought that it was spread by miasmas (bad air from decayed organic matter). Snow self-published a pamphlet that theorized that cholera was spread by contaminated water rather than miasmas, but it was not well received by the medical community. However, when a particularly bad outbreak of cholera occurred in the immediate vicinity of a certain public water pump, he canvassed the area and discovered that nearly all persons who died had consumed water from that pump. He presented his data, which demonstrated a much higher than expected incidence of the disease, to the local authorities, who immediately had the pump handle removed. As a result, the outbreak subsided very quickly. Sadly, his theory about the spread of cholera continued to be rejected by his peers. Snow was later vindicated, however, when *Vibrio cholerae* was identified as the cause of the disease. The statistical and mapping methods that he utilized during the investigation formed the foundation of epidemiology.

Measurement of Disease Frequency and Occurrence

Several measurements of disease frequency are used extensively in epidemiology to describe not only the raw number of persons having a particular disease but also the rate of occurrence. *Incidence* refers to the probability of a person being diagnosed with a disease during a specific period of time. It represents the number of newly diagnosed cases of a disease during a given time period, which is usually one year. The incidence rate may be calculated by dividing the number of new cases of a disease in a given time period by the number of persons in the population who are at risk for the disease and then multiplying the quotient by 100,000.

$$\text{Incidence} = \frac{\text{Number of } new \text{ cases in a time period}}{\text{Population}} \times 100{,}000$$

For example, in a one-year study involving 500 carpenters where 20 new cases of carpal tunnel syndrome (CTS) were diagnosed, the incidence of CTS in this population would be $20/500 = 0.04$, or 4,000 per 100,000 person-years. It is possible for some disease conditions to occur multiple times in an individual during a year (e.g., the common cold or episodes of low back pain); when calculating incidence, however, only the first occurrence is usually counted.

Measurement of Disease Frequency and Occurrence

Risk is very similar to the incidence rate; it is a measure of the occurrence of new cases of a disease within a population. The main difference is that risk provides an estimate of the proportion of unaffected persons who will develop the disease of interest over a specified period of time.[3] To estimate risk, a population must be observed over a defined period to determine the number of new cases as compared with the total number of persons who are at risk.

Prevalence is another commonly used measure of disease frequency. It is the proportion of persons in a given population who have a disease at a certain point in time. It represents the total number of cases of disease in that population, regardless of when patients were diagnosed with the condition. The prevalence rate can be calculated by dividing the total number of cases of a disease existing within a population by the total population and multiplying by 100,000.

$$\text{Incidence} = \frac{\text{Number of } \textit{existing} \text{ cases in a time period}}{\text{Population}} \times 100{,}000$$

An example of prevalence would be a study involving a community with a population of 30,000 that determined that 1,000 persons had migraine headaches. The prevalence of migraine headaches in this population would then be 1,000/30,000 = 0.33, or 3,333 per 100,000 persons. In this study, it does not matter that 200 of the cases were newly diagnosed and that 800 patients had been living with migraine headaches for some time.

The term *point prevalence* is sometimes used to represent the proportion of a population with a disease at a given point in time. In contrast, *period prevalence* is a term that corresponds to the proportion of a population that has a disease within a defined period of time. The reason for this distinction is that the point prevalence is likely to underestimate the overall frequency of certain conditions. Period prevalence, on the other hand, provides a better depiction of the overall frequency of a disease by repeatedly monitoring its occurrence within a population over time. Many conditions, such as acute low back pain, are episodic. Thus, when prevalence is measured at one point in time, only active cases will be detected in the study. Period prevalence includes all episodes of the condition that occur during a given time frame and is sometimes much higher as a result.

Occasionally a number other than 100,000 is used as a multiplier with both incidence and prevalence—for instance, 1,000. It does not matter what the multiplier is, as long as it is suitably defined, because the purpose of converting the raw numbers is simply to create a number that is more intuitive and easier to work with. Also, incidence and prevalence estimates are often reported as the *percentage* of a population with a certain condition at a specific point in time.[4] For instance, Manchikanti and coworkers[5] reported prevalence findings by means of percentages. They studied 500 consecutive chronic spine pain patients and found that the prevalence of facet joint pain among this group was 55% in the cervical spine patients, 42% in the thoracic spine pain patients, and 31% in the lumbar spine patients.

Incidence and prevalence are related to each other, differing mainly in the dimension to which they refer, with incidence being based on a defined period of time (e.g., a month or a year) and prevalence referring to a given point in time. Therefore, prevalence is essentially the incidence rate that occurred throughout the average duration of the disease.[6] This relationship is illustrated as follows:

$$\text{Prevalence} = \text{Incidence} \times \text{Duration}$$

In short-duration diseases, such as the common cold, the prevalence rate is usually much lower than the incidence rate. This is because a high proportion of the population contracts colds over a one-year period, but because the condition's duration is so short, relatively few people actually have a cold at a given point in time. Conversely, the prevalence rate of a chronic condition, such as diabetes, is usually much higher than its incidence rate. Comparatively few new cases of diabetes are diagnosed each year (1.2 million new cases in the United States in 2002), but once diagnosed, the condition remains, and each year's incidence rate is added to the overall prevalence (18.2 million cases in the United States in 2002), minus those who die having the condition (Figure 8.1).[7]

Causation in Epidemiology

Epidemiologists often attempt to determine whether exposure to a specific risk factor is a cause of a particular disease within a population. To make such a claim, three key criteria should be met: temporality, consistency, and dose-response. In this context, the first criterion, *temporality* (also known as *temporal precedence*), refers to the fact that an exposure must occur prior to the onset of a disease. Nonetheless, just because a given exposure precedes a given disease does not necessarily mean there is a cause-and-effect relationship. Alternate explanations

Causation in Epidemiology

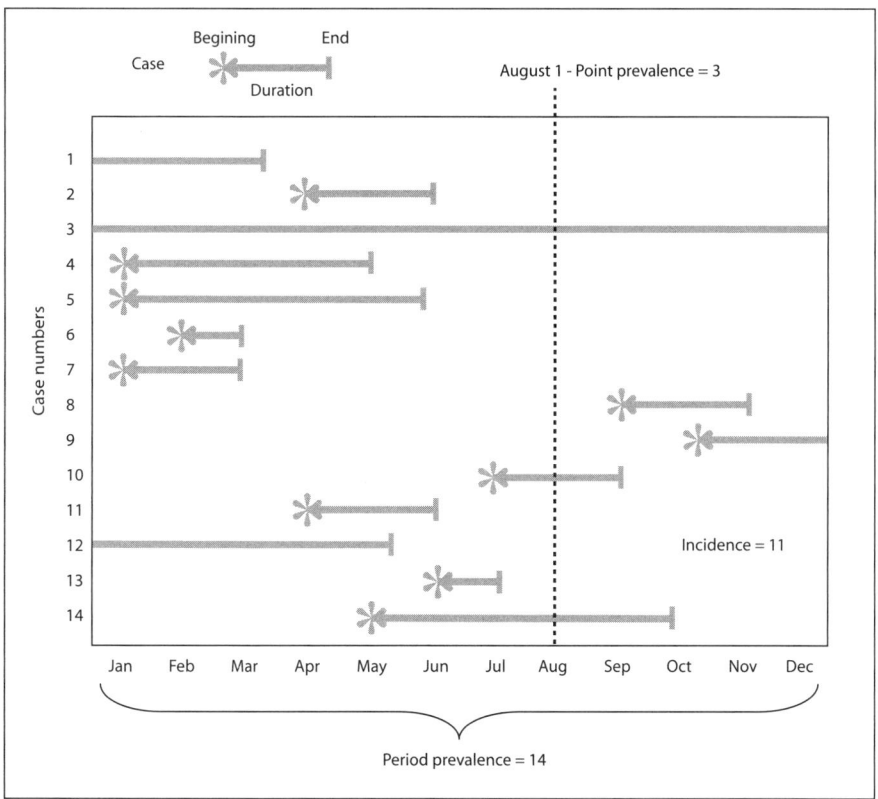

FIGURE 8.1 Fourteen cases of a disease that occurred over a one-year period. New cases are represented by an asterisk, the duration of the case by a line, and the end of a case (after a cure or death) by a bar. Cases that began or ended outside the period do not have limiters.

will always be possible when temporal relationships are used as the sole basis for supporting causation. Indeed, four interpretations are available in such cases: (1) Event A caused event B, (2) event B caused event A, (3) both events A and B were caused by a third related event, and (4) neither A nor B is related to each other or a third event, but the temporal relationship was merely by chance. As an example, consider a patient seeking chiropractic care for a lumbar disc herniation following a sports injury, where the initial symptoms did not include radicular signs or symptoms. Lumbosacral manipulation was initiated, but later on, as the condition naturally progressed, radiculopathy developed with resulting leg pain and a corresponding loss of the Achilles tendon reflex. It may appear that the disc herniation was caused by the manipulation in this case, when in fact it was present all along but was undiagnosed prior to treatment.

Consistency, the second criterion of causation, is present when studies that are reproduced by other researchers using different populations get similar results. This criterion was crucial in the effort to establish a cause-and-effect relationship between cigarette smoking and lung cancer. Tobacco companies denied the relationship for many years,[8] with the assistance of staff scientists, stating that the observational studies that had been done were not capable of establishing causation; thus, there was no "scientific proof." However, a cause-and-effect relationship is now generally accepted,[9] largely because many studies over many years have been conducted by different researchers, among different populations, all of which produced virtually the same results.[10] When based on quality observational studies, this type of consistency is capable of leading to a conclusion of causation regarding virtually any issue.

The third criterion is *dose-response*, which occurs when greater exposure to a risk factor results in a greater effect on health. Continuing on with the cigarette smoking and lung cancer example, not only have studies shown that smoking results in lung cancer, but they have also found that the more cigarettes a person smokes per day, the more likely he or she is to develop the disease.[11] Thus, as the "dose" of cigarettes increases, so does the "response" (lung cancer). Bradford Hill[12] listed six additional criteria that are often used to identify cause-and-effect relationships, but the three just mentioned are usually thought to be the most important. Table 8.1 presents the complete list of Bradford Hill's criteria for causation.

When applying the Bradford Hill criteria to issues of causation, the following advice from Hill (cited by Doll[13]) should always be taken into account.

> None of these nine viewpoints can bring indisputable evidence for or against a cause and effect hypothesis. What they can do, with greater or less strength, is to help answer the fundamental question—is there any other way of explaining the set of facts before us, is there any other answer equally, or more, likely than cause and effect?

TABLE 8.1 Bradford Hill's criteria of causation

1. **Strength of association**: The stronger the relation between the risk and the outcome is, the less likely it was caused by other factors.
2. **Consistency**: The study results should be able to be replicated by different researchers in a different setting.
3. **Specificity in the cause**: The exposure should be associated with a single specific disease.
4. **Temporality**: The exposure must precede the disease.
5. **Dose-response relationship**: Increased exposures should correspond to increased risk of disease.
6. **Plausibility**: There should be a rational scientific basis for the association.
7. **Coherence**: The association must be consistent with other knowledge on the topic.
8. **Experimental evidence**: Research that is based on experiments reinforces a causal inference.
9. **Analogy**: The association is analogous to a known causal relationship.

Source: Hill, A.B. The environment and disease: Association or causation? *Proc R Soc Med*, 1965. **58**:295–300.

Epidemiology differs from typical clinical health care practice in that its objectives are focused on prevention rather than treatment and it deals with populations rather than individual patients. Thus, when confronted with a particular disease, the epidemiologic approach is to identify subgroups that are at high risk within a population and then discover what factors caused persons in the subgroups to be at high risk. Once the likely causes of the disease are established, preventive measures can then be developed to minimize the risk factors. Finally, the effectiveness of the preventive measures that were established in response to the disease can be monitored with further epidemiologic research. The impact of this approach on the general health of the world's population has been enormous. Indeed, since environmental risk factors affect people's health more than any of the other determinants of health (i.e., heredity, biological factors, medical care, and lifestyle), epidemiologic methods are employed extensively in public health programs.[14]

Some examples of epidemiologic investigations that might be of interest to chiropractors include a study that determines whether a relationship exists between driving heavy equipment and the incidence of lower back pain,[15] a study that reports the incidence and prevalence of shoulder impingement syndrome within a population of heavy workers,[16] or one that shows that persons who consume an adequate daily supply of calcium and vitamin D are less likely to develop osteoporosis.[17]

Randomized controlled trials (RCTs) are very useful when clinical questions involve the choice of the best form of treatment. However, because of ethical concerns and feasibility, epidemiologic studies are preferred when the questions are about diagnosis, prognosis, or causation. These studies are considered *observational* or *descriptive* because variables are not manipulated; rather, subjects are merely observed in their natural settings. The findings of this type of research can be used for trend analysis, health care planning, and generating hypotheses.[18] Typically two groups are selected in epidemiologic studies, one of which is exposed to some agent or event, while the other is not. If there is a difference in the rate of disease occurrence between the groups, it may be because of the exposure. Statistical tests are then used to determine the likelihood that other persons would develop the disease given the same exposure. RCTs are generally not helpful in the investigation of causation because it is unethical to randomly assign individuals to a group that is intentionally exposed to harm.

Many of the same potential problems that negatively influence RCTs may also be present in epidemiologic studies. Moreover, because subjects are not randomly assigned to be in exposure versus no-exposure groups and because of possible differences in the baseline risk of disease between the groups, there is even more potential for bias in epidemiologic studies.[19] Ideally, subjects are randomly selected for participation in all types of epidemiologic research so that each person in the population has an equal chance of being included in the study. Random selection helps reduce the influence of a number of biases and produces a sample that is representative of the population under investigation. When less reliable selection methods are used, the credibility of the study's findings is greatly diminished.

The reliability of data sources is an important issue in all types of research, but because data in epidemiologic studies is often collected directly from people or by relying on others to provide needed information, there are some unique data reliability concerns in such studies. For instance, sometimes mail surveys are conducted on a population to determine the incidence of disease, hospital emergency room personnel are frequently utilized to collect data on certain injuries, and safety workers at job sites are asked to report occupational injuries. Researchers must depend on these individuals to perform their tasks accurately and as free from bias as possible. However, there are many potential pitfalls associated with these methods that should be considered when reading articles that report on this type of research. Clinical outcome measures that have established validity and reliability (e.g., examination findings, blood tests) are also commonly utilized in epidemiologic research.

It is important that questionnaires used in data collection be constructed correctly to ensure that the resulting information accurately reflects the features of interest in the population under study. Although survey methods and questionnaire design are rather complex topics that will not be fully covered here, there are a few basic design issues that readers of this kind of research should bear in mind. First, questions should not be double-barreled; instead, they should only inquire about one clear issue at a time. For example, a question that asks "Do you have headaches and a history of neck injury?" should be split into two questions. Second, leading questions that encourage respondents to provide a specific answer should be avoided. This problem was evident in a questionnaire used by the Canadian Stroke Consortium (CSS) to gather etiological data regarding cervical artery dissections (CADs).[20] There are a number of suspected causes for CADs, and often they are spontaneous with an unknown origin. The first question about etiology in the CSS questionnaire asked doctors participating in the study whether "cervical trauma/manipulation" was involved. Although scores of other daily occurrences have been reported to be associated with CADs, none of them were listed. Presenting cervical trauma/manipulation as the only possible choice calls for a highly biased response, thus tainting all of the data that was collected in this study. When survey questions are posed via face-to-face interviews, the likelihood of leading questions affecting the results is even higher. In addition to the wording of questions, the facial expressions, body language, and vocal inflections of the interviewer can influence the respondents' replies. Finally, respondents should be competent to answer survey questions. Persons with dementia would thus often not be capable of accurately completing a questionnaire. Another example would be patients who are asked questions about the history of their injuries in an emergency room after recently being involved in a automobile crash. They may not be able to provide accurate responses, since these patients are typically quite upset and tend to be confused. Also, mild traumatic brain injury is not uncommon after a car crash, even in minor collisions, and may result in confusion.[21]

The selection of which measures should be used in epidemiologic research is often a compromise based on the interrelationship of five factors.[6]

1. The precision of the measurement, which ideally should be as free from error as is practicable.

2. Logistical factors that have to do with matters such as cost, availability, ease of use, and so on.
3. Ethical issues, such as asking subjects to undergo tests that carry a risk of harm (e.g., x-ray or discogram).
4. Importance, which has to do with the relative value of the information that the measure produces. The primary consideration here is how important the measure is to the persons involved.
5. The sensitivity of the link between the predictor variable and the outcome variable. This link should result in a change in the outcome that corresponds to a change in the predictor variable.

Several different types of observational designs are commonly used in epidemiology: cross-sectional studies, case-control studies, and cohort studies. The type of study that is used depends on how rare the disease or condition is, as well as the availability of human and economic resources.

Cross-Sectional Studies

The first and most straightforward of the observational designs that is used extensively in epidemiology is the *cross-sectional study* (also known as *prevalence study*), which assesses both the health status and the exposure levels of individuals within a population at one point in time (Figure 8.2). However, a given cross-sectional study may span weeks or months because of the time involved in gathering the data. Since cross-sectional studies do not collect information over time, health changes that are slow to develop are not fully taken into consideration. Only patients who actively manifest the disease are included, while patients with developing conditions are ignored. An example would be a factory worker with no signs or symptoms of disease who is exposed to excessive use of the hands today, but is diagnosed with carpal tunnel syndrome five years from now. A cross-sectional study of factory workers done at present would miss this case, since the disease is only in the developmental stages. It would take a type of epidemiologic study (cohort study) that follows subjects forward in time to discover this case.

The purpose of cross-sectional studies is to try to determine whether there is an association between a suspected causal factor and a condition, for instance, a higher rate of lower back pain among a group of factory workers who are exposed

FIGURE 8.2 Cross-sectional studies evaluate the exposure level and disease status of a target population at one point in time.

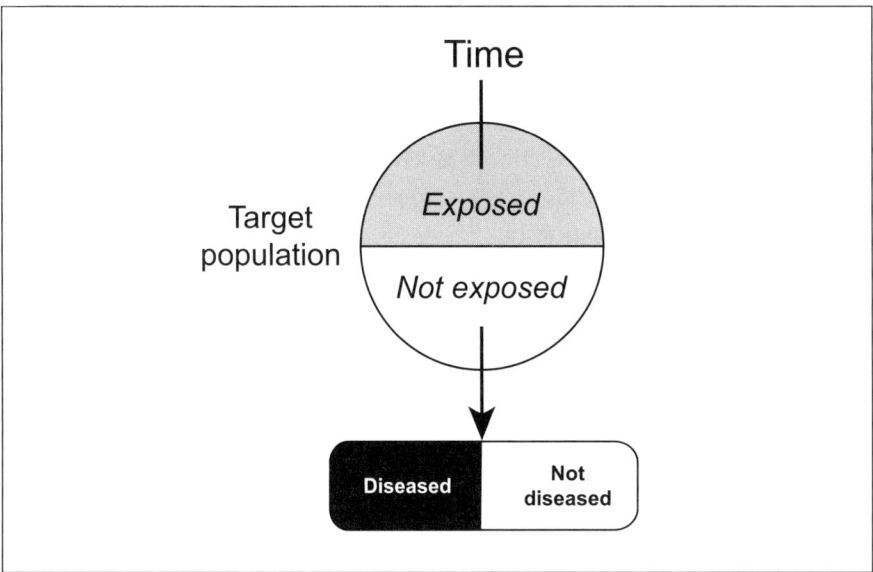

to tasks involving heavy lifting. These studies are very helpful in the discovery of such associations, but cannot establish if one caused the other. More sophisticated epidemiologic research methods, such as case-control or cohort studies, are typically used to follow up and verify their results. Cross-sectional studies are relatively easy to carry out and are inexpensive compared with other research designs because they are completed all at once, even though it may take a period of time to gather all of the information that is necessary. These studies are attractive to researchers because they do not have to wait for the health outcome to occur, nor do they have to estimate exposure levels that occurred in the past, sometimes many years previously. Additionally, cross-sectional studies are ethically acceptable, since no interventions are involved and subjects are typically only asked to answer questions via questionnaires or interviews, or their records are reviewed. Because of these advantages, they are frequently employed as the initial research tools to investigate exposures to risk factors and their relationships to disease.

An example cross-sectional study was carried out by Leboeuf-Yde and associates,[22] who were interested in finding out if there was a relationship between the educational levels of parents and the reporting of back pain in their children. The study involved interviewing 481 children aged 8 to 10 years and 325 adolescents aged 14 to 16 years. Parents' educational levels were ascertained by means of questionnaires that were administered by the children's teachers or by mail if that method was unsuccessful. The findings of the study showed that there was more back pain reported in children whose parents had the lowest educational levels than was reported in the children with higher parental education. Although these findings are interesting and may lead to future more definitive studies, only an association was established in this study, not a cause-and-effect relationship.

Case-Control Studies

A *case-control study* is a retrospective study that initially identifies two groups of subjects. All individuals in one group have the particular disease or condition under investigation (the *cases*), whereas everybody in the other group is free from the disease (the *controls*). The histories or records of potential exposures of the subjects in each group are then compared in order to discover whether any prior exposures may have influenced their probability of developing the disease. In other words, exposure is determined retrospectively by looking back in time, before the individual became a case, in order to assess exposure status (Figure 8.3). It is important that subjects selected to be controls be similar to the cases with respect to variables that could potentially influence the study's outcome. Therefore, cases and controls are typically matched on variables such as age, gender, weight, and occupation so that they are as alike as possible except for the presence of the disease under investigation.[23]

Case-control studies cannot actually determine the risk of developing a disease because of their retrospective nature, as well as the fact that their underlying populations are not adequately represented. As a result, instead of calculating risk, case-control studies estimate the odds of developing the disease given that a person was exposed to a risk factor, which is represented by the *odds ratio* (OR). It is important, however, to remember that the OR is only an estimate of risk.

The OR can be defined as the ratio of the odds of developing the disease in the exposed group divided by the odds of developing the disease in the unexposed group. If the exposure is harmful, this ratio will be greater than 1; if it is less than 1, the exposure is considered protective; and if the ratio equals 1, no risk would be attributable to the exposure. To calculate an OR and to visualize the data, it is helpful to arrange the results of a case-control study in a two-by-two contingency table (Table 8.2). Subjects are placed in the appropriate cells depending on whether they were cases or controls and whether they were exposed or not exposed. Cases that were exposed go in cell *a*, cases that were not exposed in cell *c*, controls that were exposed in cell *b*, and controls that were not exposed in cell *d*. The OR is the odds that a case was exposed, divided by the odds that a control was exposed. Referring to the two-by-two table, *a/c* is the odds that a case was

FIGURE 8.3 **Case-control studies compare two groups of subjects: one group having the disease and one group without. The purpose is to see if there is more exposure to some risk factor among the cases than the controls.**

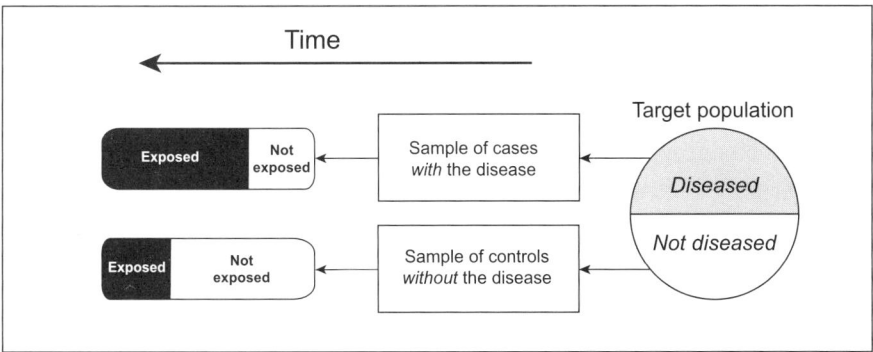

TABLE 8.2 **Two-by-two contingency table comparing exposure levels of cases versus controls in a case-control study**

	Cases	Controls
Exposed	a	b
Not exposed	c	d

exposed, and b/d is the odds that a control was exposed. The OR can then be calculated using the following formula:

$$\frac{a/c}{b/c}$$

For easier calculation, this formula can be simplified to

$$\frac{ad}{bc}$$

Case-control studies are subject to many of the same biases that were mentioned in Chapter 5, which covered experimental designs. Cases and controls are selected after both the disease outcome and the exposure have occurred, which makes this study design particularly vulnerable to a number of biases. One of them is *recall bias*, which occurs when there are systematic differences between cases and controls regarding their recall of past exposures. For instance, if a group of chronic neck pain patients were questioned about past injuries that might have contributed to their condition, they might be more likely to recall events than members of the pain-free group because they probably had to relate what happened to their doctor and insurance company after the injury, which reinforced the memory. In addition to problems with participant recall, there is a fairly high likelihood that inaccuracies or deficiencies may exist when case-control studies rely on medical records as information sources. Recall bias may also be more likely to occur with diseases that summon an emotional response in patients, such as illnesses or injuries where litigation is involved. These patients are often more motivated to recall the details of events that they think contributed to their condition than persons in the control group.

Another type of bias is *Berkson's bias* (also known as *admission rate bias*), which is actually a form of selection bias. Berkson's bias occurs when cases and controls in a hospital setting are systematically different from each other due to an increased probability among cases of being admitted to a hospital simply because the cases have a higher rate of exposure and incidence of the disease under study. Consequently, hospitalized subjects systematically report more risk factors than control subjects and therefore may not be representative of the defined population.[24]

Case-Control Studies

In spite of their limitations, case-control studies are often the best way to study rare diseases, given that more definitive prospective studies usually require many subjects, often making them impractical. It is much easier to select a group of subjects who already have the rare disease and then look back into their histories for clues than to select a huge sample of disease-free subjects and then follow them forward in time, waiting for the disease to develop in just a few. In addition, case-control studies are often preferred when the disease under study takes a long time to develop. Because prospective studies take so long to carry out and involve so many subjects when investigating rare diseases, financial costs are typically too high to be practicable. In contrast, case-control studies are relatively quick and are economical to carry out. Table 8.3 summarizes the advantages and disadvantages of case-control studies.

An example of a case-control study is one that was carried out by Carpenter and colleagues[25] to examine the relationship between developing lung cancer and alcohol consumption. They reported that there was an association between recent hard-liquor consumption and lung cancer risk, with an OR of 1.87. Thus, the odds of developing lung cancer in the drinking group was nearly twice that of the controls. Nevertheless, since smoking (a known risk factor for lung cancer) is much more common in drinkers than in nondrinkers, the authors adjusted their statistical results for smoking. Smoking was found to be a *confounding variable* in this situation that would have misrepresented the true relationship between alcohol consumption and lung cancer if its influence was not removed in the statistical analysis (Table 8.4).

TABLE 8.3 **Advantages and disadvantages of case-control studies**

Advantages	• Good for investigating rare diseases • Can be performed quickly and inexpensively • Useful for studying diseases with long latency period between exposure and manifestation • Facilitate the study of multiple potential causes at once • Existing records can often be used
Disadvantages	• Typically rely on patients' recall of past exposures • Do not permit calculation of true disease rates in the population • Difficult to validate information on exposure • Other variables that may be associated with the disease are not controlled

Chapter 8 Epidemiology

TABLE 8.4 Interpreting odds ratios

OR = 1   Disease risk is equal in the exposed and unexposed groups.
OR > 1   Exposure increases disease risk.
OR < 1   Exposure reduces disease risk.

Coffee drinking is another exposure that has been positively associated with lung cancer, although the association is spurious. Like alcohol consumption, this relationship is susceptible to confounding because coffee drinkers too are more likely to be smokers.[26] However, confounding is even more dramatic in this case: When independently considering coffee drinking and its effect on developing lung cancer, there is no relationship at all. A commonly used tool that can distinguish confounding variables from true exposure–disease associations is a *stratified analysis*, which looks at the effect each of the independent variables has on the outcome separately. This type of analysis divides a study's data into strata of homogenous subgroups to determine if an association observed in the undivided aggregate data holds true during the stratified analysis.

Consider a hypothetical case-control study investigating the relationship between coffee drinking and lung cancer that was made up of 100 cases and 100 controls. Among the cases, 70 were exposed to coffee and 30 were not, while among the controls 40 were exposed to coffee and 60 were not. These data may be arranged in a two-by-two contingency table as follows:

		Cases	Controls
Coffee drinking	Exposed	70 (a)	40 (b)
	Not exposed	30 (c)	60 (d)

Using the OR formula presented earlier, the odds of developing lung cancer among the coffee drinkers may be calculated as follows:

Case-Control Studies

$$\text{OR} = \frac{ad}{bc} = \frac{70 \times 60}{30 \times 40} = 3.5 \ (95\% \, \text{CI} = 1.95 \text{ to } 6.27)$$

When specifically looking at the groups' exposure to cigarette smoking, the odds ratio is much higher. Seventy-five of the cases were exposed to smoking and 25 were not, while only 30 controls were exposed and 70 were not:

Smokers:

		Cases	Controls
Cigarette smoking	Exposed	75 (a)	30 (b)
	Not exposed	25 (c)	70 (d)

$$\text{OR} = \frac{75 \times 70}{30 \times 25} = 7.0 \ (95\% \, \text{CI} = 3.77 \text{ to } 13.02)$$

However, when the coffee drinkers are stratified into a separate group based on their nonsmoking status, the OR becomes 1.0. Consequently, no risk would be attributable to the exposure to coffee:

Nonsmokers:

		Cases	Controls
Coffee drinking	Exposed	15 (a)	42 (b)
	Not exposed	10 (c)	28 (d)

$$\text{OR} = \frac{15 \times 28}{42 \times 10} = 1.0 \ (95\% \, \text{CI} = 0.40 \text{ to } 2.50)$$

There are two general categories of case-control studies, based on the time frame when the cases develop disease, using either the prevalence or the incidence of cases. *Prevalent case* case-control studies include all persons with the disease during the observation period. An example would be a study that included all migraine headache cases examined at a chiropractic clinic between 2000 and 2005. *Cumulative incidence* case-control studies, on the other hand, involve the selection of new (incident) cases during the period of observation.

Cohort Studies

Cohort studies follow groups of subjects forward in time and compare their outcomes after one group is exposed to some known or suspected cause of disease while the other group is not exposed. Because they follow subjects forward in time, often for years or even decades, they are sometimes called *longitudinal* or *prospective studies*. These studies begin with the identification of a population, from which two or more groups of patients are selected (the cohorts). Subjects in one of the cohorts are exposed to a factor or factors (or were exposed to it in the past), whereas those in the other group are not exposed. The supposition in cohort studies is that the factor or factors will have an effect on the likelihood of developing some outcome or disease. Outcomes are assessed for the groups prospectively during a defined period of time to determine whether any differences between the groups can be observed. If the factor or factors under study are a cause of the disease, more subjects should develop the disease in the exposed cohort than in the unexposed cohort (Figure 8.4).

Cohort studies are capable of detecting whether an exposure precedes a particular health outcome because subjects are observed prior to developing a disease; hence, they satisfy one of the main prerequisites in determining causation. Furthermore, because the exposure level is evaluated before disease develops, they are much less subject to bias than case-control studies. Consequently, cohort studies are the best available design when attempting to determine the level of risk associated with a particular exposure to a harmful substance. If the factors that increase the likelihood of developing a disease can be identified, then appropriate control measures can be devised, even if the precise etiology of the problem has not yet been established. Cohort studies are considered observational, however, because the researcher does not determine the level of exposure through

FIGURE 8.4 Cohort studies follow a disease-free group of subjects forward in time. Some in the cohort are exposed to a risk factor, while others are not. The purpose is to see if there is a greater proportion of disease among those exposed to the risk factor.

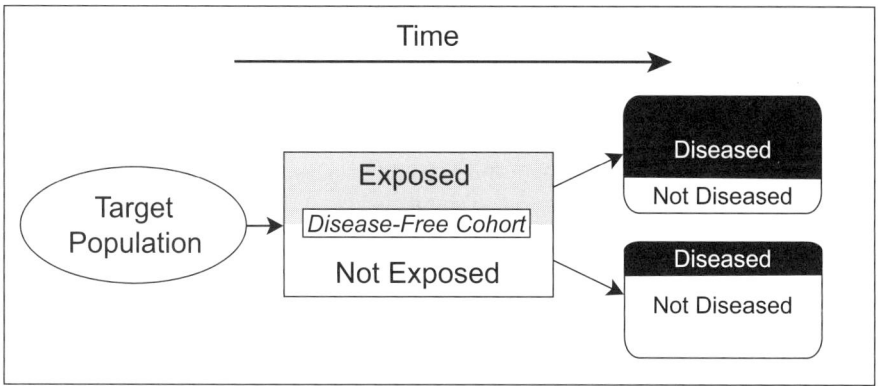

random assignment, as in experimental research, but merely observes events as they naturally unfold.[3]

Cohort studies are most useful in the investigation of reasonably common diseases because of the complexity and expense involved in assembling cohorts that are large enough to investigate rare diseases. For instance, to study an uncommon condition that has an incidence rate of 10/100,000 per year, each cohort would have to include 100,000 subjects in order to identify 100 subjects with the disease over a 10-year period. Accordingly, cohort studies are the most difficult and expensive type of epidemiologic study to carry out. On the other hand, they are generally easier to administer and less costly than RCTs. They are usually more acceptable than RCTs from an ethical perspective as well, since treatment is not withheld from one of the groups, nor is a potentially harmful treatment involved (Table 8.5).

A basic two-by-two contingency table, as was illustrated in Table 8.2, is often used to analyze the data from cohort studies. Unlike case-control studies, which calculate the odds of developing a disease in persons exposed to a risk factor in the past, cohort studies are capable of determining risk, which in this case is

TABLE 8.5	Advantages and disadvantages of cohort studies
Advantages	• Portray the natural history of disease • Do not rely on patient recall • Better for establishing a cause-and-effect relationship than case-control studies • Less vulnerability to bias or chance • Permit calculation of true disease rates in the population
Disadvantages	• Typically very expensive • Many people must be followed to obtain enough with the disease • Very time-consuming, since people start out well and one must wait for them to develop the disease • Subjects frequently drop out of the study over time • Difficult to generate a control group to study very common conditions

represented by *relative risk* (RR). RR compares the risk of some health-related event occuring in two groups that are included in a prospective study. It is the probability of disease occurrence in the exposed group, divided by the probability of disease in the unexposed group. Referring to the cells presented in Table 8.2 (although new headings must be assigned to the columns, such as "Disease" versus "No disease"), the formula for calculating RR is as follows:

$$\frac{a/(a+b)}{c/(c+d)} = \frac{\text{Probability of disease in exposed group}}{\text{Probability of disease in unexposed group}}$$

If the calculated RR is different from 1, the risk factor is considered to be associated with the risk of disease. If the RR is greater than 1, the association is positive; if it is less than 1, the association is negative or protective. For instance, RR = 2 means that the incidence rate of disease in the exposed group was twice that of the unexposed group. If RR = 0.8, there would be a 20% reduction in the incidence rate of the exposed group, as compared with the unexposed group. In other words, the factor had a protective effect on the probability of developing the disease. A good example of a protective effect was evident in a cohort study that followed 40,349 Japanese men and women over an 18-year period regarding their vegetable and fruit consumption in relation to stroke mortality.[27] The authors reported that when comparing the group of study participants who consumed vegetables and fruits once or less per week with those who consumed vegetables and fruits daily, there was a risk reduction of between 20% and 40%.

Attributable risk (AR) is another measure of association that is often presented in reports of longitudinal studies; it is the probability of disease in the exposed group *minus* the probability of disease in the unexposed group. Hence, AR represents the excess risk that is accounted for by exposure to the factor under investigation. The formula for calculating AR is

$$\frac{a}{a+b} - \frac{c}{c+d}$$

Table 8.6 is a two-by-two contingency table of the results of a hypothetical cohort study investigating the relationship between exposure to assembly line

TABLE 8.6 **Two-by-two contingency table comparing exposures in a cohort study of assembly line work and the risk of carpal tunnel syndrome**

	Carpal tunnel syndrome	
	Yes	No
Exposed (a, b)	85	500
Not exposed (c, d)	25	950

(Assembly line work)

Exposed disease rate = 85/(85 + 500) = 0.145
Unexposed disease rate = 25/(25 + 950) = 0.026

$$RR = \frac{0.145}{0.026} = 5.7 \ (95\% \, CI = 3.6 \text{ to } 9.0)$$

AR = 0.145 − 0.026 = 0.119

work and developing carpal tunnel syndrome (CTS). Based on the exposed disease rate of 0.145, the rate of disease occurrence in the exposed group would be 145/1,000. Likewise, the unexposed disease rate of 0.026 is equivalent to 26/1,000. The RR equals 5.7 in this case; thus, an assembly line worker would be 5.7 times more likely to develop CTS than those in the unexposed cohort. The AR equals 0.119 (119/1,000), which means that working on an assembly line in this study resulted in an increase of risk above the unexposed group of 119 CTS cases per 1,000 workers.

There are a few terms relating to risk that are commonly used to describe the effects of treatments utilized in either RCTs or cohort studies.[28,29] *Absolute risk reduction* (ARR) is the difference in the probability of disease between the treatment and control groups. The formula for calculating ARR is the same as the one presented earlier for attributable risk; however, in this case, the result describes how much of the difference in the reduction of disease incidence between the groups can be attributed to the treatment. *Relative risk reduction* (RRR) is the comparative reduction in rates of bad outcomes between the experimental and control groups. Although commonly reported in health care articles, RRR is not a very good way to compare outcomes because it magnifies small differences, making clinically insignificant findings appear significant.[30] RRR is calculated as follows:

$$\frac{[a/(a+b)]-[c/(c+d)]}{c/(c+d)} = \frac{\text{Absolute risk reduction}}{\text{Probability of disease in unexposed group}}$$

Another term used to describe risk in longitudinal studies that involve treatments is the *number needed to treat* (NNT), which is the number of patients who would need to be treated in order to prevent one additional bad outcome. NNT is calculated as follows:

$$\frac{1}{[a/(a+d)]-[c/(c+d)]} = \frac{1}{\text{Absolute risk rduction}}$$

For example, if an exercise program reduced the risk of construction workers developing disabling lower back injuries from 20% to 10%, then the ARR is the amount the intervention reduced the risk of the bad outcome. In this case, ARR = 10%. The NNT is 1 divided by 10%, which is 10; so, in order to save one worker from developing a disabling lower back injury, 10 of them must be involved in the intervention.

The Centre for Evidence-Based Medicine (CEBM) at the University of Toronto offers free online calculators that can easily perform these and other calculations. The web address for the CEBM calculators is http://www.cebm.utoronto.ca/practise/ca/statscal/. This web page has downloadable software for handheld computers that is capable of performing the same statistical tasks.

Some exposures are either present or absent, resulting in dichotomous exposure variables (e.g., smoker versus nonsmoker), although some exposures vary by degrees (e.g., cholesterol levels) and produce continuous variables. When continuous variables are involved, subjects are usually divided into groups for analysis based on whether their scores are high or low; mild, moderate, or severe; or some other rating scheme that is capable of categorizing continuous data. As with exposures, outcome measures and disease status are not always merely present or absent, but can also involve categorical or continuous data.

Sometimes cohort studies only involve one group of subjects, all of whom have some factor in common. These studies are referred to as *single-group cohort studies*, *longitudinal studies*, or *inception cohort studies*. Examples of factors that subjects in single group cohort studies may have in common are the early stage of a disease, exposure to a risk factor, or a positive screening test. The cohort (sometimes referred to as the inception cohort) is regularly evaluated in a longitudinal manner in order to monitor the progression of disease. In chronic diseases, these studies can also be used to observe the intervals of time that lead to changes in outcome measures. Inception cohort studies produce descriptive data that can be helpful in the analysis of trends, health care planning, and hypothesis generation.

Appraisal Tactics

Because they all deal with diseases in populations, epidemiologic study designs have many comparable features that permit a common approach to appraisal. In general, each design involves choosing a population, selecting a sample, observing the study participants, and then analyzing the data to determine the rates of disease and any relationships with risk factors that may exist.

As mentioned earlier, random selection diminishes the influence of a number of potential biases and is therefore preferred. Nevertheless, even when random selection is employed, there are still factors that can methodologically weaken an epidemiologic study. For instance, the response rate to follow-up evaluations or questionnaires is sometimes low. A low response rate may be because responders are different from nonresponders in some meaningful way. An example would be a questionnaire about occupational risk factors that was mailed to participants in a study that involved a cohort of former workers at a given factory. Employees who were out of work because of work-related disabilities might be more likely to respond to the questionnaire for several reasons. They would most likely have more time to complete the questionnaire, since they would not be working; also, because they acquired their disability at work, they might be displeased with the former employer and more motivated to reply. These disabled persons would likely report more exposures to occupational risk factors than nonresponders, thus providing a skewed representation of the workplace.

Articles that deal with epidemiologic methods contain some unique elements that should be considered when reading them and assessing their quality. Please refer to the *checklist for the appraisal of epidemiologic articles* in Appendix 6, which will facilitate the appraisal of these articles. As with other study designs, there are some specific questions that the reader should ask, which are as follows:

- *What is the study's main objective?* An article reporting on an epidemiologic study should clearly state the primary reason why it was carried out. Without a stated objective, the reader can never be certain that the authors conducted the research with a purpose or whether they were in reality conducting a fishing expedition. Stating research objectives is often accomplished by posing a study question in the Introduction section of the article. For example, the objective of an epidemiologic study might be as follows: "Is there a positive relationship between a history of wearing shoes with high heels and low back pain in middle aged females?" Another example of a study objective would be "To identify the risk factors for lumbar degenerative disc disease in factory workers."

- *Was the study population clearly identified?* Some articles describe the sampling methods that were employed, the inclusion and exclusion criteria that were applied, and features of the resulting sample, but fail to provide adequate details about the study population. This information is vital to the external validity of the study, however, and represents a flaw when missing or deficient. An example would be a study that derived participants from a senior citizen center. This population source would result in a very limited capacity to generalize the study's findings to the general population. Any risk factors identified in this group may not apply to other age groups or in other settings, or both.

- *Did cases and controls originate from the same population?* Study participants should be comparable on as many factors as is feasible, other than the exposure or exposures at question. Indeed, many times cases and controls (or cohorts) are matched with regard to factors such as age, gender, health status, and so forth. Consider a study investigating risk factors for developing low back pain among factory workers, where cases were selected from employees at the factory, while controls originated from food service employees of a restaurant chain. This design would be problematic because there are two distinct populations involved and each would be exposed to unique risk factors that could contribute to low back pain in either group. Furthermore, differences in outcomes could merely be the result of the dissimilar work environments involving factors such as the amount of time spent walking, job stress, or exposure to heavy lifting. In contrast, if both the cases and controls were chosen from among the population of factory workers, it would be much easier to distinguish exposure levels.

- *Did sufficient numbers of subjects complete the study?* A high dropout rate may introduce bias into the study because subjects who dropped out may have somehow been different from those who completed the study. For example, in a hypothetical cohort study investigating the relationship between heavy labor and back problems, suppose many in the cohort of laborers quit work due to back pain. They would therefore be lost to follow-up, since they were no longer employed, which would result in a flawed estimate of risk.

- *Was the appropriate study design used?* To a large extent, the appropriate study design in epidemiologic research depends on the rarity of the disease being studied. Case-control designs can be suitably used with common diseases, but they are best utilized with rare conditions, since persons who already have the disease are selected at the beginning of the study. Cohort designs, on the other hand, are not feasible with rare conditions because very large cohorts are required in order to accumulate enough cases for the results to be statistically meaningful. Consequently, cohort studies are best suited to investigate factors associated with more common diseases.

When there is a very long interval between the exposure and the outcome, case-control designs are preferred over cohort designs, essentially because they are less demanding to carry out. Also, cohorts would have to be followed throughout this long interval to wait for the condition to develop. Since people are exposed to a variety of risks, it may be very difficult to discern which factors are truly related to the condition.

Another consideration regarding appropriate study design is that there is a much greater potential for bias in case-control and cross-sectional studies than with cohort studies. This is the primary reason cohort studies were placed above case-control studies in the hierarchy of study designs that was presented in Chapter 1. As a result, cohort studies come closer to establishing cause-and-effect relationships, although consistent findings between other studies are still necessary. Keep this in mind when authors of cohort studies suggest that certain risk factors actually caused related outcomes.

- *Were the exposures adequately described?* Authors should list all of the exposures/factors that are to be studied and provide information on how they will be measured. They should also discuss the accuracy and precision of the measurement methods and demonstrate that they can reliably be used to assess the exposure variables. Accurate measurement of exposure and outcome variables is very important when attempting to identify associations in epidemiologic studies. Better studies characterize the magnitude or duration of the exposures, or both, which can provide information needed to determine dose-response relationships.

- *Was the outcome clearly defined?* An epidemiologic article should explain how the presence or absence of the outcome was determined, and the same method of measurement should be used in both groups. The method of measurement that is utilized should also have established validity and reliability. Studies should only investigate one outcome at a time because each outcome is likely to have a variety of associated risk factors, often making it difficult to identify which risk specific factor corresponds to which outcome.

- *Is it readily apparent that the exposure preceded the outcome?* This question applies especially to case-control studies where the temporality of exposures is determined retrospectively, and it is not always as straightforward as one would think. For instance, a relationship between depression and chronic pain following whiplash injuries is often cited in the literature, but there is debate about whether depressed patients are more likely to develop chronic whiplash pain[31] or whether patients become depressed as a result of the chronic pain.[32] This type of problem is also challenging when attempting to determine the temporal relationship between cervical manipulation and vertebral artery dissection.[33] The symptoms of spontaneous vertebral artery dissection include neck pain and headache, which prompt patients to seek chiropractic treatment. When the dissection progresses to ischemic stroke following the cervical manipulation, the relationship may have been merely temporal, not causal. There is no good way to make that kind of determination at this time.

- *Was an association observed? If so, how strong is it?* If a study reports an association between a factor and an outcome, the strength of the association will be reported as a RR in cohort studies or an OR in case-control studies. To decide whether these results are meaningful, consider the relative strength of the association and whether it is statistically significant. To determine whether the RR or OR is statistically significant, check to see if their reported confidence intervals include the value 1, which corresponds to no association. If the confidence interval does include 1, then the results would not be considered statistically significant. Alternatively, p values may be reported, which should be less than or equal to 0.05 to reach statistical significance. A weak association that does not quite reach statistical significance will not be very useful to a clinician, but may point to the need for further research using larger samples or better methodology or both. When a statistically significant relationship between factors and an outcome is presented, one must also determine whether it is clinically important. For instance, suppose a study reported that a 50% reduction in fat consumption resulted in statistically significant reduction in the incidence of colon cancer, but the latter reduction was only 5%. The major lifestyle changes involved would not be reasonable, given the very small reduction in risk. Furthermore, there may be additional risks that negatively affect health that result from the very low fat diet.

    Another thing to consider about the strength of an association is that it is one of the key criteria for determining causation. The stronger an association is, the less likely it is to be due to chance or bias. Conversely, weak associations sometimes occur in small studies just by chance, although the results will usually fail to reach statistical significance.

- *What biases potentially influenced the results of the study?* There are many possible sources of error in epidemiologic research, which can be classified into two main categories of bias: *selection bias*, which is the result of errors that occur in the process of selecting participants, and *observation bias* (also known as *information bias*), which has to do with errors that occur during data collection. Another potential source of error has to do with confounding, which is the result of extraneous variables affecting the observed association. Extraneous variables are variables that were not included in the study design but are associated with the exposure and outcome, affecting the results of the study one way or the other.

  Several types of observation bias should be considered when reading epidemiologic articles. *Recall bias* is of particular concern in case-control studies and occurs when persons in each group report their prior exposures differently. It occurs in cohort studies when participants report ensuing exposures differently. Another type of bias is the use of outcome measures that lack reliability or validity or both, which seriously weakens the authority of the study's results. Accordingly, articles should be examined to verify that the reliability and validity of outcome measures have been addressed. *Evaluator bias* occurs when there are systematic differences in the way information is gathered from study participants. This bias is suspected especially when evaluators know the status of patients' exposures or conditions prior to assessing outcomes. Cohort studies are subject to *follow-up bias*, which occurs when some of the study participants are lost to follow-up. As a result, their outcomes are not measured. Because dropouts may be different from those who remain in the study, loss of participants to follow-up can be a major source of bias.

- *Was the statistical analysis appropriate?* Confirm that the relationship between exposures and outcome is presented appropriately; that is, RR is utilized with prospective studies, and OR with retrospective. All variables presented in the Methods section of the article should be included in the statistical analysis; if not, there is no way for readers to determine whether important findings have been obscured.

- *Were the study's conclusions supported by the evidence that was presented?* Conclusions should be logically derived from the study's results, without speculation or unsupported statements. Nonetheless, authors of epidemiologic research reports sometimes overstep their bounds and suggest such things as cause-and-effect relationships, overgeneralization of findings, or expecting patients to change behaviors based on weak associations. In general, authors should not attempt to make inferences about associations without experimental studies that include randomization and comparison groups. Findings should also be in agreement with what was proposed in the introduction and discussion.
- *Should patients modify their behaviors to avoid the risk factors that were presented?* If the results of just one small case-control study suggested that the odds of developing carpal tunnel syndrome increased by 10% after prolonged exposure to keyboard work, practitioners would probably not take any action. Furthermore, most individuals would not make the effort to restrict their activities just to reduce their risk by 10%. However, if several case-control studies and a large cohort study showed that persons exposed to prolonged keyboard work were nearly five times as likely to develop carpal tunnel syndrome, practitioners should urge their patients to modify or limit their keyboard use, and many would be compliant.

A number of other considerations must be taken into account before a practitioner should apply the findings of epidemiologic research to his or her patients. The utility of such research depends on (1) the appropriateness of the research design, (2) the clinical and biological plausibility of the results, (3) the validity of the research methodology, (4) the representativeness and size of the sample, (5) the strength and significance of relationships that are presented, and (6) the consistency of the results with other research. This last point is probably the most important issue regarding the ability to generalize results to patients in your practice.

References

1. Green, L.W., and J.M. Ottoson. *Community and Population Health*. 8th ed. 1999. Boston: WCB/McGraw-Hill.
2. Stolley, P.D., and T. Lasky. *Investigating Disease Patterns: The Science of Epidemiology*. 1995. New York: Scientific American Library.

3. Greenberg, R. *Medical Epidemiology*. 1993. Norwalk: Appleton & Lange, 146.
4. Coggon, D., G. Rose, and D. Barker. *Epidemiology for the Uninitiated*. 4th ed. 1997. London: BMJ Publishing Group.
5. Manchikanti, L., et al. *Prevalence of facet joint pain in chronic spinal pain of cervical, thoracic, and lumbar regions*. BMC Musculoskeletal Disorders, 2004. **5**(1):15.
6. Streiner, D.L., G.R. Norman, and H.M. Blum. *PDQ Epidemiology*. 1989. Philadelphia.
7. Centers for Disease Control and Prevention. *National Diabetes Fact sheet: General Information and National Estimates on Diabetes in the United States, 2003*. Rev ed. 2004. Atlanta: U.S. Department of Health and Human Services.
8. Warner, K.E. *What's a cigarette company to do?* Am J Public Health, 2002. **92**(6):897–900.
9. Ruano-Ravina, A., A. Figueiras, and J.M. Barros-Dios. *Lung cancer and related risk factors: An update of the literature*. Public Health, 2003. **117**(3):149–56.
10. Warner, K.E. *The role of research in international tobacco control*. Am J Public Health, 2005. **95**(6):976–84.
11. Ruano-Ravina, A., et al. *Dose-response relationship between tobacco and lung cancer: New findings*. Eur J Cancer Prev, 2003. **12**(4):257–63.
12. Hill, A.B., *The environment and disease: Association or causation?* Proc R Soc Med, 1965. **58**(?):295–300.
13. Doll, R. *Sir Austin Bradford Hill and the progress of medical science*. BMJ, 1992. **305**(6868):1521–6.
14. Morgan, M.T. *Environmental Health*. 2nd ed. 1997. Belmont: Wadworth Group.
15. Pope, M., K. Goh, and M. Magnusson. *Spine ergonomics*. Annu Rev Biomed Eng, 2002. **4**:49–68.
16. Frost, P., and J. Andersen. *Shoulder impingement syndrome in relation to shoulder intensive work*. Occup Environ Med, 1999. **56**(7):494–8.
17. Feskanich, D., W.C. Willett, and G.A. Colditz. *Calcium, vitamin D, milk consumption, and hip fractures: A prospective study among postmenopausal women*. Am J Clin Nutr, 2003. **77**(2):504–11.
18. Grimes, D.A., and K.F. Schulz. *Descriptive studies: What they can and cannot do*. Lancet, 2002. **359**(9301):145–9.
19. Pearce, N. *Introduction*. In *A Short Introduction to Epidemiology*. 2005. Wellington, NZ: Massey University, 9.
20. *Canadian Stroke Consortium*. 2002. http://www.strokeconsortium.ca/.
21. Packard, R.C. *Epidemiology and pathogenesis of posttraumatic headache*. J Head Trauma Rehabil, 1999. **14**(1):9–21.
22. Leboeuf-Yde, C., et al. *Back pain reporting in children and adolescents: The impact of parents' educational level*. J Manipulative Physiol Ther, 2002. **25**(4):216–20.
23. Sorensen, H.T., and M.W. Gillman. *Matching in case-control studies*. BMJ, 1995. **310**(6975):329–30.
24. Evans, S.J. *Good surveys guide*. BMJ, 1991. **302**(6772):302–3.
25. Carpenter, C.L., H. Morgenstern, and S.J. London. *Alcoholic beverage consumption and lung cancer risk among residents of Los Angeles County*. J Nutr, 1998. **128**(4):694–700.
26. Stensvold, I., and B.K. Jacobsen. *Coffee and cancer: A prospective study of 43,000 Norwegian men and women*. Cancer Causes Control, 1994. **5**(5):401–8.

27. Sauvaget, C., et al. *Vegetable and fruit intake and stroke mortality in the Hiroshima/Nagasaki life span study. Stroke*, 2003. **34**(10):2355–60.
28. Barratt, A., et al. *Tips for learners of evidence-based medicine: 1. Relative risk reduction, absolute risk reduction and number needed to treat. CMAJ*, 2004. **171**(4):353–8.
29. Sackett, D.L., et al. *Evidence-Based Medicine: How to Practice and Teach EBM*. 2nd ed. 2000. Edinburgh: Churchill Livingstone.
30. Flaherty, R.J. *A simple method for evaluating the clinical literature. Fam Pract Manag*, 2004. **11**(5):47–52.
31. Kivioja, J., M. Sjalin, and U. Lindgren. *Psychiatric morbidity in patients with chronic whiplash-associated disorder. Spine*, 2004. **29**(11):1235–9.
32. Wallis, B.J., et al. *The psychological profiles of patients with whiplash-associated headache. Cephalalgia*, 1998. **18**(2):101–5; discussion 72–3.
33. Haldeman, S., F.J. Kohlbeck, and M. McGregor. *Stroke, cerebral artery dissection, and cervical spine manipulation therapy. J Neurol*, 2002. **249**(8):1098–104.

NINE

Reliability and Validity Designs

The ability to measure phenomena accurately and consistently is extremely important in research, as well as in clinical practice. Without accurate and consistent measures, it would be virtually impossible to make the kind of comparisons that are needed to monitor patients' progress in practice or to accurately assess differences between groups in clinical trials. The *reliability* of a test refers to its ability to provide consistent results when repeated by the same examiner or when more than one examiner tests the same attribute in the same group of subjects. The type of test involved may be a physical observation, a questionnaire, or some kind of measuring device. To illustrate the importance of reliability, think of a weight-loss study that measured patients' progress using an unreliable scale that registered a different reading, varying by 10 to 20 pounds, each time the same subject stepped on. The results of the study would undoubtedly be invalid, and if that unreliable scale were used in a clinical setting, patients' progress could not be evaluated accurately.

A scale with an error of this magnitude would most likely be obvious to the examiner and a correction would be made promptly, but some flawed measures are not so noticeable. To cite an example, motion palpation is used by thousands of chiropractors in both clinical and research settings, although several studies have pointed out that it does not produce especially consistent findings when different doctors examine the same patients.[1-3] Even though speaking from personal experience, the test surely gives the impression of being reproducible to the examiner. Also, certain motion palpation procedures have fared better under scrutiny than others,[4] and the regions of the spine differ in their amenability to examination by this procedure. Fortunately, there are specific research designs available that can determine the degree of reliability of tests and measures to help researchers and practitioners choose the best investigative tools.

Tests should also be valid in order to be useful to practitioners or researchers. The *validity* of a test or measuring device refers to the degree to which it actually measures what it is intended to measure. If a test is valid, changes in the characteristic that is being measured will result in corresponding changes in the measurement that represent true differences among the persons being tested. On the other hand, if a test does not reflect changes in patients very well, its validity will be diminished.

All measurements are subject to some degree of error. Even a test that seems outwardly simple, such as checking leg lengths, does not produce the same results each time it is repeated.[2] In fact, it has been recommended that differences in leg lengths should exceed about 4 mm before an examiner confidently concludes that a real change has occurred.[5] This unreliability may occur as a result of the different ways examiners move the legs about during the test or the perspective from which they observe the heels. There may also be variability of the subject being tested due to positioning on the table, reflex muscle contractions, and so on.

Since all measurements have some degree of error, any given test score will actually be composed of a true score plus an error component. Thus,

$$\text{Observed score} = \text{True score} + \text{Error}$$

If it were obtainable, a true score would be the result of a measurement derived from a perfect instrument in an ideal environment. True score theory considers that when observing the scores of a group of subjects, there will be variation of the true scores that is related to individual differences of the subjects and there will be variation that is due to an error component. Thus, the scores derived from a group of individuals will always be variable, and the variability will generate a distribution of true scores and error that approximates the normal curve when the sample size is large enough. Because variability of test scores conforms to the normal curve, groups in a study designed to establish the reliability of a test can be compared using various parametric statistical tests.

Reliability and Validity Designs

Errors can occur randomly, due to chance variation, or systematically because of factors that are constant. *Random errors* are caused by fluctuations of measurement that can be attributable to the examiner, the subject, or the measuring instrument that is utilized. Random errors are just as likely to bring about higher scores as they are lower scores; hence, they do not have an effect on a group's mean score. For instance, blood pressure readings are rarely the same when repeated on the same subject, which may be due to factors such as arm positioning, stethoscope placement, background noise, emotional disposition of the patient, time of day, and so forth. The subject's blood pressure may go up or down in response to any of these factors. *Systematic errors*, on the other hand, move scores in one direction, either higher or lower, in response to a factor that is having a constant effect on the measurement system (Figure 9.1). Accordingly, systematic error is considered to be a form of bias. Continuing with the blood pressure example, if the sphygmomanometer was out of calibration so that it

FIGURE 9.1 Systematic error shifts the mean of a group's observed scores higher or lower than the true score. Random error affects the variability of scores.

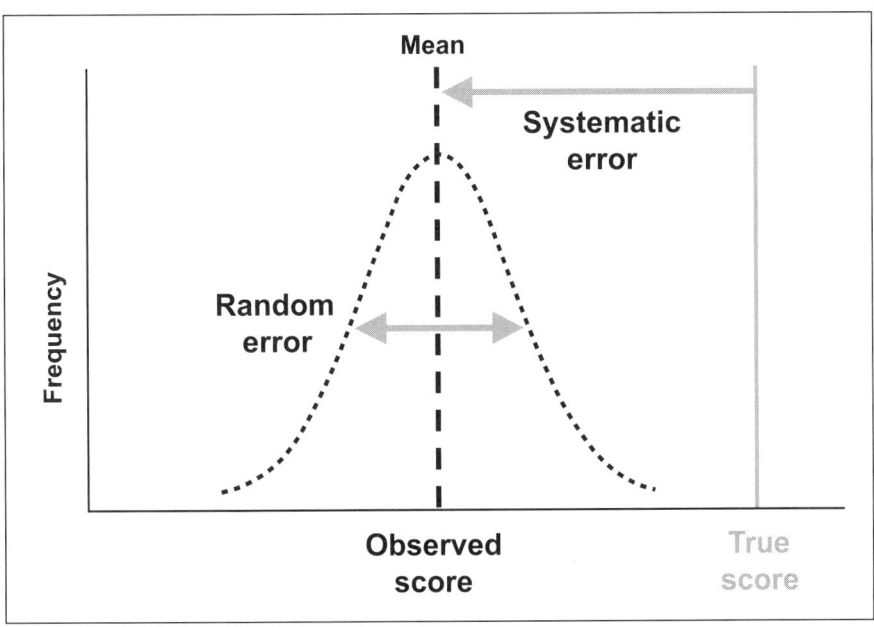

always generated elevated readings, the subject's score would predictably be high. Another example of systematic error would be a blood pressure study where patients were required to climb four flights of stairs to reach the examination site prior to each test. Subjects' overall scores would systematically be elevated as a result, which would be especially detrimental to the study's conclusions if subjects in the comparison group had their blood pressure taken on the ground floor.

Estimating Reliability

Reliability can be quantified in several different ways, depending on the type of reliability being tested as well as whether continuous, categorical, or dichotomous data is involved. The basis of calculating the reliability coefficient is similar for them all, however. One way of defining reliability is as the proportion of true score variance divided by the observed score variance. The observed score variance includes error variance in addition to the true score variance (Figure 9.2). *Error variance* is the portion of variability that is due to faults in measurement. *True score variance* is the result of real differences between subjects' scores that occur because people are biologically different or that occur when repeated measures are taken on an individual (e.g., fluctuations of blood pressure).

FIGURE 9.2 The observed score is comprised of the true score variance plus the error variance.

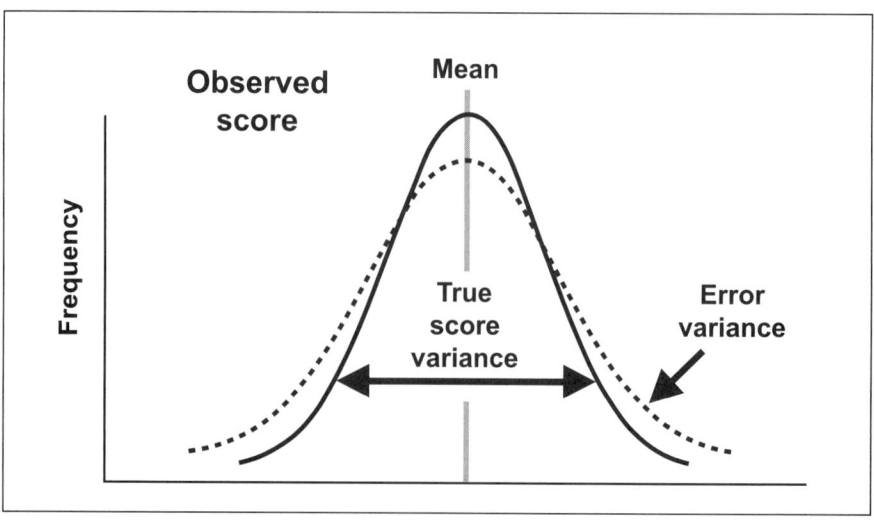

Estimates of reliability are often represented by the *reliability coefficient*, which may be calculated as follows:

$$\text{Reliability coefficient} = \frac{\text{True score variance}}{\text{True score variance} + \text{Error variance}}$$

Notice from this equation that the reliability coefficient gets larger as the error variance gets smaller, signifying increased reliability, and is equal to 1.0 when the error variance is 0.0. Conversely, the larger the error variance is, the smaller and less reliable the reliability coefficient is. Thus, the reliability coefficient ranges from 0.0 to 1.0, with 0.0 representing no reliability and 1.0 representing perfect reliability. A reliability coefficient of 0.75 means that 75% of the variance in the scores is due to the true variance of the trait being measured and 25% is due to the error variance. When the reliability coefficient is 0.75 or better, it is generally considered to indicate good reliability, whereas 0.5 to 0.75 points to moderate reliability, and less than 0.5 indicates poor reliability.

Establishing the reliability of a test often involves two or more examiners testing the same subjects for the same characteristic using the same measure and then ascertaining the degree to which their findings agree. If different examiners use the same instrument to score the same thing, their scores should match. This is called *interexaminer reliability* when comparisons are between different examiners. Another commonly used method to ascertain the reliability of a test is to have the same examiner test the same subjects on two or more occasions and then determine the degree to which the examiner agrees with himself or herself, which is called *intraexaminer reliability*. One way to quantify inter- or intraexaminer reliability is to compute the degree to which sets of scores are correlated. Correlation was covered in Chapter 4; briefly, it is a measure of the relationship that may exist between two or more variables. Thus, as two examiners perform the same test on the same group of subjects, there should be a high degree of correlation between their findings. In a reliable test, if one examiner finds subject's scores to be high, scores from the other examiner on the same subjects should also be high, and likewise if low. The problem with this method of ascertaining examiner reliability is that it is possible to have good correlation while there is concurrent poor agreement between the examiners. This occurs when one examiner consistently scores subjects higher or lower than the other examiner. As a result, correlation is rarely used by itself in reliability studies, although statistical tests that consider the degree of *agreement* between examiners are common (Table 9.1).

Tests should be reliable and produce consistent results when repeated, assuming there has been no change in whatever is being measured. To assess the *test-retest reliability* of a measure, a test is administered to the same group of individuals on more than one occasion to determine the degree of correlation between the test scores. Some conditions are changeable over time (e.g., pain) and are not good candidates for test-retest reliability studies. Therefore, when test-retest reliability is investigated, it is assumed that no change has occurred in the condition being considered between tests. Test-retest reliability is commonly used to assess questionnaires or instruments that operate automatically and are not directly controlled by the examiner.

Questionnaires are regularly used in clinical practice and research to assess patients' pain levels, disability status, satisfaction with treatment, and so on. Before using one of these questionnaires, practitioners and researchers need to know whether test-retest reliability has been established. An example study was carried out to document the test-retest reliability of a questionnaire designed to assess physical environmental factors that might be associated with physical activity in adults.[6] Subjects were asked questions about their access to exercise facilities, the facilitites' functionality and safety, aesthetics, and natural environment. The questionnaires were administered by telephone interviews and were given to the same group of subjects on two occasions, with an average of 16.8 days between interviews. The authors reported high reliability for some of the

TABLE 9.1 Types of test reliability

Interexaminer: Results of a measure are consistent between different examiners who are evaluating the same information.

Intraexaminer: Results of a measure are consistent when repeated by the same examiner.

Test-retest: Measures taken on two different occasions with no intervention in between will produce similar results.

Parallel forms: Two tests of different forms that theoretically test similar constructs will provide similar results.

Split-half reliability: Items in a questionnaire are divided in half and then the two halves are compared, which should give similar results.

questions and low reliability for others. This kind of information can be used to modify questionnaires for future use so that only questions with higher reliability are included.

Another estimate of reliability is *parallel-forms reliability* (also known as *alternate-forms reliability*), which compares two versions of a questionnaire or test that measure the same constructs. Both tests are administered to the same sample of subjects, and then the scores on the two forms are compared to determine the level of correlation between the two. When scores are similar, the parallel forms reliability is considered good and a correspondingly high correlation coefficient will be present. For example, a study might compare different devices used to measure cervical range of motion to determine the degree to which their findings correlate.

Internal consistency reliability is an estimate of the ability of each of the items in a questionnaire to actually measure the construct that is being targeted. Ideally, all questions should measure various characteristics of the construct and nothing else. The questionnaire is administered to a single group of people on one occasion, and then the results are examined to see how well questions that deal with the same construct correlate. A reliable instrument would incorporate questions that all contribute in a similar way to the questionnaire's overall score. For example, the Neck Disability Index (NDI) was developed to assess disability levels in neck pain patients.[7] The internal consistency reliability of the instrument was tested by administering it to 52 subjects and then calculating an alpha coefficient (also known as Cronbach's coefficient alpha) to test its internal consistency. Cronbach's coefficient alpha evaluates items in a questionnaire to determine whether they measure the same construct or if they are superfluous. Essentially, it is the mean correlation between each of a set of items. The maximum value for coefficient alpha is 1; at the other extreme, it can have a value that is less than 0 when a lot of negatively correlating items are included in a questionnaire. An instrument with a reliability coefficient value that is 0.70 or greater is generally considered to be acceptable. A study carried out by Vernon and Mior[7] concluded that the NDI was reliable because the coefficient alpha value was 0.80.

Kappa Statistic

When verifying the reliability of different tests and measures, a two-by-two contingency table can be very helpful to visualize the results of two examiners who

Chapter 9 Reliability and Validity Designs

are evaluating the same group of patients (Table 9.2). Referring to Table 9.2, the findings of rater 1 and rater 2 are in agreement in cells a and d, whereas they are in disagreement in cells b and c. Quite often journal articles that deal with interexaminer reliability will present their findings in the form of a two-by-two contingency table; if not, such tables are fairly easy to create from the data that is presented.

Agreement between two examiners can be represented by the overall percentage of agreement of paired ratings, although this quantity does not account for the amount of agreement that would be expected to occur merely by chance. Moreover, it is normally expected that when two examiners evaluate the same patients, there will be occasional agreements just by chance, even when using unreliable measures. Thus, only agreement that occurs beyond chance levels can be considered to represent true agreement. The *kappa statistic* is capable of quantifying the amount of true agreement that exists between two examiners because it considers the proportion of agreement that would be expected beyond chance.[8] Kappa is an appropriate statistic to use when dealing with dichotomous or nominal data.

TABLE 9.2 **A two-by-two contingency table comparing the findings of two examiners evaluating the same group of patients**

		Rater 2		
		Test +	Test −	Row Total
Rater 1	Test +	a (agree)	b (disagree)	$a + b$
	Test −	c (disagree)	d (agree)	$c + d$
	Column Total	$a + c$	$b + d$	$a + b + c + d$ Grand Total

Estimating Reliability 283

The basis for calculating the kappa statistic is as follows:

$$\text{Kappa} = \frac{\text{Observed agreement} - \text{Chance agreement}}{1 - \text{Chance agreement}}$$

In this formula, *observed agreement* is represented by P_O, which is the total proportion of observations where there is agreement. The definition of P_O and the formula for its calculation that is based on the two-by-two contingency table found in Table 9.2 are as follows:

$$P_O = \frac{\text{Number of } exact \text{ agreements}}{\text{Number of possible agreements}} \text{ or } \frac{a+d}{a+b+c+d}$$

Chance agreement is represented by P_C, which is the proportion of agreements that would be expected by chance. The definition of P_C is as follows:

$$P_C = \frac{\text{Number of } expected \text{ agreements}}{\text{Number of possible agreements}} \text{ or } \frac{a_{\text{expected}} + d_{\text{expected}}}{a+b+c+d}$$

The expected values are also found by using the two-by-two contingency table and applying the same procedure that was used for calculating expected cell values in the chi-square test presented in Chapter 4. Briefly, the expected value for each cell is found by multiplying the row total by the column total and then dividing by the grand total.

After the values of P_O and P_C have been calculated, they are utilized in the following formula to calculate the kappa statistic:

$$\text{Kappa} = \frac{P_O - P_C}{1 - P_C}$$

Referring to this equation, when the amount of observed agreement exceeds chance agreement, the resulting kappa will be positive. The magnitude of the calculated kappa statistic reflects the strength of agreement that is present. If the calculated kappa statistic is negative, it is an indication that the observed agreement between raters is less than what would be expected by chance. Perfect agreement is represented by a kappa value of 1, and chance agreement by a kappa value of 0,[9] although perfect agreement is very rare in the kinds of tests used by chiropractors. Various interpretations as to what represents a good level of agreement have been suggested for the calculated kappa statistic.[10,11] An interpretation of the kappa statistic is provided in Table 9.3.

Intraclass Correlation Coefficient

The kappa statistic is not appropriate when test results involve continuous variables; instead, the *intraclass correlation coefficient* (ICC) should be used to assess interexaminer reliability. The ICC is an index of reliability that ranges from below 0.0 to +1.0, with 1.0 representing strong reliability and 0.0 representing weak reliability. Table 9.4 presents several interpretations for ranges of calculated ICC values. Keep in mind, however, that these interpretations are merely suggestions and that the meaning of reliability that a particular ICC value points to depends on the nature of the measurement involved as well as the condition it is used to detect.

The most straightforward way to think of the ICC is as the ratio of between-groups variance to total variance, where between-groups variance is related to the

TABLE 9.3 Degree of agreement beyond chance for kappa values

Kappa Value	Agreement Beyond Chance
0	None
0–0.2	Slight
0.2–0.4	Moderate
0.4–0.6	Fair
0.6–0.8	Substantial
0.8–1.0	Almost perfect

Source: Adapted from Maclure, M., and W.C. Willett. Misinterpretation and misuse of the kappa statistic. *Am J Epidemiol*, 1987. **126**(2):161–9.

TABLE 9.4 Interpretation of intraclass correlation coefficient (ICC) values

ICC Value	Degree of Reliability
>0.75	Excellent
0.40–0.75	Fair to good
<0.40	Poor

fact that different subjects will have scores on the test that truly differ, and total variance is related to score differences attributed to the interrater unreliability of two or more examiners rating the same person.

The ICC is calculated using a two-way ANOVA test utilizing one of three possible models, the three models each utilize one of two different forms. Thus, there are six types of ICC, with six different corresponding formulas, that may be used. Determining which model to employ depends on how raters are chosen and how subjects are assigned. Computation of the ICC is rather complex; consequently, it will not be covered in this text. The reader is referred to Portney and Watkins' excellent book, *Foundations of Clinical Research: Applications to Practice*,[12] for a straightforward explanation.

When the ICC is used, the type of ICC should always be presented in research papers, along with a notation as to which model and form was employed. The first number represents the ICC model, and the second represents the form that was used. An example of how the ICC should be reported comes from a study that investigated the interexaminer reliability of the detection of lumbar lateral shift. Reliability of shift judgments was moderate ($ICC^{2,1}$ values ranging from 0.48 to 0.64).[13]

Validity

Tests and measurements used in research, as well as in clinical practice, should actually evaluate the traits they were intended to evaluate. The greater the degree of validity that a test has, the more likely it is that the resulting measures will represent real differences between subjects' scores and not systematic error. Hence, the level of test validity depends on the degree to which constant error has been controlled for.

The validity of a test depends to a great extent on its purpose. For instance, a sphygmomanometer is a valid instrument for measuring blood pressure but is not valid for measuring cerebrospinal fluid pressure. A chiropractic example would be leg length inequality, which has not been shown to be valid to predict the incidence of lower back pain,[14] although it is a reliable test when done on patients in the prone position.[15] Moreover, it is possible for a test to be reliable and at the same time be invalid. Consider a test that involves measurement of skull circumference to determine subjects' intelligence. The test would probably demonstrate excellent reliability, but it would not be a valid predictor of intelligence. Thus, to say it another way, an invalid test may be reliable. On the other hand, an unreliable test can never be considered valid.

The validity of a test is not an absolute judgment; rather, it is a matter of degrees. Accordingly, it is technically incorrect to refer to a test as being either "valid" or "invalid," although it is commonly done. A more logical way to refer to validity is based on categories that reflect the degree of validity for a given test (e.g., highly valid, moderately valid, or marginally valid), which can be established via evidence derived from studies that are capable of determining validity.

A number of different methods can be used to estimate the extent of validity for tests and measures; these can be divided into three major categories: self-evident, pragmatic, and construct validity. The *self-evident* methods involve a basic understanding of a test's apparent value as a measurement tool rather than its relative value. In other words, self-evident methods of assessing validity refer to whether the test appears to measure what it is supposed to measure.

The first self-evident method of establishing validity is *face validity*, which simply involves deciding whether the test appears to have merit "on face value." For example, a questionnaire that was designed to measure headache intensity could be considered to have face validity if it included questions about the location of head pain. Face validity is the lowest level of test validation and is used only at the beginning of inquiry, when very little is known about the variable being measured. If research has been carried out on the variable in question, then face validity is no longer adequate and more advanced methods of establishing validity are required. However, when researchers are exploring a new topic, discussion of face validity will likely be included.

The second self-evident validation method is *content validity*, which refers to the ability of a test to include or represent all of the content of a construct. For example, a new test designed to assess the level of radicular neurological involvement that only deals with muscle strength would have poor content validity. This is because tendon reflexes and superficial sensations are also major considerations in the construct of assessing radicular neurological involvement that must be included in the test; if they are left out, content validity would be lacking.

Another type of content validity involves comparing the content of the measurement technique under consideration with the literature that is available on the topic and then deciding whether the test accurately reflects what is in the literature. Therefore, content validity is usually assessed by means of a literature review or consultation with known experts in the field. The assembled information is critically reviewed and then compared with the measure under consideration to ensure that the content of the literature and the measure are in agreement. Hence, when developing new tests, the estimation of content validity is a vital part of the formative process.

The *pragmatic* methods of estimating the degree of test validity explore the practical value of a new test and consider whether it actually works as hypothesized. In other words, in practice, is the test capable of detecting which patients have or do not have the disease or condition? *Criterion-related validity* refers to how well a test corresponds with an external criterion that is an independent measure of the characteristic being tested. A *criterion* is the standard by which a measure is judged; thus, if a test is valid, it should correlate well with or predict some relevant criterion.

Concurrent and predictive validity are subgroups of criterion-related validity that compare a new test with another test either concurrently or in the future. *Concurrent validity* is a pragmatic method of evaluating a test that involves comparing the results of a new test with an established test, both given at the same point in time, to determine if there is an adequate degree of correlation. An established test is often referred to as a *gold standard* test (also known as *reference standard*), which can be defined as a test that is commonly acknowledged to be the best available. A few examples of typical gold standard measures are the results of blood tests, x-rays, and biopsies. For example, a new procedure to measure leg length could be tested for concurrent validity by comparing the results of the new method with scanogram x-rays (the gold standard), or a study that compares a clinical test to detect spondylolisthesis with x-ray findings. The use of high-quality gold standards in concurrent validity studies improves the legitimacy of the study's results.

Another pragmatic method of evaluating tests is *predictive validity*, which determines the extent to which a test can accurately predict some future event. Studies that are capable of ascertaining predictive validity measure some characteristic on one occasion and then wait to see if the projected outcome actually occurs at some time in the future. For example, Axen and associates[16] carried out a study to determine whether low back pain patients undergoing chiropractic care who reported improvements early in the course of treatment would have better outcomes than patients who showed little improvement by their fourth visit. They found that they could predict more favorable treatment outcomes in those who improved early. Thus, the "test" (early improvement) had predictive validity regarding the outcome (a favorable outcome). Tests that have good predictive validity are useful to practitioners in planning treatment and communicating prognostic information to patients.

Construct validity is essentially the extent to which a test adequately measures a theoretical construct (e.g., pain, disability). In construct validity, the characteristic being investigated is not observed directly; instead, an abstraction of the characteristic is observed (e.g., pain scale, disability questionnaire) that effectively corresponds to the construct being considered. Construct validity does not actually involve a specific type of research design or statistical test, but rather the amassing of evidence by establishing some of the other types of validity (e.g., convergent validity, discriminant validity, criterion-related validity. Construct validity, then, can be thought of as the accumulation of evidence that points to the ability of a test to actually measure what it claims to be measuring. Hence, several approaches using different methods to consider the same construct are used to evaluate construct validity. The validity of a test is supported if the results of these approaches are in agreement with one another. On the other hand, if they are contradictory, the validity of the test under consideration would be in doubt.

The construct validity of a test or measure is determined by comparing the test under consideration with other tests that measure a similar construct. Research designs that are capable of assessing construct validity examine other measures of the same construct that should correlate well with the new test. Another way to assess construct validity is to compare the new test with other measures that are different, but related, which should not correlate well.

Convergent validity refers to the degree of correlation that exists between a new test and another measure of the same or similar constructs. To say that something has good convergent validity, there should be a relatively high correlation between the new test and another measure of the same construct. Thus, if a questionnaire were developed that measured the functional ability of patients to move their necks during daily activities, it should correlate well with their clinical range of motion evaluations.

Discriminant validity (also known as *divergent validity*) is the extent to which the new test is found to be unrelated to another measure that it should actually be different from. Discriminant validity can thus be thought of as the opposite of convergent validity. For example, a measure of visual acuity and a measure of knee function should be independent of one another. An estimation of discriminant validity was present in a study that assessed the Motion Sensitivity Test (MST), which is used to evaluate dizziness in subjects during a series of rapid changes of head or body positions. The test is used by practitioners to develop exercise programs for patients with motion-provoked dizziness and to monitor their progress while receiving vestibular rehabilitation therapy. A study designed to assess the discriminant validity of the MST compared its ability to detect patients known to have motion-provoked dizziness against control subjects without the condition.[17]

An example of a study that investigated both the convergent and discriminant validity of a test is one by Gagnon and colleagues that dealt with the Standardized Finger-Nose Test (SFNT) in ataxic neuromuscular disorders.[18] The SFNT was compared with other upper extremity function tests, a functional independence measure, and social participation. The authors concluded that convergent validity was moderate to strong, based on positive correlations with gross and fine finger dexterity ($r = 0.82–0.84$), global upper extremity performance ($0.74–0.79$), functional independence ($r = 0.74$), and social participation ($r = 0.78$). They thought that discriminant validity was supported because there was a difference in upper extremity coordination between the older and younger age groups, with the older subjects performing significantly worse than those in the younger group. This suggested that the SFNT was able to discriminate between the different levels of function.

There are a number of different ways to present and classify the various types of validity. Table 9.5 consists of self-evident and pragmatic methods as major headings, with construct validity as a co-heading. Concurrent and predictive validity are subgroups of criterion-related validity.

The concept of the validity and reliability of measures can be compared with scores on a target (Figure 9.3). Errors of measurement occur either because the scores systematically miss the bull's-eye in one particular direction or because

TABLE 9.5 Types of validity for tests or measures

Self-evident
- *Face validity:* Whether the test appears to measure what it was intended to measure.
- *Content validity:* The test fully measures the construct of what it is supposed to measure.

Pragmatic
- *Construct validity*: The ability of a test to measure concepts or ideas that cannot be observed directly.
  - *Criterion-related validity:* The results of the test correlate well with the results of another test designed to measure the same thing.
    - *Concurrent validity:* The test correlates well with an established test that measures the same phenomenon.
    - *Predictive validity:* The test is capable of measuring a trait and then predicting an outcome.
  - *Convergent validity:* The extent to which a test correlates well with another measure of the same construct.
  - *Discriminant validity:* The extent to which a test does not correlate well with another test that it should not be related to.

FIGURE 9.3 The validity and reliability of tests and measures can be compared to the pattern of scores on a target. (A) When scores of a test are close to the bull's-eye, the test is considered to be valid. When scores are arranged in tight formation, the test is considered to be reliable. (B) When scores are off-center, the test is less valid. (C) When scores are scattered, the test is less reliable.

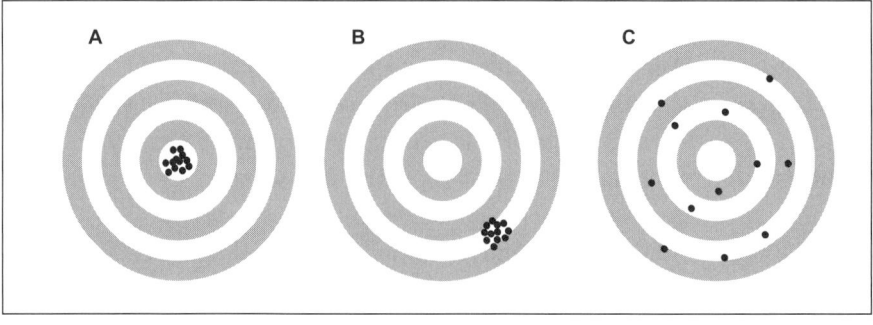

they are randomly scattered across the target. When scores are systematically off-center in one direction, it is the result of bias. Something has gone wrong with the test environment to cause all scores to be inaccurate. For instance, a scale used in a weight-loss study that is out of calibration and weighs everyone heavy by 15 pounds. When test scores are randomly off-center in any direction, it is the result of random error. Some subjects will be affected and others will not. When a test or measure is free from bias, it is considered to be *accurate*; when a test is free from random error, it is considered to be *precise*.[19]

Sensitivity and Specificity

A common way of establishing the validity of a test is to ascertain its *sensitivity* (the ability of a test to correctly identify people who have the target disorder), its *specificity* (the ability of a test to correctly identify people who do not have the target disorder), its *positive predictive value* (the probability that a positive test will correctly predict that the target disorder is present), and its *negative predictive value* (the probability that a negative test will correctly predict that the target disorder is not present).

Sensitivity provides information to clinicians on how good a test is at correctly identifying patients with the condition of interest. Specificity, on the other hand, provides information on how good the test is at correctly identifying patients who do *not* have the condition of interest.[20] Sensitivity and specificity are expressed as a percentage, with 0% corresponding to the absence of sensitivity or specificity and 100% to perfect sensitivity or specificity. These test indices can easily be calculated using a two-by-two contingency table, as depicted in Table 9.6. The appropriate formulas, along with several others, are presented in Table 9.7.

The results of many clinical tests are dichotomous, such as "positive" or "negative" findings, although ordinal and continuous scales are also commonly encountered. Moreover, the four levels of measurement that were mentioned in Chapter 4 (nominal, ordinal, interval, and ratio) are relevant to test outcomes. An example of a test that involves an ordinal scale is a pain scale that rates the level of pain as mild, moderate, or severe. Examples of tests that utilize a continuous scale are blood pressure and lifting capacity. To calculate sensitivity, specificity, and predictive values, the results of tests that involve ordinal and continuous measures must first be converted to a dichotomous scale. This dichotomization is accomplished by

TABLE 9.6 A two-by-two contingency table that depicts the relationship between rest results and a condition

		Condition (per "gold standard")		Row Total
		Present	Absent	
Test Result	Positive	a (True +)	b (False +)	$a + b$
	Negative	c (False −)	d (True −)	$c + d$
	Column Total	$a + c$	$b + d$	$a + b + c + d$ Grand Total

establishing a *cutoff point* so that scores above a specified value are considered positive and scores below that value are considered negative. Important information about the test may be lost when this is done, but it is necessary to facilitate the analysis of the test for sensitivity and specificity (Figure 9.4).

The cutoff point that is chosen has a direct influence on the test's sensitivity, specificity, and positive and negative predictive values. Changes in the cutoff point will cause one of these validity indices to increase while at the same time causing the value of the other one to decrease. Thus, if sensitivity rises, specificity will decrease, and vice versa.[21] This model is true for positive and negative predictive values as well, resulting in a similar inverse relationship. The precise value that is set for the cutoff point depends on whether it is desirable to maximize sensitivity at the expense of specificity or to maximize specificity at the expense of sensitivity. If sensitivity is maximized, the chance of a false negative increases, whereas if specificity is maximized, the chance of a false positive increases (Figure 9.5).

In the process of using tests to make clinical decisions, the comparative value of sensitivity and specificity should be taken into consideration. When a given test lacks sensitivity, people with the target disorder will be missed (false negatives). When a test lacks specificity, people who do not actually have the target

TABLE 9.7 Attributes derived from the comparison of a new test against a gold standard test in validation studies

Attribute	Formula*	Definition
Sensitivity	$a/(a+c)$	The ability of a test to identify persons who have the condition
Specificity	$d/(b+d)$	The ability of a test to identify persons who do not have the condition
Positive predictive value	$a/(a+b)$	The probability that a person with a positive test actually has the condition
Negative predictive value	$d/(c+d)$	The probability that a person with a negative test does not have the condition
Likelihood ratio of a positive test	$\dfrac{a/(a+c)}{(1-d)/b+d}$	A ratio of the probability of a positive test in a person with the condition compared with the probability of a positive test in a person without the condition
Likelihood ratio of a negative test	$\dfrac{1-a/(a+c)}{d/(b+d)}$	A ratio of the probability of a negative test in a person with the condition compared with the probability of a negative test in a person without the condition
Prevalence	$\dfrac{a+c}{a+b+c+d}$	The proportion of people in the sample who have the condition
Accuracy	$\dfrac{a+d}{a+b+c+d}$	The proportion of people correctly identified as either having or not having the condition

*Letters refer to the cells in Table 9.6.

disorder will be identified as having it (false positives). When the consequences of reporting false positive findings to a patient are insignificant, such as incorrectly reporting to a patient that his or her triglyceride levels are elevated (which results in the patient shifting to a healthier lifestyle), a test that emphasizes sensitivity may be appropriate. However, when a positive test leads to painful or

FIGURE 9:4 The ideal test would clearly segregate those with the condition into the group that tests positive and those without the condition into the group that tests negative. In the real world, however, many tests generate false positives and false negatives.

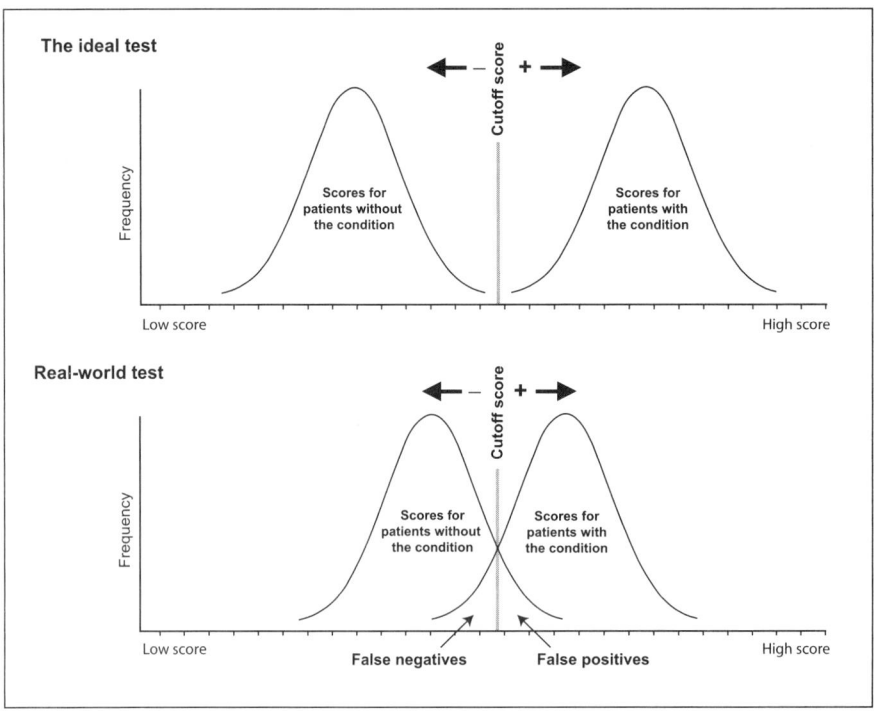

expensive treatment, then false positive tests must be minimized by using tests with high specificity. On the other hand, when a positive test points to serious illness in a patient that could possibly be resolved if detected in time, such as cancer, false negatives must be minimized and more sensitive tests should be used. When the consequences of false positives and false negatives are about equal, both sensitivity and specificity may be maximized.

When a test's sensitivity is very high, a negative test will rule out the condition that is under consideration, since there will be very few false negatives. Thus, if a test with very high sensitivity is negative, it is highly likely that it will be a true negative. A helpful mnemonic for this relationship is SnOUT (Sensitivity

Validity 295

FIGURE 9.5 When higher scores point to a worsening condition, raising the cutoff score increases the specificity, but there will be more false negatives. Lowering the cutoff score increases the sensitivity, but there will be more false positives.

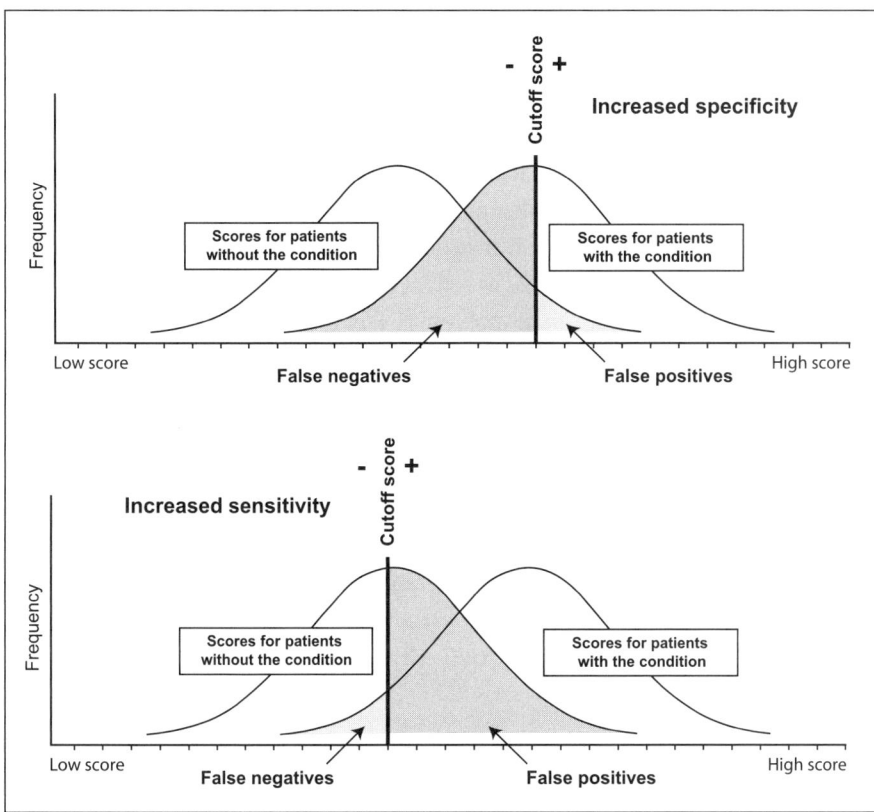

rules OUT). Likewise, when a test with very high specificity is positive, the disorder can be ruled in, since there will be very few false positives. In a positive test, it is highly likely that the test result will be a true positive. The mnemonic in this case is SpIN (Specificity rules IN).

There is no widespread agreement about what represents an acceptable level of sensitivity or specificity for a given diagnostic test. Furthermore, what constitutes an acceptable value for sensitivity or specificity is changeable, depending on the clinical situation. For instance, acceptable levels may be different when the intent of the test or the setting of the test changes. Acceptable levels also may differ when the condition's prevalence is dissimilar in the group being tested or when alternate methods of testing are available.

The relative magnitude of sensitivity versus specificity is an important consideration when selecting tests for screening purposes, which is dependent, to a large extent, upon the prevalence of the target condition. When the condition is rare, very few cases have the potential to be detected within the population. Accordingly, many false positives may be generated through screening, even when tests with high specificity are utilized. This is not a serious problem, however, if positive screening tests lead to further testing to confirm results. In contrast, screening for conditions that are very common may overlook many cases, even when a highly sensitive test is used. With these factors in mind, screening tests with high specificity relative to sensitivity should be utilized when the harm related to additional diagnostic testing or mislabeling is sizeable, whereas screening tests with high sensitivity in relation to specificity should be used when the cost of missing a case is high, such as with serious conditions and where highly effective treatment exists.[22]

A *likelihood ratio* (LR) is the probability that the results of a diagnostic test would be expected in a patient with the condition of interest (sensitivity) compared with the expected results of the same test in a patient without the condition (specificity). The LR of a positive test is represented by

$$sensitivity/(1 - Specificity)$$

The LR of a negative test is

$$(1 - Sensitivity)/Specificity$$

These ratios are easily calculated using values for sensitivity and specificity, which are often provided in journal articles.

Given a positive test, when the calculated LR is greater than 1, the probability that the condition is present is increased; when the LR is less than 1, the probability that the condition is present is decreased; and when the LR is equal to 1, the probability that the condition is present versus not being present is the same.[23]

Jaeschke and coworkers[24] categorized the ranges of possible LR values and described the implications for each category (Table 9.8 and Figure 9.6).

The *pretest probability* of a particular condition is a value that is usually estimated by the practitioner after the patient's initial assessment. It represents the probability that the patient has the condition under consideration before the test is actually carried out. Pretest probability is typically based on the clinician's experience, the prevalence of the condition being considered, and published literature. It may be modified up or down for a particular patient in the presence of risk factors. The pretest probability can be combined with the LR to generate a *posttest probability* of having the condition. A high *pretest* probability coupled with a high likelihood ratio will generate a very high *posttest* probability. Thus, a practitioner who was reasonably confident about a correct diagnosis prior to the test would be much more confident after obtaining the positive results of a test that had a high LR. The opposite of this scenario would occur if low pretest probabilities and low LRs were involved.

LRs have been referred to as the most useful single indicator of a test's diagnostic strength.[25] They can be used by clinicians to facilitate making decisions about the necessity of further testing and when to begin appropriate treatment. If the posttest probability of a test is very high, it is very likely that the condition is present, and treatment should be initiated. On the other hand, if the posttest probability is very low, the condition may be ruled out and no further diagnostic or

TABLE 9.8 **Meanings of the various ranges of possible likelihood ratio values**

LR > 10 or < 0.1
Generates large and conclusive changes in the probability of a given diagnosis

LR in the range of 5 to 10 or 0.1 to 0.2
Generates a moderate and usually important change in the probability of a given diagnosis

LR in the range of 2 to 5 or 0.5 to 0.2
Generates a small but sometimes important change in the probability of a given diagnosis

LR in the range of 1 to 2 or 0.5 to 1
Changes the probability of a given diagnosis to a small and rarely important degree

Source: Adapted from Jaeschke, R.Z., et al. How to use diagnostic test articles in the intensive care unit: Diagnosing weanability using f/Vt. *Crit Care Med*, 1997. **25**(9):1514–21

FIGURE 9.6 High or low likelihood ratios help rule a condition in or out, but mid-range values provide little information to help make this decision.

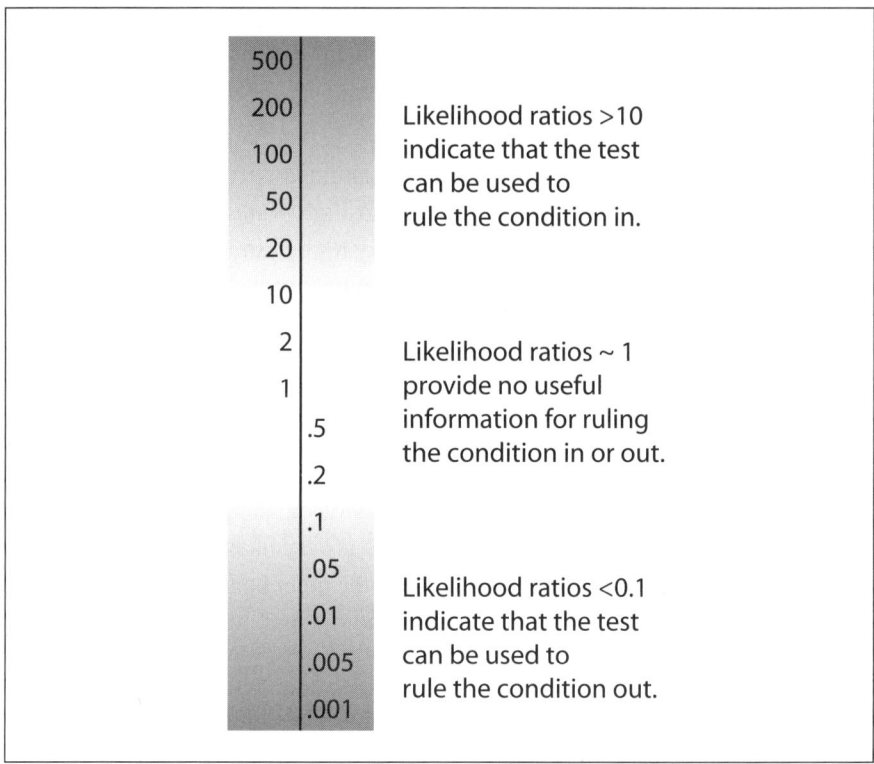

therapeutic action would be necessary. LRs can also be used serially, so that the posttest probability derived from one diagnostic test can be used as a pretest probability for the next.

Fagan[26] devised a nomogram that can be used by clinicians to quickly and easily convert pretest to posttest probabilities using LRs (Figure 9.7). To use the nomogram, first locate the patient's pretest probability for having the condition under consideration, and then locate the value of the LR of the test that is being used. Draw a line between the located pretest probability and the LR and extend this line until it passes through the posttest probability. This point becomes the new estimate of the probability that the patient has the condition.

Validity 299

FIGURE 9.7 Nomogram for finding the posttest probability of disease. A straight line is drawn from the patient's pretest probability of disease through the likelihood ratio of the test that is to be used. The line will point to the posttest probability of disease.

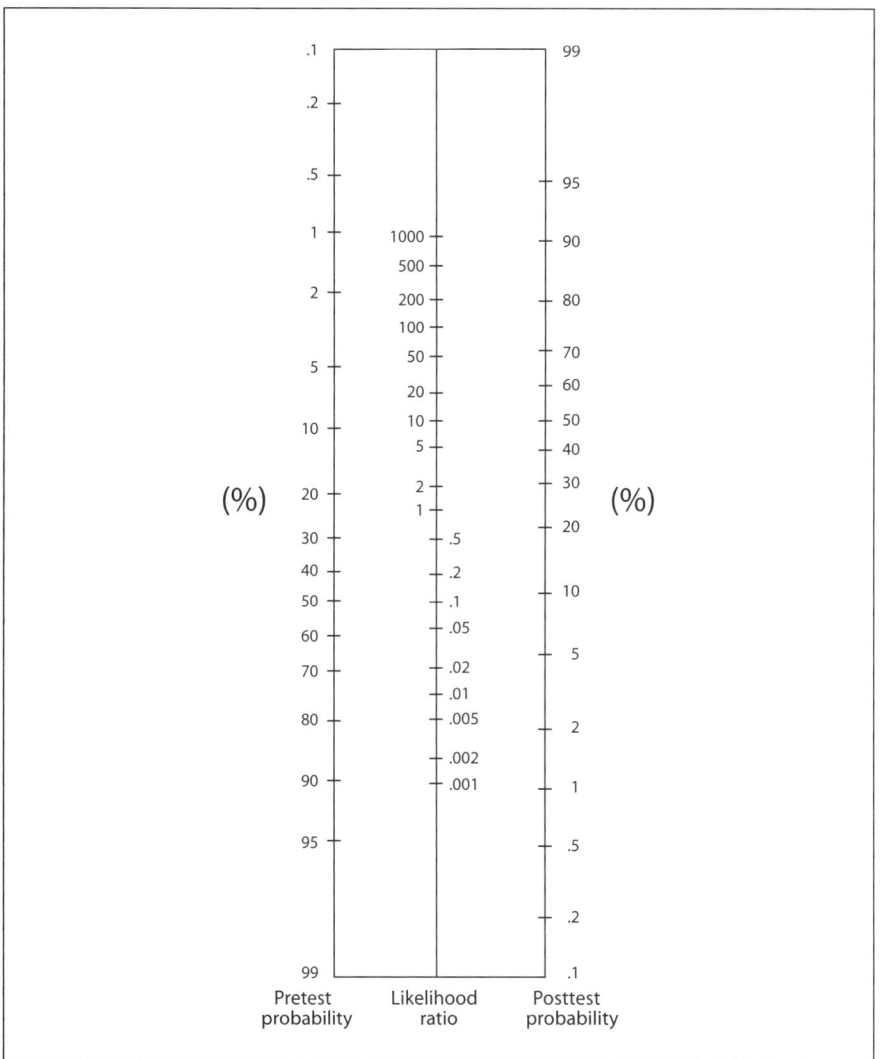

Source: Massachusetts Medical Society. Copyright © 1975. All rights reserved. Used with permission.

Clinical Disagreement

It is possible for practitioners to disagree about clinical findings, even when valid and reliable tests have been utilized. Indeed, Sackett and associates[27] pointed out three sources of clinical disagreement: the examiner, the examined, and the examination. In the case of the examiner (practitioner), there may be disagreement about the findings derived from tests due to biological variation in the senses—for example, a hearing-impaired examiner reporting an inaccurate blood pressure measurement. Another source of disagreement is the tendency to record inference rather than evidence, which occurs when practitioners make assumptions about the patient's symptoms and examination findings rather than simply recording what was observed. This can lead to a wrong diagnosis and may close the door to further investigation because of misplaced confidence in the assumption. The examiner can also be ensnared by diagnostic classification schemes, which occurs when the criteria about what constitutes "abnormal" are arbitrary. This is evident in the chiropractic profession because the diagnostic criteria for a manipulable lesion have not been clarified in the literature, which may lead to arbitrary classification by individual practitioners as to what constitutes the presence of a manipulable lesion in the spine.[1] Examiners can also be led astray by prior expectation, which refers to practitioners having a tendency to find what they hope and expect to find. For instance, if a chiropractor has a particular interest in carpal tunnel syndrome (CTS), he or she might hope for and expect to find CTS diagnostic indicators in all patients with upper extremity complaints. Another reason for disagreement due to the examiner is simple incompetence. This could be due to the examiner's inadequate training, impairment (e.g., due to fatigue or substance abuse), lack of concern for the patient, or any other factor that lowers his or her capacity to examine patients.

The second source of clinical disagreement, the examined, can also be related to several different issues. First, biologic variation may occur in the system being examined: Many signs and symptoms vary over time, such as pain levels, muscle spasm, and blood pressure which leads to disagreement among practitioners. Second, the effects of illness and medications can distort the findings of clinical examination because the signs or symptoms of the target disorder may be altered. An example is a lower back pain patient who has taken medication for pain prior to chiropractic evaluation. Third, there may be selective recall of past events by patients, particularly those who have chronic or serious conditions. These patients may tend to key in on a particular event that they think was the underlying cause of their condition. The fourth issue related to the examined is toss-ups, which has to do with disagreement among clinicians due to diverse opinions about the best options for patient care.

The examination itself is also a potential source of clinical disagreement. This can be related to disruptive environments, which can interfere with the ability of the practitioner to perform a reliable examination. Examples of disruptive environments are an athletic field or a patient's child crying during an examination. Another cause of examination-related disagreement is when disruptive interactions between examiners and the examined exist, which has the potential to form barriers to communication between the doctor and patient. These barriers may be due to patient apprehension, distrust of the doctor, or anything else that could worsen communication. The final reason for clinical disagreement is incorrect function or use of diagnostic tools. If a diagnostic instrument is used improperly, inaccurate results will no doubt follow. Furthermore, some instruments must be calibrated periodically to work properly or may be damaged when physically abused.

Appraisal Tactics

Like other research designs, the validity and clinical relevance of studies that evaluate diagnostic tests are important. However, additional unique concerns involved in the critical appraisal of these studies must be taken into consideration. One of these unique concerns arises because there will always be a degree of uncertainty associated with diagnostic tests. This uncertainty is caused by several factors:

- The assignment of normal and abnormal values is usually done somewhat arbitrarily, which leads to uncertainty about a patient's positive versus negative status.
- A trade-off occurs when either sensitivity or specificity is emphasized. Moreover, if the cutoff point is positioned so as to identify more patients with the condition, more false positives will be found, and the opposite will occur if the cutoff point is positioned so that fewer patients with the condition are identified.

- Biological variation of the individuals within the population can lead to patients with the same level of disease having different test results.
- The course of the disease can vary (e.g., patients are at different stages of the disease process or have different degrees of severity).
- Variation can be caused by the fact that clinical tests are not perfectly reliable and valid, which produces varied scores even in repeat tests of identical patients (i.e., the same patient being tested multiple times).
- Uncertainty also may exist when a test deals with an intermediate outcome, but no information is available about its connection to an important clinical outcome.

The initial step in appraising an article that deals with the evaluation of tests is to determine whether its purpose is to establish the reliability or validity (or both) of the test. Reliability studies consider the reproducibility of tests by comparing scores within and/or between examiners or within and/or between questionnaires. Validity studies, on the other hand, compare test results with those of established tests or determine if the test is capable of accurately predicting a particular outcome. Some specific questions that the reader should ask when assessing articles that deal with test validity and reliability are listed here. A *checklist for the appraisal of diagnostic accuracy articles* is provided in Appendix 7.

- *Was the test adequately described?* Authors of articles about diagnostic tests should describe the procedures involved in the test in enough detail so that the study could be replicated.[28] Items that should be covered include how patients must prepare for the test (e.g., fasting prior to certain blood tests), what patients must endure while going through the test (e.g., the medications that are administered for routine colonoscopy), and how the results are analyzed and interpreted. Knowledge of patient inconveniences, cost, and the potential for harm must be weighed against the need for information that initially prompted the test. Hence, the necessity for including this kind of information in articles that deal with diagnostic tests.
- *Did the study sample include a full range of subjects with and without the condition?* It is important for studies that assess the quality of diagnostic

tests to include all types of patients in their sample, such as one would see in everyday clinical practice. If a higher than normal proportion of patients who obviously have the condition is included in the study, there is a greater likelihood that those with the disease will test positive. The test may not perform very well in the general population, however, since it includes more people presenting earlier in the course of the disease. In practice, although a test is capable of identifying obviously ill patients, it may not effectively discriminate the mildly ill. Sackett and colleagues[27] also suggested that both treated and untreated subjects be included in these studies. Nonetheless, it has been reported that only 27% of studies that deal with diagnostic tests actually specify the spectrum of included subjects in terms of symptoms or disease severity, eligibility criteria, or even basic demographic information.[29]

- *If the study utilized a gold standard for comparison, was it an acceptable one?* The credibility of a study that compares a new test with a gold standard depends to a great extent on the soundness of the gold standard used. Unfortunately, it is rare for a test to be both highly sensitive and highly specific, which means that an ideal gold standard is often difficult to find. Ideally a gold standard test would comprise the results of biopsy, or long-term follow-up to confirm the presence or absence of the disease. This is frequently not possible, however, and less rigorous comparisons are used instead. Nevertheless, if the gold standard that was used is not acceptable, the article may not be usable.

- *Were the test results and the gold standard assessed independently in a blinded fashion?* Raters should be unaware of the results of previous testing, since this information has the potential to greatly affect the interpretation of tests. For instance, pathology becomes much more noticeable on an x-ray once the abnormality has been pointed out. If raters are aware of certain aspects of a patient's health, their interpretation of test results will often be swayed one way or the other, depending on whether or not raters think the patient has the condition under investigation. Greenhalgh[30] refers to "expectation bias," which occurs when raters are influenced by the knowledge of certain features of the case. She gives the example of the knowledge of the presence of chest pain when interpreting a patient's electrocardiogram.

The decision to carry out the gold standard test should not influenced by the results of the test that is being evaluated. When the decision is influenced one way or the other, ensuing *verification* (also known as *work-up) bias* comes into play. For instance, if the gold standard test was only carried out on subjects who tested positive to the index test, false negatives would not be given the confirmatory test, even though they would be expected to test positive. In better-quality studies, all patients who are tested with the index test are also tested with the gold standard test. Information about negative tests is often not present in these studies, however, because patients are not usually exposed to further inconvenient testing subsequent to a negative test. This often leaves the reader wondering whether negative test results are valid. One more caution about studies that judge a test against a gold standard is to be wary when more than one type of gold standard test is utilized—for instance, some patients in a study receiving a biopsy for confirmation of the new test, while others have to wait for the condition to develop.

- *Do the results of this study apply to the patient before me?* A good test will perform well with patients both within and outside the original study group.[31,32] For a test to apply to patients in your practice, it should have been carried out in a population comparable to the kinds of patients you see. The study's population should be composed of age and gender distributions similar to the composition of your practice, as well as having a comparable severity level of the condition in question. Often the prevalence of a condition or its severity is higher in an academic environment than in the general population. This overrepresentation of affected patients may influence the sensitivity of the test, making it higher than what would be expected if it were studied in the general population.

- *Will patients benefit as a result of being tested?* There are probably other tests available that a new test is replacing, and you should determine whether this new test is preferable to the old ones. It may be that the new test is less convenient, more expensive, and provides little or no additional information. Be especially aware of articles about diagnostic tests that are connected in any way with business interests that may have concerns related to the study's outcome.

The information derived from a test should be beneficial to patients and have the potential to result in a change in the way their condition is managed. Some tests, on the other hand, do not really add any new information above what was found during the patient's examination or from other tests. Consequently, the new test would be unnecessary and should not be administered. In another patient with a different case presentation, however, the same test might be useful.

Another thing to consider regarding the benefit of a test to patients is the consequences of not performing the test. For instance, a test that is designed to detect a condition that is potentially very harmful if left undiagnosed (e.g., abdominal aneurysm) would be very beneficial when indicated. There should also be an acceptable level of risk associated with the test that is proportional to the importance of the information to be derived. An example would be angiography of the vertebral artery for a patient with symptoms of cerebellar ischemia. Angiography of the cervical arteries has more risk than magnetic resonance angiography (MRA) because arterial catheterization is required for angiography, yet some experts consider that the tests provide comparable information.[33] In this situation, clinicians may opt for the less risky test.

- *Is the test reliable?* The results of reliability studies should reflect an adequate degree of consistency between different examiners and repeat tests by the same examiner. When questionnaires are involved, they too should produce consistent results when repeated. Refer to Tables 9.3 and 9.4 for an interpretation of reported kappa and ICC values. Not only should the appropriate coefficients of agreement be within acceptable ranges, but also the associated confidence intervals should point to findings that are statistically significant.

- *Is the test valid?* Depending on the type of validity study carried out (e.g., concurrent, predictive, convergent validity), diverse statistical tests may be used to portray the characteristics of the groups, such as the degree of correlation (e.g., Pearson's correlation), differences between groups (e.g., *t*-test or ANOVA), and analysis of frequencies (e.g., chi-square), as well as sensitivity and specificity. The results of the statistical tests should be significant, and accompanying *P* values or confidence intervals should be reported. Confidence intervals are more likely to be wide and less likely to point to statistical significance when a study's sample size is relatively small. Thus, it is very important to examine reported confidence intervals in reports of smaller studies.

Sensitivity and specificity, when reported, should be relatively high and appropriate for the intended use of the test. Also, the gold standard comparison being used in the study should itself be a valid marker for the particular feature being tested.

References

1. French, S.D., S. Green, and A. Forbes. *Reliability of chiropractic methods commonly used to detect manipulable lesions in patients with chronic low-back pain. J Manipulative Physiol Ther*, 2000. **23**(4):231–8.
2. Hestbaek, L., and C. Leboeuf-Yde. *Are chiropractic tests for the lumbo-pelvic spine reliable and valid? A systematic critical literature review. J Manipulative Physiol Ther*, 2000. **23**(4):258–75.
3. Christensen, H.W., et al. *Palpation of the upper thoracic spine: An observer reliability study. J Manipulative Physiol Ther*, 2002. **25**(5):285–92.
4. Marcotte, J., M.C. Normand, and P. Black. *The kinematics of motion palpation and its effect on the reliability for cervical spine rotation. J Manipulative Physiol Ther*, 2002. **25**(7):E7.
5. Cooperstein, R., et al. *Validity of compressive leg checking in measuring artificial leg-length inequality. J Manipulative Physiol Ther*, 2003. **26**(9):557–66.
6. Evenson, K., and A. McGinn. *Test-retest reliability of a questionnaire to assess physical environmental factors pertaining to physical activity. Int J Behavioral Nutrition Physical Activity*, 2005. **2**(1):7.
7. Vernon, H., and S. Mior. *The Neck Disability Index: A study of reliability and validity. J Manipulative Physiol Ther*, 1991. **14**(7):409–15.
8. McGinn, T., et al. *Tips for learners of evidence-based medicine: 3. Measures of observer variability (kappa statistic). CMAJ*, 2004. **171**(11):1369–73.
9. Viera, A.J., and J.M. Garrett. *Understanding interobserver agreement: The kappa statistic. Fam Med*, 2005. **37**(5):360–3.
10. Maclure, M., and W.C. Willett. *Misinterpretation and misuse of the kappa statistic. Am J Epidemiol*, 1987. **126**(2):161–9.
11. Landis, J., and G. Koch. *The measurement of observer agreement for categorical data. Biometrics*, 1977. **33**:159–74.
12. Portney, L.G., and M.P. Watkins. *Foundations of Clinical Research : Applications to Practice*. 2nd ed. 2000. Upper Saddle River, NJ: Prentice Hall.
13. Clare, H.A., R. Adams, and C.G. Maher. *Reliability of detection of lumbar lateral shift. J Manipulative Physiol Ther*, 2003. **26**(8):476–80.
14. Nourbakhsh, M.R., and A.M. Arab. *Relationship between mechanical factors and incidence of low back pain. J Orthop Sports Phys Ther*, 2002. **32**(9):447–60.
15. Nguyen, H.T., et al. *Interexaminer reliability of activator methods' relative leg-length evaluation in the prone extended position. J Manipulative Physiol Ther*, 1999. **22**(9):565–9.

16. Axen, I., et al. *The Nordic Back Pain Subpopulation Program: Can patient reactions to the first chiropractic treatment predict early favorable treatment outcome in nonpersistent low back pain? J Manipulative Physiol Ther*, 2005. **28**(3):153–8.
17. Akin, F.W., and M.J. Davenport. *Validity and reliability of the Motion Sensitivity Test. J Rehabil Res Dev*, 2003. **40**(5):415–21.
18. Gagnon, C., J. Mathieu, and J. Desrosiers. *Standardized finger-nose test validity for coordination assessment in an ataxic disorder. Can J Neurol Sci*, 2004. **31**(4):484–9.
19. Riegelman, R.K. *Studying a Study and Testing a Test: How to Read the Medical Evidence.* 4th ed. Philadelphia: Lippincott Williams & Wilkins. 2000.
20. Sackett, D.L. *The rational clinical examination. A primer on the precision and accuracy of the clinical examination. JAMA*, 1992. **267**(19):2638–44.
21. Riddle, D., and P. Stratford. *Interpreting validity indexes for diagnostic tests: An illustration using the Berg Balance Test. Phys Ther*, 1999. **79**(10):939–48.
22. Gaeta, T. *Screening and Diagnostic Tests.* 2005. http://www.emedicine.com/emerg/topic779.htm. Accessed June 8, 2005.
23. Strauss, S.E. *Evidence-Based Medicine: How to Practice and Teach EBM.* 3rd ed. Edinburgh and New York: Elsevier/Churchill Livingstone. 2005.
24. Jaeschke, R.Z., et al. *How to use diagnostic test articles in the intensive care unit: Diagnosing weanability using f/Vt. Crit Care Med*, 1997. **25**(9):1514–21.
25. Worster, A., G. Innes, and R. Abu-Laban. *Diagnostic testing: An emergency medicine perspective. Can J Emerg Med*, 2002. **4**(5).
26. Fagan, T.J. *Nomogram for Bayes theorem* [Letter]. *N Engl J Med*, 1975. **293**(5):257.
27. Sackett, D.L., et al. *Clinical Epidemiology: A Basic Science for Clinical Medicine.* 2nd ed. 1991. Boston: Little, Brown & Company.
28. West, S., et al. *Systems to Rate the Strength of Scientific Evidence (Evidence Report/Technology Assessment No. 47; AHRQ Publication No. 02–E016).* Rockville, MD: Agency for Healthcare Research and Quality, 2002. 204.
29. Reid, M.C., M.S. Lachs, and A.R. Feinstein. *Use of methodological standards in diagnostic test research. Getting better but still not good. JAMA*, 1995. **274**(8):645–51.
30. Greenhalgh, T. *How to read a paper: Papers that report diagnostic or screening tests. BMJ*, 1997. **315**(7107):540–3.
31. Jaeschke, R., G. Guyatt, and D.L. Sackett. *Users' guides to the medical literature. III. How to use an article about a diagnostic test. A. Are the results of the study valid? Evidence-Based Medicine Working Group. JAMA*, 1994. **271**(5):389–91.
32. Jaeschke, R., G.H. Guyatt, and D.L. Sackett. *Users' guides to the medical literature. III. How to use an article about a diagnostic test. B. What are the results and will they help me in caring for my patients? The Evidence-Based Medicine Working Group. JAMA*, 1994. **271**(9):703–7.
33. Kirsch, E., et al. *MR angiography in internal carotid artery dissection: Improvement of diagnosis by selective demonstration of the intramural haematoma. Neuroradiology*, 1998. **40**(11):704–9.

PART III

Practical Applications of Evidence-Based Chiropractic

CHAPTER TEN

Evidence-Based Chiropractic and Documentation

Evidence-based chiropractic (EBC) is a process that entails locating the best evidence that is available, appraising the validity of that evidence, and then applying it to the individual patient, along with the clinical expertise of the practitioner. Indeed, Sackett[1] defined evidence-based practice as "the conscientious, explicit, and judicious use of the current best evidence in making decisions about the care of individual patients." Although the primary purpose of EBC involves the care of individual patients, it has other uses that can be applied to patient care and practice management in general. Moreover, the process of finding the best evidence for an individual patient can be applied to nearly every aspect of clinical practice. Using EBC methods, practitioners can discover the best treatments for managing commonly encountered conditions, as well as appropriate diagnostic tests. It can even provide evidence-based direction for equipment purchases and decisions about which seminars to attend.[2]

Supporting Diagnostic and Treatment Protocols Through Good Documentation

In clinical practice, documentation essentially consists of recording the subjective complaints of patients, the objective findings, one's assessment, and the plan for case management. The focus of this chapter is on objective findings, which, for the most part, involve the reporting of observations and test results. Regrettably, many common clinical tests used to evaluate spinal conditions have been poorly standardized, so that even if a test is called by the same name, it may be performed and evaluated differently by different examiners.[3] This creates a problem that, in addition to raising issues about reliability and validity, may lead to erroneous test results.

Good clinical documentation should be a reflection of the thought processes involved in patient management and provide evidence of the patient's progress while under care. This type of record keeping enables practitioners to accurately monitor patient progress so that they are able to make the best possible clinical decisions. It may also allay some of the problems associated with third-party record reviews and medicolegal issues,[4] because the patient's clinical record is generally the only evidence taken into consideration when such entities make decisions.

The use of valid and reliable outcome measures (OMs) in chiropractic practice has a number of benefits to various interested parties. They are beneficial to patients because appropriate care will be much more likely to ensue when clinical progress is carefully monitored and recorded. They also are of benefit to practitioners, who will have the best information possible with which to formulate diagnoses and plan care. Furthermore, patients and third-party payers will be more likely to receive a legitimate service in return for their monetary expenditures. The beneficial qualities of OMs are often referred to as *utility*, which essentially refers to the usefulness of a test in meeting the needs of the patient, referrer, and payer.[5] OMs should also be sensitive to change, which means that they should change in direct association with actual changes that occur in the patient characteristic being measured.

In the clinical setting, OMs are administered to patients before treatment is given and then afterward, with the assumption that any changes in the measures are attributable to the treatment. This may not be true, however, because intervening events may occur that also have an effect on the OM and obscure before-and-after comparisons. Patients may receive treatment from other providers while under care; they may reinjure themselves or attempt to self-treat themselves. However, numerous sequential evaluations may alleviate some of these problems and help to identify trends that are attributable to the intervention.

Evidence-based methods are often utilized by health care purchasers and managers in an attempt to control costs, although some feel that this is an exploitation of the system.[1] Nonetheless, the practice continues. Accordingly, practitioners should be aware of and utilize the best available evidence to support the procedures utilized in their practices. This will facilitate better interactions with all parties and ultimately may result in improved reimbursement rates. Providing the appropriate level of evidence-based care may at times result in lower health care costs, since unnecessary therapies and diagnostic tests may be avoided. Patients should also improve faster when they receive appropriate care.

Guidelines

Clinical practice guidelines have been defined as "systematically developed statements to assist practitioner and patient decisions about appropriate health care for specific clinical circumstances."[6] Guidelines have the potential to make health care more efficient and consistent among practitioners, as well as to diminish the gap between what clinicians actually do in practice and what is supported by the scientific evidence.[7] In addition to assisting practitioners and patients in making appropriate health care decisions, four additional uses for guidelines have been suggested: (1) educating individuals or groups, (2) assessing and assuring the quality of care, (3) guiding the distribution of health care resources, and (4) reducing the risk of legal liability for negligent care.[6]

Guidelines are typically produced by representative experts in a particular field through an organized process that involves assembling the available evidence regarding conditions and their treatments that are normally handled by members of that field. The object of developing guidelines is to locate the best available evidence, which can then be used by clinicians to provide optimal patient care. Guidelines development is a five-step process:[7]

1. Identifying the subject area of the guideline.
2. Assembling and running guideline development groups.
3. Obtaining and assessing the evidence about the clinical question.
4. Transforming the evidence into a clinical guideline.
5. Arranging for external review of the guideline.

The evidence assessment process involved in the development of high-quality guidelines is similar to that of a systematic review, following a strict protocol and assessing each article using consistent scoring methods. Consequently, high-quality guidelines are generally a reliable source of clinical information, and treating patients according to their recommendations will typically provide the best likelihood for clinicians to achieve desired outcomes (Figure 10.1).[8]

Some guidelines may be referred to as being "evidence-based," which means that a rigorous process was followed during their development and that they are based on the highest-quality scientific evidence. Nonetheless, guidelines differ in quality, primarily in relation to the rigor of the development methods that were employed. For instance, in the chiropractic profession, the Guidelines for Chiropractic Quality Assurance and Practice Parameters (Mercy guidelines)[9] were recommended for application, in preference to the Vertebral Subluxation in Chiropractic Practice (Council on Chiropractic Practice) and the Recommended Clinical Protocols and Guidelines for the Practice of Chiropractic (International Chiropractor's Association guidelines).[10,11]

Even high-quality guidelines may have disadvantages. For example, evidence is sometimes unavailable or is of low quality regarding a particular condi-

FIGURE 10.1 **Process involved in the development of guideline recommendations.**

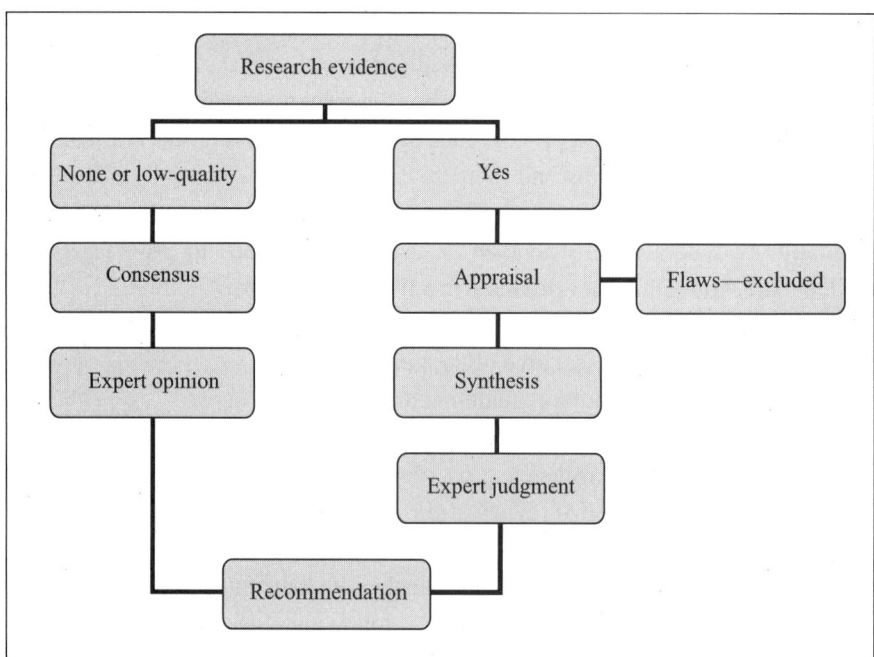

tion or treatment. In these cases, guidelines may only serve to inform clinicians about the lack of evidence. Another disadvantage of guidelines is that they only address one condition at a time, whereas patients often present with several complaints at a time in clinical practice. Thus, a clinician using a guideline for a specific patient must select the recommendations that will be most helpful and disregard those that do not apply. Also, each patient is unique in many respects, which means that guideline-recommended treatment options may not always be appropriate. Clinicians may therefore be obligated to withhold treatment in these instances due to contraindications. Because of these limitations, guidelines should never be utilized carte blanche as a treatment cookbook.[12]

Guidelines development primarily involves the use of research evidence, although the process is not always entirely successful. There are numerous instances where little or no scientific evidence exists on a given topic and alternate strategies are required in order to produce recommendations. In these cases, guidelines developers incorporate the consensus views of experts.[13] This approach, however, is not wholly reliable since it merely represents the opinions of a panel of experts. Nonetheless, the experts are typically leaders in the field and are likely to generate more trustworthy information than an individual practitioner.

The Delphi method is a technique that is frequently used in guidelines development to establish a group position about an issue. The method involves repeated questioning of a group of panel members whose opinions are being sought, usually via questionnaires. After each panel member has responded to the initial questionnaire, the results from that round of questions are sent to all members, along with subsequent questionnaires. This information is typically presented anonymously. Members are able to consider the opinions of other panel members and then are encouraged to modify their previous replies if they deem it appropriate after reading the information from the others. Generally, after two or three rounds, a group consensus is established by averaging all of the information that has been gathered.

Guidelines should be updated periodically as new information becomes available. The time frame for needed updates is variable, depending on how rapidly change occurs on a particular topic or within a given field.[14] The Mercy guidelines, which were published in 1993, stipulated that they should be updated at a later date.[9] However, that update has not taken place, and no plans for updating them in the future are known to this author. Accordingly, and in spite of the superior methods that were involved in their creation, this deficiency limits the current validity of the Mercy guidelines.

When making a decision about whether to make use of recommendations from a particular practice guideline, a number of factors should be considered.[15–17] First, the guideline recommendations should be valid, which can be determined by ascertaining the extent to which proper methods were utilized in their development. Developers should describe their methods, which should reflect rigorous systematic methods regarding how the evidence was selected and appraised. If this information is not included, either in a policy statement or supporting article, one must question whether systematic methods were actually employed. Second, one must consider whether the guideline recommendations will actually be helpful in the care of your patients. Conditions that are addressed in the guidelines should be applicable to the chiropractic setting, and the recommendations should be applicable to chiropractic patients. Guidelines may not apply to patients in patient populations that differ from the source articles. For instance, the rate of disease prevalence or certain risk factors may differ between the populations.

The term *best practice* depicts the organizational use of evidence to improve practice. It has been defined as "activities, disciplines and methods that are available to identify, implement and monitor the available evidence in health care."[18] Best practice may at times be referenced in conjunction with clinical guidelines, since the concept refers to their use in improving practice. Sometimes the concept of best practice is confused with clinical guidelines, but they are distinct topics. Best practice is built on a foundation of evidence-based practice and the need for its implementation in clinical practice.[19]

Guidelines are frequently utilized by entities other than practitioners and patients, such as health care payers and regulatory agencies. Guideline recommendations may be used by these entities to oversee patient care, either retrospectively or prospectively. Repercussions may result from care that is provided outside these recommendations (e.g., reduced insurance reimbursements and state board disciplinary actions). Health care payers may at times exploit clinical guidelines in an effort to limit patient care by citing portions of the document that support restricted services. However, even though a scientific process is involved in the development of guidelines, they are only capable of providing assistance and direction and are not prescriptive statements. Accordingly, this practice has been criticized.[12] Sackett[1] made a perceptive statement on this issue:

External clinical evidence can inform, but can never replace, individual clinical expertise, and it is this expertise that decides whether the external evidence applies to the individual patient at all and, if so, how it should be integrated into a clinical decision. Similarly, any external guideline must be integrated with individual clinical expertise in deciding whether and how it matches the patient's clinical state, predicament, and preferences, and thereby whether it should be applied.

Outcome Measures Commonly Used in Chiropractic

The choice of which OMs to use in a given clinical situation is not fixed. It depends on what the objectives are for that particular patient and, to a certain extent, the party or stakeholder that is targeted to receive the information. The definition of what constitutes successful treatment differs somewhat, depending on the perspective of the stakeholder involved.[20] As far as the clinician and the patient are concerned, an acceptable clinical outcome may merely consist of pain relief. Health care payers, on the other hand, consider cost-efficient patient management and patient satisfaction to be the most important criteria in defining successful outcomes.[21] Employers may define successful outcomes as a return to work for their injured employees. Consequently, the selection of OMs may differ according to the needs of the entity that is to receive the information. In addition, just because an OM is deemed appropriate in one situation, does not mean that it will be appropriate in another. For instance, anteroposterior and lateral lumbar x-rays are appropriate in the evaluation of patients with acute lower back pain only when certain red flags are present (e.g., over 50 years of age, unrelenting night pain, pain at rest, fever above 100.4°F, serious injury). In the absence of these red flags, x-rays may not be useful as a diagnostic tool.[22]

There are many different valid and reliable OMs to choose from for use in a chiropractic practice, although only a small percentage of them are consistently used by practitioners. These commonly used OMs are recognized by fellow practitioners and health care payers and are typically more useful to support care than those that are less familiar. Some of the more common OMs that are used not only in practice but also in research are presented in this chapter. The reader is referred to a book titled *The Clinical Application of Outcomes Assessment* by Steven Yeomans,[5] for a description of additional OMs.

Health-related quality of life (HRQL) measures are typically self-administered questionnaires that are designed to assess patients' physical, psychological, emotional, and social well-being.[23] HRQL measures facilitate patients in reporting, from their perspective, information about what activities they can and cannot do, how frequently they can do them, and the degree of difficulty they experience while performing them. Because patients are allowed to report their personal experiences from their own perspective, HRQL questionnaires are sometimes criticized by practitioners as being subjective and unreliable. Some practitioners consider "objective" clinical measures to be more reliable, but it is usually the other way around: HRQL measures are more reliable. Some of the "objective" OMs are also problematic because they are usually not very meaningful to patients. HRQL measures are indeed capable of assessing patients' functional limitations and are quite suitable and useful in monitoring the effects of treatment.[24]

There are two basic categories of HRQL measures: generic instruments, which are designed to evaluate patients' overall health status, and specific instruments, which are intended to assess particular conditions, patient groups, or areas of function.[25] Specific instruments are capable of estimating the impact of a particular disease or condition on patients' capacity to function. Two very commonly encountered generic HRQL measures are the SF-36 health survey[26] and the Sickness Impact Profile.[27] These instruments are able to quantify patients' overall level of health to enable tracking of their progress over time. In chiropractic practice, the Oswestry Disability Index and Neck Disability Index are two commonly used specific instruments that deal with disability due to low back and neck pain, respectively. Condition-specific instruments such as these have certain advantages over the generic variety, because they evaluate the elements of function that are germane to the condition at issue. Thus, they are typically more responsive to changes in patients' primary conditions than generic instruments.

When reading the literature dealing with chiropractic therapies, measures of pain and function are the most commonly utilized OMs. These types of measures are used frequently in spine-related research because valid and reliable instruments are available to reproducibly quantify these constructs. Instruments that measure pain typically invite patients to mark down their perceived level of pain on a scale ranging from no pain to severe pain. Numerical scales may range from 0 to 10 or from 0 to 100, or patients may be asked to place a mark representing their pain level on a 100-mm line. Measures of function include questionnaires designed to assess activity limitations that are attributable to a specific condition, general health assessment questionnaires, and tests to evaluate motion. For example, Boline and colleagues[28] conducted a randomized clinical trial that compared spinal manipulation with amitriptyline for the treatment of chronic tension-type headaches. The OMs used by the authors included changes in patient-reported daily headache intensity, weekly headache frequency, over-the-counter medication usage, and functional health status as reported by means of the SF-36 health survey.

Measures of Pain

Pain cannot be measured directly; rather, it must be estimated from replies to oral or written patient queries. The process of gathering information on pain is highly susceptible to influence by the culture, conditioning, education, and so forth of the involved patient. Furthermore, after being expressed by the patient, the pain information must then be interpreted by the clinician. This lack of objective measurement may be frustrating to some clinicians; however, a number of readily available tools are capable of translating the subjective experience of pain into valid and reliable measures that are very useful in clinical practice and research. It does not really matter which of the scales is chosen, but once selected, the same scale should be consistently used for subsequent evaluations.

Pain Scales

The *Numeric Rating Scale* (NRS; also known as the numeric pain scale or 11-point pain scale) is very commonly used in both the research and practice settings. Patients are asked to estimate the severity of their pain using a 0 to 10 scale, where 0 represents "no pain" and 10 represents the "worst possible pain" (Figure 10.2). This type of pain measure may be used either verbally or visually. When

FIGURE 10.2 **The Numeric Rating Scale of pain. The patient is instructed to circle the number that best represents his or her pain level.**

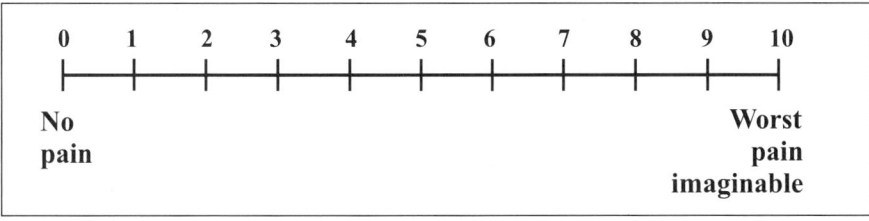

used to verbally assess pain, the patient is asked, "On a scale of 0 to 10, where 0 means no pain and 10 is the worst possible pain, what is your current level of pain?" It is generally agreed that scores ranging from 1 to 4 suggest a mild level of pain intensity, scores in the 5 to 6 range point to a moderate level of pain, and scores of 7 or higher indicate pain that is considered to be severe. A closely related scale, the *101-point numeric rating scale* (NRS-101), may occasionally be encountered when reading the literature, although the added number of levels in the NRS 101 provides very little information over the 11-point scale.

Another pain assessment OM is the *Visual Analogue Scale* (VAS), which is made up of a 10-centimeter line with descriptive phrases at each end that depict the extremes of pain (Figure 10.3). The left end of the scale typically uses the wording "No Pain," and the right end, "Severe Pain" or "Worst Pain Ever." No intermediate marks are placed along the line. The patient is instructed to draw a vertical line through the scale to represent the intensity of his or her pain. The distance of the mark from the left end of the line (in millimeters) represents the level of the patient's pain. Be advised that the use of different printers and copiers will likely produce lines of differing lengths.

The NRS and VAS are not limited exclusively to measuring pain. For instance, they can be used to assess the impact that pain has on various aspects of daily living. Patients are asked to rate the extent to which pain affects or interferes with items such as their activities, sleep, ability to lift, or personal care. Suitable anchors would be 0, signifying "does not interfere," and 10, signifying "completely interferes." The NRS and VAS can also be adapted to assess the level of anxiety or depression in pain patients.[29]

FIGURE 10.3 **The Visual Analogue Scale. The patient's pain level is determined by measuring the distance from the beginning of a 10-centimeter line to the patient's mark.**

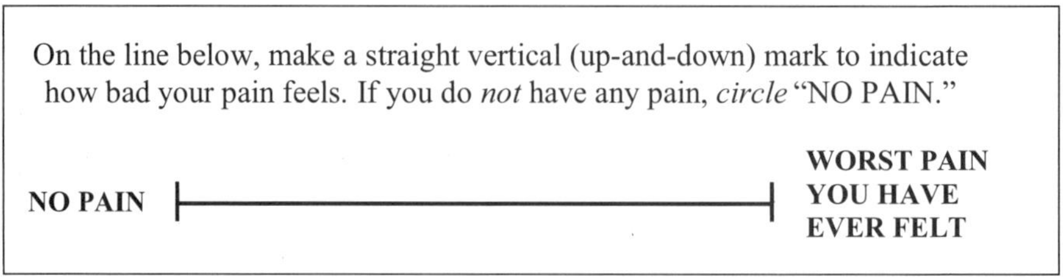

On the line below, make a straight vertical (up-and-down) mark to indicate how bad your pain feels. If you do *not* have any pain, *circle* "NO PAIN."

NO PAIN ├──────────────────────────────────┤ WORST PAIN YOU HAVE EVER FELT

One important advantage of the VAS over the NRS pain scale is that VAS scores are considered to be ratio rather than ordinal measurements, since there are equal intervals and there is a true zero. Moreover, there is no fixed relationship between scores when the NRS scale is used, so that a pain score of 4 is not necessarily twice as severe as a score of 2. This is important in the research setting because the statistical analysis of ordinal data is restricted to chi-square tests, which are not as robust as the parametric tests (i.e., *t*-test or ANOVA). This means that statistically significant differences are not as likely to be detected between groups when studies use the NRS scale.

The *Characteristic Pain Intensity* (CPI) score[30] is an average of the patient's pain levels "right now, typical or on average, and when it is at its worst" (see Appendix 8). This scale can provide valuable information about the true character of pain, especially in cases where pain intensity varies.[31] Without such a measure, patients presenting for evaluation at a particularly good or bad time would not be able to convey their true pain level. The CPI uses three VAS pain intensity ratings that represent different points in time: right now, on average, and when the pain is at its worst. An average of these three scores has several advantages over merely considering pain at one point in time. Moreover, the CPI correlated better with measures of pain-related disability, pain medication use, and standard pain measures than individual ratings. Also, distributions of CPI scores were more normally distributed.

The *Verbal Rating Scale* (VRS) of pain intensity consists of a series of adjectives that reflect the extremes of pain (e.g., "no pain" to "intense pain"). Patients choose the adjective that they think effectively characterizes their pain level, selecting from a list of possibilities. For example, the five-point VRS assigns scores as follows: "no pain" receives a score of 0, "mild pain" a score of 1, "moderate pain" a score of 2, "severe pain" a score of 3, and "very severe pain" a score of 4 (Table 10.1). The single number that corresponds to the adjective chosen by the patient would constitute the VRS pain intensity score. More or fewer adjectives may be used with the VRS to represent the preferred intervals of pain. Patients prefer the simplicity of the VRS; however, it lacks sensitivity, may be less reliable, and is easily misinterpreted, since adjectives do not necessarily mean the same thing to different persons.[32]

Tenderness rating scales are helpful to quantify the discomfort levels associated with the palpation of myofascial tissues. Hubbard and Berkoff[33] used the scale presented in Table 10.2 to portray tenderness associated with trigger points.

TABLE 10.1 Five-point Verbal Rating Scale of pain intensity

Score	Description
0	No pain
1	Mild pain
2	Moderate pain
3	Severe pain
4	Very severe pain

TABLE 10.2 Tenderness rating of soft tissue

Grade	Definition
0	No tenderness
1	Mild tenderness without grimace or flinch
2	Moderate tenderness with grimace or flinch
3	Severe tenderness with marked flinch or withdrawal
4	Unbearable tenderness; patient withdraws with light touch

Source: Adapted from Hubbard, D.R., and G.M. Berkoff. Myofascial trigger points show spontaneous needle EMG activity. *Spine*, 1993. **18**(13):1803–7.

The correlation of the patient's interpretation of tenderness with the examiner's observation of the patient's reaction to pain stimulus can help objectify the information obtained from palpation evaluation.

A similar tenderness scale that was developed primarily for use with fibromyalgia patients[34] is as follows:

0: No pain or grimace response
1 (mild): Pain without grimace, flinch, or withdrawal
2 (moderate): Pain with grimace or flinch
3 (severe): Pain with marked flinch or withdrawal
4 (unbearable): Patient is untouchable at that site and withdraws without palpation.

In this context, *grimace* was defined as a "facial expression," *flinch* as "a slight body movement," *marked flinch* as an "exaggerated body movement," and *withdrawal* as "moving the body part away from the examiner."

Pain Drawings

Pain drawings are commonly used both in clinical practice and in research to assess the intensity of and location of patients' pain. The process typically involves patients shading regions in which they are experiencing pain within the outlines of a blank body image (Figure 10.4). Pain drawings can be used by themselves or incorporated into self-report health surveys, although their utility is enhanced when they are used in combination with other OMs.

FIGURE 10.4 Body image with five areas of possible pain that indicate the extent of low back involvement.

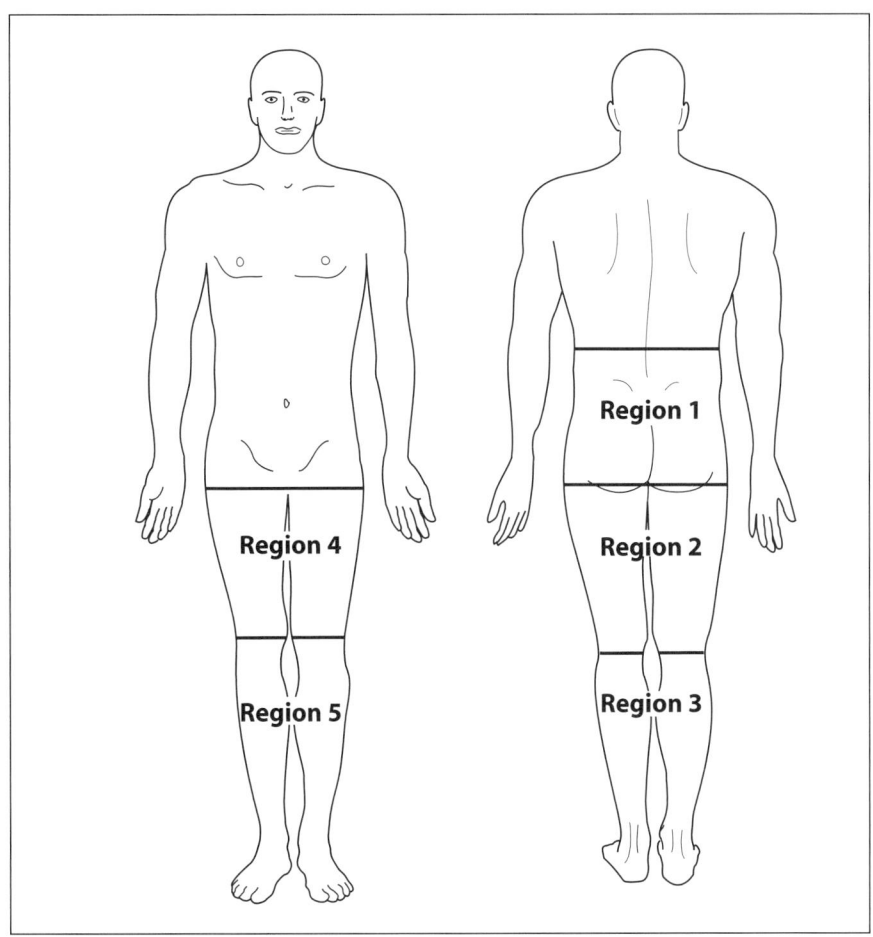

Margolis and associates[35] developed a system whereby patients mark their areas of pain on a blank body image, and then a transparent grid depicting 45 regions of the body is superimposed over the completed image (Figure 10.5). The

FIGURE 10.5 Margolis and associates developed a coding system based on a grid of regions on a body image, which may be useful in detecting changes in multiple areas over time.

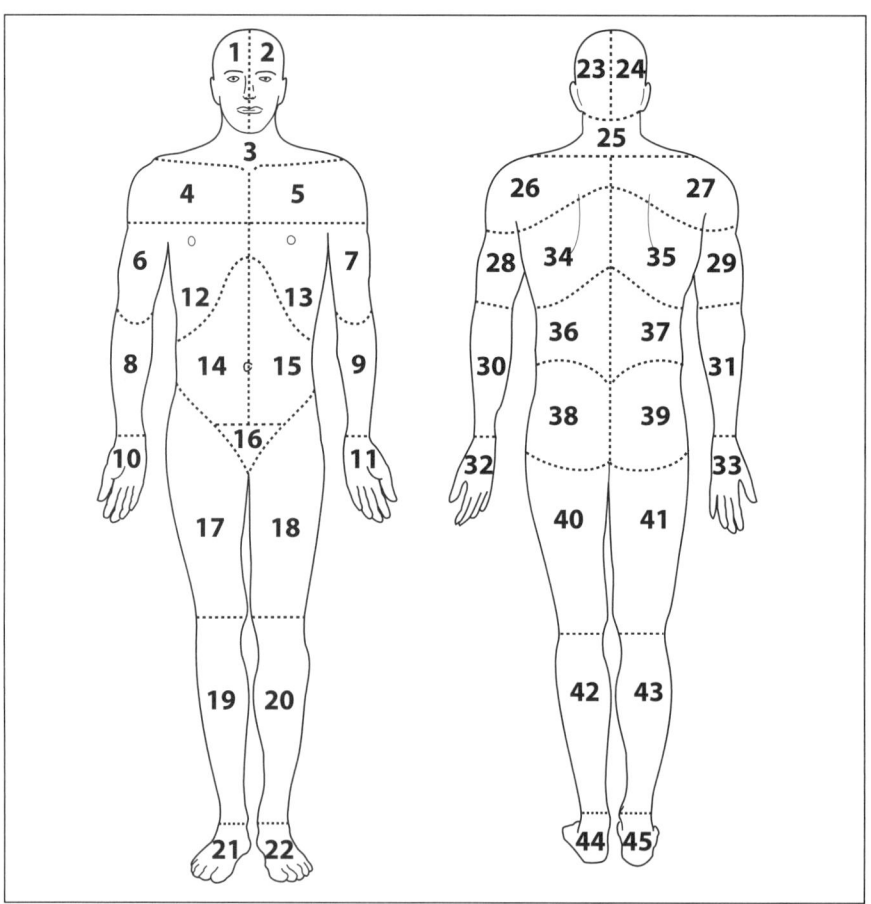

Source: Reprinted with permission from the International Association for the Study of Pain from Margolis, R.B., R.C. Tait, and S.J. Krause. A rating system for use with patient pain drawings. *Pain*, 1986. **24**:60.

drawings can be scored as to the percentage of body surface in the shaded regions by referring to a list of weighted values, shown in Table 10.3.

The test-retest reliability of pain drawings has been established in previous studies, even when administered in diverse settings.[35-37] Pain drawings are sometimes used in clinical practice to identify psychological disturbances in patients.[38] However, this method has demonstrated low sensitivity and positive predictive value,[39,40] suggesting pain drawings they have limited utility for this purpose, especially when used alone.

Pain Questionnaires

The *McGill Pain Questionnaire* (MPQ) was developed in 1975 by Melzak[41] to provide a quantitative measure of clinical pain. It is probably the most comprehensively tested pain measure of all time, and it has fared very well. Moreover, the MPQ has become the gold standard of pain measures, against which newly developed instruments are often tested. The MPQ is composed of three major classes of word descriptors that can be used by patients to identify their subjective pain experience. The three major classes are words that describe the sensory qualities of the experience; words that describe the affective aspects, in terms of

TABLE 10.3 Percentage of the body surface represented by the regions described by Margolis and colleagues

Area Numbers	Percentage
25, 26, 27	0.50
4, 5, 16	1.00
3, 8, 9, 10, 11, 30, 31, 32, 33	1.50
1, 2, 21, 23, 24, 44, 45	1.75
6, 7, 12, 13, 28, 29, 36, 37	2.00
38, 39	2.50
14, 15	3.00
19, 20, 42, 43	3.50
34, 35	4.00
17, 18, 40, 41	4.75

Source: Reprinted with permission from the International Association for the Study of Pain from Margolis, R.B., R.C. Tait, and S.J. Krause. A rating system for use with patient pain drawings. *Pain*, 1986. **24**:60.

tension, fear, and autonomic responses to the pain experience; and evaluative words that describe the intensity of the pain experience.

The four major parts of the MPQ are as follows: (1) a pain drawing on which patients mark the location of their pain; (2) pain descriptors that span 20 categories and 78 total possibilities (e.g., "sharp," "intense," "pinching," "aching"), with each descriptor having a rank value that signifies the relative intensity of pain; (3) several questions that assess how the pain changes over time and what relieves or increases it; and (4) a section that measures pain intensity.

A short form of the McGill Pain Questionnaire (SF-MPQ) performs comparably to the standard MPQ, yet takes less time to administer.[42] Hence, it is a practical option for office use that will generate nearly the same information as the standard MPQ (see Appendix 9). The SF-MPQ is scored as follows: mild = 1, moderate = 2, severe = 3; a value of 0 is assigned if an item is left unchecked. The mean score for sensory pain is the total of scores for items 1 through 11, divided by 11. The mean score for affective pain is the total of scores for items 12 through 15, divided by 4. The overall mean pain score is obtained by totaling scores for all 15 items and then dividing by 15.

Psychometric Measures

A relationship exists between the occurrence of pain, especially chronic pain, and patients' emotional and psychological state. Moreover, chronic pain may lead to anxiety, depression, and a feeling of hopelessness. Pain may exacerbate existing depression, and some patients may actually develop chronic pain as a result of depression.[43] Many chiropractors screen their pain patients using self-administered psychometric questionnaires, which can be helpful in identifying those who may need psychological referral.

The *Beck Depression Inventory* (BDI) is a frequently used depression screening test that can easily be integrated into a busy clinical practice. It has been reported to be the most commonly used self-administered scale for measuring depression worldwide.[44] Administering the BDI to chiropractic patients does not require any special training, and patients can usually complete the form in less than 10 minutes. Patients are simply asked to complete a 21-item instrument by marking a number ranging from 0 to 3 that corresponds with statements about how they perceive themselves. Each of the four statements is arranged in increasing levels of depression symptoms. An example of one of the BDI graded items"is as follows: 0, "I don't feel disappointed in myself" 1, "I am disappointed in myself"; 2, "I am disgusted with myself"; and 3, "I hate myself." Patients with BDI scores in the range 10 to 18 are considered to be mildly depressed, while those with scores ranging from 19 to 21 may be experiencing borderline clinical depression. Chiropractic patients consistently scoring above 18 on the BDI may need to be referred for evaluation by a psychologist.

The BDI has been tested numerous times for validity and reliability and has performed quite well. A systematic review of the BDI reported that the BDI had high internal consistency, high content validity, and good discriminant validity in being able to differentiate between depressed and nondepressed subjects, and that it was sensitive to change.[44] The BDI is copyrighted by the Psychological Corporation and may be purchased for use in clinical practice by contacting the company at http://www.psychcorp.com.

Another psychometric instrument that can be used to assess musculoskeletal pain patients is the *Symptom Checklist-90-Revised* (SCL-90-R). Originally published as the SCL-90,[45] it was modified slightly by the original author in 1983 to become the revised version.[46] The questionnaire contains 90 items that patients can typically complete in 12 to 15 minutes. Each of the included items is graded on a five-point (0–4) scale of distress that ranges from "not at all" to "extremely." The test measures nine primary symptom dimensions and three global indices. The Global Severity Index provides an overall summary of the test.

The reliability, validity, and utility of the SCL-90-R have been well established in many studies. It is commonly used for research purposes, as well as in clinical practice by psychologists and psychiatrists for assessment and for monitoring progress. The SCL-90-R can also be used by other health care professionals to screen patients for psychological involvement. The test must be purchased and is available in kit form from Pearson Assessments at http://www.pearsonassessments.com. The kit comes with a manual that includes published norms for comparison with patient scores.

Measures of Function

As mentioned earlier, there are many measures of function including questionnaires to evaluate activity limitations associated with a variety of conditions (e.g., knee pain, asthma, temporomandibular joint disorder, etc.). General health assessment questionnaires are also considered measures of function, as are physical tests that evaluate traits such as strength and range of motion.

Low Back–Specific Questionnaires

The *Oswestry Disability Index* (ODI) (also known as the Oswestry low back pain disability questionnaire) is one of the most commonly used condition-specific OMs in the management of spinal disorders.[47] The ODI was originally introduced by Fairbank and coworkers[48] in 1980 and has been used extensively in both research and clinical practice. Its validity and reliability has been well established,[49–51] and it compares favorably against other low back questionnaires.[52] Furthermore, a reliability coefficient (r) of 0.89 for same-day test-retest reliability was reported for the modified version of the ODI.[53]

The questionnaire includes 10 sections of six statements each that deal with activities of daily living and pain. At least four versions are available; however, the original authors recommended that their ODI 2.0 version should be used.[54] The Revised ODI omitted the original Section 8 that dealt with sex, replacing it with a section about the changing degree of pain[55] (see Appendix 10 and Table 10.4).

The ODI is self-administered by the patient and can usually be completed in less than five minutes. Scoring of the questionnaire is straightforward and can be performed by the doctor or a staff member. Each section of the ODI consists of six statements that describe an increasing level of disability associated with various activities. The last statement has the highest possible score, which is 5, and the first statement is valued at 0. The statements in between 0 and 5 are assigned ranked scores from 1 to 4. Sometimes patients choose more than one box in each section, in which case the highest score taken. The formula for calculating the ODI score is as follows:

TABLE 10.4 Question about sex that was omitted in the Revised Oswestry Disability Index

Section 8: Sex Life
- My sex life is normal and causes no extra pain.
- My sex life is normal but causes some extra pain.
- My sex life is nearly normal but is very painful.
- My sex life is severely restricted by pain.
- My sex life is nearly absent because of pain.
- Pain prevents any sex life at all.

Source: Reprinted with permission from Jeremy Fairbank, MD.

$$\text{ODI score (\%)} = \frac{\text{Total scored}}{\text{Total possible score}} \times 100$$

where the "total scored" is the total of all the statements selected by the patient, and the "total possible score" is the number of sections completed by the patient times 5. For example, if a patient with a raw score of 18 completed all 10 sections of the ODI, his or her percentage score would be calculated as follows:

$$\text{ODI score (\%)} = \frac{18 \text{ (total scored)}}{50 \text{ (total possible score)}} \times 100 = 36\%$$

If another patient also had a raw score of 18, but neglected to complete one section, his or her final score would be calculated as follows:

$$\text{ODI score (\%)} = \frac{18 \text{ (total scored)}}{45 \text{ (total possible score)}} \times 100 = 40\%$$

Alternatively, if patients complete all 10 sections of the ODI, their raw scores can simply be multiplied by 2 to convert to a percentage.

The minimum clinically important difference needed to distinguish patients who have improved from those who have not using the modified ODI has been estimated as 6 points.[56] Other researchers, however, have calculated it to be as high as 15 points.[52] The interpretation of given ODI scores was supplied by Fairbank and associates and is presented in Table 10.5.

The ODI and Visual Analogue Scale for pain were found to be the most reliable and responsive to clinical change for musculoskeletal disorders when compared with four other commonly used questionnaires.[52,57] As summarized by Fairbank and Pynsent,[47] "The ODI has stood the test of time and many reviews. It is usable in a wide variety of applications as a condition-specific outcome measure of spine-related disability."

Another frequently used OM that deals with low back pain is the *Roland-Morris Questionnaire* (RMQ).[58] Like the ODI, this questionnaire has been evaluated in a number of studies and shown to be valid and reliable for the assessment of low back disability. Moreover, Roland and Morris reported a same-day test-retest

TABLE 10.5 Interpretation of Oswestry Disability Index scores

ODI Score	Disability Level	Interpretation
0–20%	Minimal disability	This group can cope with most living activities. Usually no treatment is indicated, apart from advice on lifting, sitting posture, physical fitness, and diet. In this group, some patients have particular difficulty with sitting, and this may be important if their occupation is sedentary (e.g., a typist or driver).
20–40%	Moderate disability	This group experiences more pain and problems with sitting, lifting, and standing. Travel and social life are more difficult, and patients well be off work. Personal care, sexual activity, and sleeping are not grossly, affected and the back condition can usually be managed by conservative means.
40–60%	Severe disability	Pain remains the main problem in this group of patients, but travel, personal care, social life, sexual activity, and sleep are also affected. These patients require detailed investigation.
60–80%	Crippled	Back pain impinges on all aspects of these patients' lives both at home and at work, and positive intervention is required.
80–100%		These patients are either bed-bound or exaggerating their symptoms. This can be evaluated by careful observation of the patient during the medical examination.

Source: Reprinted with permission from Jeremy Fairbank, MD, from Fairbank, J.C., et al. The Oswestry low back pain disability questionnaires. *Physiotherapy*, 1980. **66**(8):271–3.

reliability value of $r = 0.91$, and Kopec and colleagues[59] reported an intraclass correlation coefficient (ICC) value of 0.93 for administration over 1 to 14 days. The RMQ has also been shown to be sensitive to change over time for low back pain patients.[60]

The RMQ is comprised of 24 questions that deal with low back pain and function, which patients can complete in approximately five minutes. The questionnaire can easily be scored in about one minute, either by the practitioner or a staff member. Scores range from 0, indicating no pain and normal function, to 24, pointing to the highest level of pain and diminished function. Patients are instructed to check the boxes next to the questions that describe themselves relative to their back pain (see Appendix 11). A pain rating scale that incorporated a thermometer to portray the various levels of pain accompanied the RMQ in the original article (Figure 10.6).

FIGURE 10.6 **Pain rating scale from Roland and Morris. Patients are instructed to put a cross by the words that best describe their level of pain. The thermometer provides patients with a visual clue as to the degree of pain.**

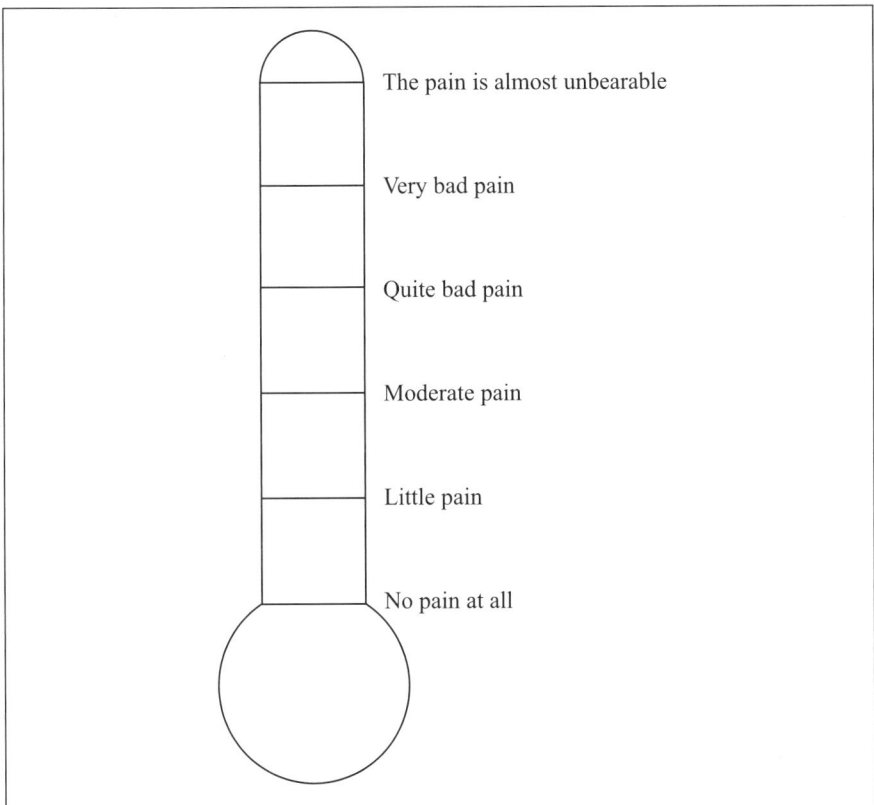

Source: From Roland, M., and R. Morris. A study of the natural history of back pain. Part I: development of a reliable and sensitive measure of disability in low-back pain. *Spine*, 1983. **8**(2):141–4. Reprinted with permission, Wolters Kluwer Health, LWW.

Roland and Morris did not provide an interpretation for the various levels of possible RMQ scores, although patient progress can be monitored by noting changes over time. Von Korff and Saunders[61] reported that scores of 13 or higher denoted significant disability that was associated with an unfavorable outcome. The percentage of improvement can be calculated as follows:

$$\text{RMQ improvement (\%)} = \frac{\text{Baseline RMQ score} - \text{Follow-up RMQ score}}{\text{Baseline RMQ score}} \times 100$$

For example, if a patient's initial RMQ score was 20 and his or her follow-up RMQ score was 6, the percentage of improvement would be calculated as follows:

$$\text{RMQ improvement (\%)} = \frac{20 - 6}{20} \times 100 = 70\%$$

Stratford and associates[60] reported that the minimum clinically important difference for RMQ evaluations was in the range of 4 to 5 points, while Davidson and Keating[52] reported its range as 8.6 to 9.5 points. Thus, patients would have to improve by at least 4 points on reevaluation in order to consider their condition as being improved. In a cross-sectional study that compared the ODI and RMQ scores in groups of patients with different levels of clinical severity, those with acute conditions and those with radiculopathy had higher scores than simple low back pain patients.[50] Several researchers have reported that the magnitude of the minimum clinically important difference appears to be dependent on the patient's initial RMQ score. It is lower (i.e., less than 5 points) for patients with low initial RMQ scores and higher (i.e., more than 5 points) for those with high initial scores.[60,62]

Neck-Specific Questionnaires

A commonly used instrument for assessing functional limitations associated with neck pain is the *Neck Disability Index* (NDI) (see Appendix 12). The instrument was developed in 1991 by Vernon and Mior as a modification of the Oswestry low back pain disability questionnaire.[63] Like the ODI, the NDI has 10 sections, and each of the sections has six related statements with ranked values ranging from 0 to 5. In their original article, the authors assessed concurrent validity by comparing the results of scored NDI questionnaires with both VAS and MPQ scores that were derived from the same groups of subjects. Correlation coefficients were moderately high in both instances (0.60 with the VAS, and 0.69–0.70 with the MPQ). Test-retest reliability was found to be very good ($r = 0.89$), and internal consistency was found to be good, with an overall Cronbach's coefficient alpha of 0.80. A subsequent study found the internal consistency of the NDI to be even higher, with a Cronbach's coefficient alpha of 0.92.[64] The minimal clinically important difference for the NDI is a five-point change in the raw score. The NDI is scored the same as the ODI (see earlier in the chapter), although the interpretation of NDI scores is somewhat different (Table 10.6).[63]

Neck pain is an almost universal complaint among whiplash patients; thus, questionnaires that deal with neck pain disability are commonly used to measure the functional limitations that are experienced by this population of patients. Because of the special needs of this population, the *Whiplash Disability Questionnaire* (WDQ) was developed to specifically address the functional impact of whiplash[65] (see Appendix 13).

The WDQ was constructed by using the basic components of the NDI and adding several questions designed to evaluate patients' emotional health, social activity, and fatigue.[66] Rather than a series of statements in each section, as in the NDI, the WDQ uses an 11-point (0–10) numerical scale for the patients' responses. Cronbach's coefficient alpha for the WDQ was 0.96, pointing to excellent internal consistency; there was also excellent short-term and one-month test-retest reliability (ICC = 0.96 and 0.93, respectively).[67] The minimum clinically important difference needed for the WDQ was determined to be 15 points.

Some of the other neck-specific questionnaires that one might encounter include the Copenhagen Neck Functional Disability Scale,[68] Northwick Park Neck Pain Questionnaire.[69] Neck Pain and Disability Scale,[70] and Patient-

TABLE 10.6 Interpretation of Neck Disability Index scores

NDI Score (Raw)	Disability Level
0–4	No disability
5–14	Mild disability
15–24	Moderate disability
25–34	Severe disability
≥ 35	Complete disability

Specific Functional Scale.[71] The first three of these instruments are very similar; however, only the NDI has been revalidated in diverse study populations,[72] and it is much more commonly encountered than the others.

Headache-Specific Questionnaires

The *Headache Disability Inventory* (HDI) was developed to assess the impact of headache on daily living[73] (see Appendix 14). The instrument consists of 25 questions, with 12 emotional and 13 functional subscales. Construct validity and internal reliability were found to be strong, and the test-retest reliability was acceptable. Test-retest reliability for the HDI was reevaluated by the original authors in a later study and found to be good.[74] Patients answer each question by choosing between the following responses: "yes" (a value of 4 points), "sometimes" (2 points), or "no" (0 points). Accordingly, the maximum possible HDI score is 100 points. Jacobson and associates[73,74] did not provide an interpretation for HDI scores, although they did report that when HDI scores were within the range of 2 to 32, self-perceived headache severity was mild; within the range of 33 to 59, moderate; and when 60 or greater, severe. At least a 29-point change in the total HDI score must occur from test to retest before the changes can be attributed to a patient's treatment. This requirement may be seen as a weakness of the HDI, since it is not possible to determine whether a patient's improvement is significant if his or her initial score was 29 or below.

The *Migraine Disability Assessment* Score (MIDAS) is another self-administered measure of disability associated with headache. The MIDAS questionnaire is very short, consisting of seven items, with only five items contributing to the overall score[75] (see Appendix 15). It was developed based on the Headache Impact Questionnaire (HIQ),[76] although with MIDAS, the method used to calculate the overall disability score is easier. Also, MIDAS scores are more intuitively meaningful than HIQ scores. Both of these properties enhance the questionnaire's clinical utility. Test-retest reliability was high for the MIDAS questionnaire, with reported correlation coefficients as follows: Spearman's rho = 0.84, and Pearson's r = 0.75. Internal consistency was also good, with a reported Cronbach's coefficient alpha of 0.83.

MIDAS scores are derived from three domains of activity: lost time from (1) work for pay, (2) housework or chores, and (3) leisure activities. The total number of headache-related missed days from school, paid work, or household work, and from family, social, or leisure activities over the previous three months contribute to the MIDAS score. The number of days where at least 50% reduced productivity was incurred is taken into consideration in questions 2 and 4. Questions A and B do not contribute to the MIDAS score, but are used to assess the frequency and intensity of the headaches. MIDAS scores have been divided into four grades that correspond to levels of headache disability, ranging from minimal or infrequent to severe (Table 10.7).

General Health Questionnaires

The *36-item short-form* (SF-36)[26] (also known as the RAND 36-Item Health Survey) is a general health questionnaire that assesses patients' health status from their point of view (see Appendix 16). The instrument is extensively used, both in research and clinical practice, and has been translated into a number of different languages. It can be used with patients experiencing diverse conditions[77–80] and among diverse populations.[81,82] One of the advantages of the SF-36 is that it can be self-administered by patients who are at least 14 years old by simply answering 36 straightforward questions. It typically takes patients about 5 to 10 minutes to complete and can also be administered via face-to-face interview or by telephone.

The SF-36 assesses eight concepts of health that are generally classified as being related to physical, emotional, or psychological distress. The eight health concepts or scales are as follows: (1) limitations in physical activities because of health problems, (2) limitations in usual role activities because of physical health problems, (3) bodily pain, (4) general health perceptions, (5) vitality, (6) limitations in social activities because of physical or emotional problems, (7) limitations in usual role activities because of emotional problems, and (8) mental health. When graded, the SF-36 generates a standardized score that reports on eight health scales, two summary measures, and self-perceived changes in health status.

TABLE 10.7 Grading system for the MIDAS questionnaire

Grade	Definition	Score
I	Minimal or infrequent disability	0–5
I	Mild or infrequent disability	6–10
III	Moderate disability	11–20
IV	Severe disability	>20

There is a distinction between the SF-36 and the RAND 36-Item Health Survey. They were both developed as part of the Medical Outcomes Study (a two-year study of patients with chronic conditions) and they both contain the same series of questions; however, the recommended scoring procedures are different.[83] Moreover, two of the eight scales (pain and general health) are scored differently; thus, the results for those scales are not comparable between the RAND and the standard SF-36. The reader is referred to the RAND Health website at http://www.rand.org/health/surveys/sf36item for further information and permissions on using the RAND 36-Item Health Survey in clinical practice at no cost.[84] The SF-36 is available for a fee through a licensing program from Quality Metric Incorporated. More information may be obtained at the SF-36 website: http://www.sf-36.org.

Scoring of the RAND 36-Item Health Survey involves two steps, which produce scores for each of the eight scales. The first step is to assign recorded values from the key presented in Table 10.8 to each of the patient's categorical responses. For instance, if the patient responded to item 21 by choosing selection 2, a value of 80 would be recorded. Higher recorded values correspond to a more favorable health status. The second step is to average the scores for each item in each of the eight scales to determine the scale scores. Table 10.9 identifies which items should be averaged for each scale. If an item is unanswered, it is eliminated from the calculation. Thus, only completed items should be used to calculate scale averages.

The internal consistency of the SF-36 has been reported to be high,[85] with Cronbach's coefficient alpha exceeding 0.8 on all of the included scales except social functioning, which had an alpha of 0.76. Other studies have also found the SF-36 to have excellent reliability,[86,87] and the physical functioning dimension has exceeded alpha = 0.90 in several studies.

An even shorter version of the SF-36 is the SF-12, which is a valid alternative to the longer version for assessing general health outcomes. The SF-12 incorporates only 12 of the SF-36 items, with one or two items from each of the eight health concepts being included. SF-12 scores have been shown to correlate well with those of the 36-item version.[88] Like the SF-36, the SF-12 must be purchased from Quality Metric Incorporated.

The *Dartmouth Primary Care Cooperative Information Project (COOP) chart system* is a patient-friendly measure of functional health status for adults and adolescents that is simple to administer and score.[89] The original Dartmouth

TABLE 10.8 Scoring the RAND 36 Item-Health Survey—Step 1: change categorical responses to recorded values

Item Numbers	Original Response*	Recorded Value
1, 2, 20, 22, 34, 36	1	100
	2	75
	3	50
	4	25
	5	0
3, 4, 5, 6, 7, 8, 9, 10, 11, 12	1	0
	2	50
	3	100
13, 14, 15, 16, 17, 18, 19	1	0
	2	100
21, 23, 26, 27, 30	1	100
	2	80
	3	60
	4	40
	5	20
	6	0
24, 25, 28, 29, 31	1	0
	2	20
	3	40
	4	60
	5	80
	6	100
32, 33, 35	1	0
	2	25
	3	50
	4	75
	5	100

*Precoded choices as presented in questionnaire.

COOP charts were slightly revised in the COOP/WONCA version, which queries patients about their function in the preceding two weeks instead of four weeks. The COOP charts measure the following dimensions of health: physical, emotional, daily activities, social activities, social support, pain, and overall health. The instrument is composed of a series of nine separate charts, with each one

TABLE 10.9 Scoring the RAND 36 Item Health Survey—Step 2: average items to form scales

Scale	Number of Items	Items to Average*
Physical functioning	10	3, 4, 5, 6, 7, 8, 9, 10, 11, 12
Role limitations due to physical health	4	13, 14, 15, 16,
Role limitations due to emotional problems	3	17, 18, 19
Energy/fatigue	4	23, 27, 29, 31
Emotional well-being	5	24, 25, 26, 28, 30
Social functioning	2	20, 32
Pain	2	21, 22
General health	5	1, 33, 34, 35, 36

*After recording their score according to Table 10.8.

having a title, a question about the functional status of the patient, and five responses for patients to choose from. A drawing accompanies each response that portrays an appropriate level of functioning or well-being.[90]

The COOP charts were found to be reliable and valid in a study involving over 2,000 patients that was carried out in four dissimilar clinical settings.[91] Short-term test-retest reliability resulted in ICCs that ranged from 0.73 to 0.98. The COOP charts were also correlated well with longer previously validated measures of function. This study also reported that the COOP charts were rated as being easy to use, both by patients as well as most clinicians. They can be self-administered by the patient or administered by the clinician or staff member. Scoring of the instrument is also reported to be easy. A high score (4 or 5) on any of the charts is considered to be abnormal.

There is no fee for their use, but the COOP charts are copyrighted, so practitioners must obtain permission before using them by contacting Debbie Johnson at the Dartmouth COOP Project, Dartmouth Medical School, Butler Building, HB 7265, Hanover, New Hampshire 03756 (telephone, 603-650-1220; e-mail, Deborah.Johnson@Dartmouth.edu).

The *Sickness Impact Profile* (SIP) is another general health questionnaire[92] that is commonly used in research; it is less often used in clinical practice, primarily due to its lengthiness. It is especially appropriate in conjunction with pain management,[93-95] and its validity and reliability have been established as acceptable for its use an OM for low back pain patients.[96,97] The SIP consists of 136 items that are capable of measuring patients' perceived level of impairment. There are 14 included subscales that deal with illness and the associated activity levels of those who are ill. Patients are asked to respond to statements only when they apply to them that day. The SIP deals with the physical as well as the psychosocial domains of health and assesses the limiting effects of pain across a wide range. Because of its widespread use in research, as well as the fact that its reliability and validity are so well established, it can be considered to be a gold standard OM for the self-reported features of pain.[98]

One thing to consider when patients are asked to complete multiple questionnaires is that an obvious break between each measure or topic should be provided to avoid confusion. Also, the use of similar presentation styles (i.e., font and layout of the forms) across measures can reduce errors.

Physiologic Measures

Physiologic OMs are direct examiner assessments that include the evaluation of such characteristics as range of motion, muscle strength and endurance testing, electromyography, postural analysis, algometry, and x-ray analysis. Physiologic OMs are objective and are often considered by practitioners to be more reliable than qualitative measures. However, the health-related quality of life measures are generally more reliable, as was stated earlier.

Range of motion (ROM) assessment is very common in clinical practice, although the validity and reliability are variable, depending on the region being examined and the evaluation method employed. The dual inclinometry method of examining lumbar ROM has been shown to be valid and reliable, especially regarding forward flexion. Moreover, Sauer and associates[99] reported that when measurements were taken radiographically, as compared with inclinometry, the correlation coefficient for pure flexion was $r = 0.98$ and for extension was $r = 0.75$.

Reliability has also been established for lumbar ROM testing in other studies, but the measurements were always done in isolation from other physical examination procedures. However, one study had examiners carry out lumbar ROM evaluations within a typical physical examination, as would be encountered in clinical practice. The results showed that most scores were not reliable in that setting.[100] The accuracy and clinical utility of lumbar ROM measurement also depend, to a great extent, on the training of the examiner.[101] Results are also influenced by the time of day that measurements are taken, making it important for comparative evaluations to be taken at the same time of day.[102] Considering the findings of these studies, lumbar ROM scores derived from the clinical environment may not actually be reliable, even though ample experimental evidence exists pointing to reliability.

In a meta-analysis that dealt with cervical ROM, Chen and coworkers[103] reported that intraexaminer ICC values in half-cycle single inclinometry studies ranged from 0.4 to 0.9, and interexaminer ICCs ranged from 0.7 to 0.9. The authors also reported that interexaminer r^2 values ranged from 0.2 for compass evaluation, to 0.96 for single inclinometry of cervical active total motions. Dual inclinometry of the cervical spine was shown to be highly reliable after a one-week interval, with ICC values ranging from 0.86 to 0.92.[103] On the other hand, visual observation of ROM is generally not reliable, with reported errors as high as 45 degrees. Selection of an appropriate method of ROM evaluation is therefore an important decision for clinicians. Chen and colleagues[103] concluded that dual inclinometry was the best available method to assess cervical ROM in clinical practice.

Some measures of impairment do not correlate well with patient function or disability, making their usefulness as outcome measures questionable. Indeed, Nattrass and associates[104] reported that range of motion and straight leg raise tests correlated poorly with spine-related impairment. These authors also pointed out that there was poor reliability using the American Medical Association guides' spinal range of motion model, which resulted in marked variation in the percentage of whole-body impairment that was reported between examiners, ranging from 0% to 18%.[104]

In spite of the limitations and controversies associated with measuring ROM, the procedure does provide important clinical information and has been shown to be an objective OM. Furthermore, it is widely used, both in clinical practice as well as in research.

Algometry involves the use of an instrument known as an *algometer* (also known as a *pain threshold meter*) that can be used to quantify the amount of surface pressure that is associated with subjective pain tolerance or tenderness at various points on the body. An algometer is simply a handheld rubber-tipped force gauge that registers the kilograms per square centimeter or pounds per square inch when pressure is applied. It is utilized by placing the rubber tip over the point to be examined (e.g., trigger point, tendon insertion, fibromyalgia test point) and applying an escalating amount of pressure. The patient is instructed to report the ensuing level of pain. Patients may be asked to report their pressure threshold or pressure tolerance. *Pressure threshold* is the minimum amount of pressure needed to cause pain.[105] *Pressure tolerance* is the maximum amount of pressure the patient can tolerate.[106] Pressure threshold measurement is typically used when testing over tender areas, whereas pressure tolerance is utilized with normal tissues. The tenderness rating scale that was presented in Table 10.2 can also be used to describe levels of pain associated with pressures applied during algometry.

Numerous studies have investigated the reliability and validity of algometry and have generally been favorable. Furthermore, the procedure has been tested in a variety of settings and on different tissues of the body.[105,107–110]

An international group of back pain researchers made recommendations for standardized measurement of outcomes to assess in patients with back pain.[111] They concluded that the key elements of assessment would include measures of pain symptoms, function, well-being, disability, and satisfaction with care. They indicated that back pain–related symptoms are best assessed by use of the following OMs:

1. VAS
2. Roland-Morris scale or Oswestry questionnaire
3. SF-12 or SF-36
4. Days off work or activity intolerances to reflect disability
5. A single question regarding overall satisfaction with care

It is important for clinicians to use the validated form of a test, without modifying any of the information from what was presented in the original literature. If pain scales, questionnaires, or physiologic tests are modified, even something as minor as changing the order of questions, the results may be affected; thus, the altered measure can no longer be considered to be valid or reliable. The instruments provided in the appendices are replicated as accurately as possible and should be functional in clinical practice.

References

1. Sackett, D.L. *Evidence-based medicine. Spine*, 1998. **23**(10):1085–6.
2. Green, B.N., C.D. Johnson, and A. Adams. *Caveat emptor! Evaluate and maximize your technique seminar experience. Topics in Clinical Chiropractic*, 1998. **5**(2):19–26.

Chapter 10 Evidence-Based Chiropractic and Documentation

3. Strender, L.E., et al. *Interexaminer reliability in physical examination of patients with low back pain. Spine,* 1997. **22**(7):814–20.
4. Mootz, R.D. *Maximizing the effectiveness of clinical documentation. Topics in Clinical Chiropractic*, 1994. **1**(1):60–5.
5. Yeomans, S.G. *The Clinical Application of Outcomes Assessment.* Stamford, Conn: Appleton & Lang. 2000.
6. Field, M., and K.N. Lohr, eds. *Guidelines for Clinical Practice. From Development to Use.* Institute of Medicine. Washington, DC: National Academy Press. 1992.
7. Eccles, M., and J. Mason. *How to develop cost-conscious guidelines. Health Technology Assessment*, 2001. **5**(16). 1–16.
8. Shekelle, P.G., et al. *Clinical guidelines: Developing guidelines. BMJ,* 1999. **318**(7183): 593–6.
9. Haldeman, S., D. Chapman-Smith, and D.M. Petersen. *Guidelines for Chiropractic Quality Assurance and Practice Parameters : Proceedings of the Mercy Center Consensus Conference.* Gaithersburg, Md: Aspen Publishers. 1993.
10. Cates, J.R., et al. *An independent assessment of chiropractic practice guidelines. J Manipulative Physiol Ther*, 2003. **26**(5):282–6.
11. Cates, J.R., et al. *Evaluating the quality of clinical practice guidelines. J Manipulative Physiol Ther*, 2001. **24**(3):170–6.
12. Mottur-Pilson, C. *Clinical practice guidelines: Friend or foe?* 2005. American College of Physicians. http://www.acponline.org/sci-policy/guidelines/friendorfoe.htm.
13. Raine, R., C. Sanderson, and N. Black. *Developing clinical guidelines: A challenge to current methods. BMJ*, 2005. **331**(7517):631–33.
14. Shekelle, P., et al. *When should clinical guidelines be updated? BMJ*, 2001. **323**(7305): 155–7.
15. Hayward, R.S., et al. *Users' guides to the medical literature. VIII. How to use clinical practice guidelines. A. Are the recommendations valid? The Evidence-Based Medicine Working Group. JAMA*, 1995. **274**(7):570–4.
16. Wilson, M.C., et al. *Users' guides to the medical literature. VIII. How to use clinical practice guidelines. B. What are the recommendations and will they help you in caring for your patients? The Evidence-Based Medicine Working Group. JAMA*, 1995. **274**(20):1630–2.
17. Basinski, A.S. *Evaluation of clinical practice guidelines. CMAJ*, 1995. **153**(11):1575–81.
18. Perleth, M., E. Jakubowski, and R. Busse. *What is 'best practice' in health care? State of the art and perspectives in improving the effectiveness and efficiency of the European health care systems. Health Policy*, 2001. **56**(3):235–50.
19. Driever, M.J. *Are evidenced-based practice and best practice the same? West J Nurs Res*, 2002. **24**(5):591–7.
20. Resnik, L., and E. Dobrykowski. *Outcomes measurement for patients with low back pain. Orthop Nurs*, 2005. **24**(1):14–24.
21. Grimmer, K., et al. *Differences in stakeholder expectations in the outcome of physiotherapy management of acute low back pain. Int J Qual Health Care*, 1999. **11**(2):155–62.
22. Institute for Clinical Systems Improvement. *Adult Low Back Pain.* Bloomington, Minn: Institute for Clinical Systems Improvement. 2004.
23. Jette, A.M. *Using health-related quality of life measures in physical therapy outcomes research. Phys Ther*, 1993. **73**(8):528–37.

24. Beattie, P., and C. Maher. *The role of functional status questionnaires for low back pain.* Aust J Physiother, 1997. **43**(1):29–38.
25. Guyatt, G.H., D.H. Feeny, and D.L. Patrick. *Measuring health-related quality of life.* Ann Intern Med, 1993. **118**(8):622–9.
26. Ware, J.E., Jr., and C.D. Sherbourne. *The MOS 36–item short-form health survey (SF-36). I. Conceptual framework and item selection.* Med Care, 1992. **30**(6):473–83.
27. Bergner, M., et al. *The Sickness Impact Profile: Validation of a Health Status Measure.* Med Care, 1976. **14**(1):57–67.
28. Boline, P.D., et al. *Spinal manipulation vs. amitriptyline for the treatment of chronic tension-type headaches: A randomized clinical trial.* J Manipulative Physiol Ther, 1995. **18**(3):148–54.
29. Bradley, L.A., N.L. McKendree-Smith, and G.S. Alarcon. *Pain complaints in patients with fibromyalgia versus chronic fatigue syndrome.* Curr Rev Pain, 2000. **4**(2):148–57.
30. Bijur, P.E., C.T. Latimer, and E.J. Gallagher. *Validation of a verbally administered numerical rating scale of acute pain for use in the emergency department.* Acad Emerg Med, 2003. **10**(4):390–2.
31. Von Korff, M., et al. *Back pain in primary care. Outcomes at 1 year.* Spine, 1993. **18**(7):855–62.
32. Williamson, A., and B. Hoggart. *Pain: A review of three commonly used pain rating scales.* J Clin Nurs, 2005. **14**(7):798–804.
33. Hubbard, D.R., and G.M. Berkoff. *Myofascial trigger points show spontaneous needle EMG activity.* Spine, 1993. **18**(13):1803–7.
34. Wolfe, F., et al. *The American College of Rheumatology 1990 criteria for the classification of fibromyalgia. Report of the Multicenter Criteria Committee.* Arthritis Rheum, 1990. **33**(2):160–72.
35. Margolis, R.B., R.C. Tait, and S.J. Krause. *A rating system for use with patient pain drawings.* Pain, 1986. **24**(1):57–65.
36. Margolis, R.B., J.T. Chibnall, and R.C. Tait. *Test-retest reliability of the pain drawing instrument.* Pain, 1988. **33**(1):49–51.
37. Lacey, R.J., et al. *Interrater reliability of scoring of pain drawings in a self-report health survey.* Spine, 2005. **30**(16):E455–8.
38. Hildebrandt, J., et al. *The use of pain drawings in screening for psychological involvement in complaints of low-back pain.* Spine, 1988. **13**(6):681–5.
39. Pande, K.C., S. Tripathi, and R. Kanoi. *Limited clinical utility of pain drawing in assessing patients with low back pain.* J Spinal Disord Tech, 2005. **18**(2):160–2.
40. Parker, H., P.L. Wood, and C.J. Main. *The use of the pain drawing as a screening measure to predict psychological distress in chronic low back pain.* Spine, 1995. **20**(2):236–43.
41. Melzack, R. *The McGill Pain Questionnaire: Major properties and scoring methods.* Pain, 1975. **1**(3):277–99.
42. Melzack, R. *The short-form McGill Pain Questionnaire.* Pain, 1987. **30**(2):191–7.
43. Rush, A.J., P. Polatin, and R.J. Gatchel. *Depression and chronic low back pain: Establishing priorities in treatment.* Spine, 2000. **25**(20):2566–71.
44. Richter, P., et al. *On the validity of the Beck Depression Inventory. A review.* Psychopathology, 1998. **31**(3):160–8.
45. Derogatis, L.R., K. Rickels, and A.F. Rock. *The SCL-90 and the MMPI: A step in the validation of a new self-report scale.* Br J Psychiatry, 1976. **128**:280–9.

46. Derogatis, L.R. *SCL-90–R: Administration, Scoring and Procedures Manual Vol. II.* 1983. Towson, Md: Clinical Psychometric Research.
47. Fairbank, J.C., and P.B. Pynsent. *The Oswestry Disability Index. Spine,* 2000. **25**(22):2940–52; discussion 2952.
48. Fairbank, J.C., et al. *The Oswestry low back pain disability questionnaire. Physiotherapy,* 1980. **66**(8):271–3.
49. Beurskens, A.J., H.C. de Vet, and A.J. Koke. *Responsiveness of functional status in low back pain: A comparison of different instruments. Pain,* 1996. **65**(1):71–6.
50. Leclaire, R., et al. *A cross-sectional study comparing the Oswestry and Roland-Morris functional disability scales in two populations of patients with low back pain of different levels of severity. Spine,* 1997. **22**(1):68–71.
51. Loisel, P., et al. *Is work status of low back pain patients best described by an automated device or by a questionnaire?* Spine, 1998. **23**(14):1588–94; discussion 1595.
52. Davidson, M. and J.L. Keating. *A comparison of five low back disability questionnaires: Reliability and responsiveness. Phys Ther,* 2002. **82**(1):8–24.
53. Baker, D., P.B. Pynsent, and J. Fairbank. *The Oswestry Disability Index revisited: Its reliability, repeatability, and validity, and a comparison with the St Thomas Disability Index.* In *Back Pain: New Approaches to Rehabilitation and Education,* M. Roland and J.R. Jenner, eds. 1989. Manchester, United Kingdom: Manchester University Press, 174–86.
54. Fairbank, J. *Revised Oswestry disability questionnaire. Spine,* 2000. **25**(19):2552.
55. Hudson-Cook, N., K. Tomes-Nicholson, and A. Breen. *A revised Oswestry disability questionnaire.* In: *Back Pain: New Approaches to Rehabilitation and Education,* M.O. Roland and J.R. Jenner, eds. 1989. Manchester, United Kingdom: Manchester University Press, 187–204.
56. Fritz, J.M. and J.J. Irrgang. *A comparison of a modified Oswestry low back pain disability questionnaire and the Quebec Back Pain Disability Scale. Phys Ther,* 2001. **81**(2):776–88.
57. Triano, J.J., et al. *A comparison of outcome measures for use with back pain patients: Results of a feasibility study. J Manipulative Physiol Ther,* 1993. **16**(2):67–73.
58. Roland, M. and R. Morris. *A study of the natural history of back pain. Part I: development of a reliable and sensitive measure of disability in low-back pain. Spine,* 1983. **8**(2):141–4.
59. Kopec, J.A., et al. *The Quebec Back Pain Disability Scale. Measurement properties. Spine,* 1995. **20**(3):341–52.
60. Stratford, P.W., et al. *Defining the minimum level of detectable change for the Roland-Morris questionnaire. Phys Ther,* 1996. **76**(4):359–65; discussion 366–8.
61. Von Korff, M., and K. Saunders. *The course of back pain in primary care. Spine,* 1996. **21**(24):2833–7; discussion 2838–9.
62. Riddle, D.L., P.W. Stratford, and J.M. Binkley. *Sensitivity to change of the Roland-Morris Back Pain Questionnaire: Part 2. Phys Ther,* 1998. **78**(11):1197–207.
63. Vernon, H., and S. Mior. *The Neck Disability Index: A study of reliability and validity. J Manipulative Physiol Ther,* 1991. **14**(7):409–15.
64. Hains, F., J. Waalen, and S. Mior. *Psychometric properties of the Neck Disability Index. J Manipulative Physiol Ther,* 1998. **21**(2):75–80.
65. Pinfold, M., et al. *Validity and internal consistency of a whiplash-specific disability measure. Spine,* 2004. **29**(3):263–8.

66. Hoving, J.L., et al. *Validity of the Neck Disability Index, Northwick Park Neck Pain Questionnaire, and problem elicitation technique for measuring disability associated with whiplash-associated disorders. Pain*, 2003. **102**(3):273–81.
67. Willis, C., et al. *Reproducibility and responsiveness of the Whiplash Disability Questionnaire. Pain*, 2004. **110**(3):681–8.
68. Jordan, A., et al. *The Copenhagen Neck Functional Disability Scale: A study of reliability and validity. J Manipulative Physiol Ther*, 1998. **21**(8):520–7.
69. Leak, A.M., et al. *The Northwick Park Neck Pain Questionnaire, devised to measure neck pain and disability. Br J Rheumatol*, 1994. **33**(5):469–74.
70. Wheeler, A.H., et al. *Development of the Neck Pain and Disability Scale. Item analysis, face, and criterion-related validity. Spine*, 1999. **24**(13):1290–4.
71. Westaway, M.D., P.W. Stratford, and J.M. Binkley. *The Patient-Specific Functional Scale: Validation of its use in persons with neck dysfunction. J Orthop Sports Phys Ther*, 1998. **27**(5):331–8.
72. Pietrobon, R., et al. *Standard scales for measurement of functional outcome for cervical pain or dysfunction: A systematic review. Spine*, 2002. **27**(5):515–22.
73. Jacobson, G.P., et al. *The Henry Ford Hospital Headache Disability Inventory (HDI). Neurology*, 1994. **44**(5):837–42.
74. Jacobson, G.P., et al. *Headache Disability Inventory (HDI): Short-term test-retest reliability and spouse perceptions. Headache*, 1995. **35**(9):534–9.
75. Stewart, W.F., et al. *Reliability of the migraine disability assessment score in a population-based sample of headache sufferers. Cephalalgia*, 1999. **19**(2):107–14; discussion 74.
76. Stewart, W.F., et al. *Reliability of an illness severity measure for headache in a population sample of migraine sufferers. Cephalalgia*, 1998. **18**(1):44–51.
77. Stoll, T., et al. *Consistency and validity of patient administered assessment of quality of life by the MOS SF-36; its association with disease activity and damage in patients with systemic lupus erythematosus. J Rheumatol*, 1997. **24**(8):1608–14.
78. Anderson, C., S. Laubscher, and R. Burns. *Validation of the Short Form 36 (SF-36) health survey questionnaire among stroke patients. Stroke*, 1996. **27**(10):1812–6.
79. Johnson, P.A., et al. *Comparison of the Medical Outcomes Study Short-Form 36–Item Health Survey in black patients and white patients with acute chest pain. Med Care*, 1995. **33**(2):145–60.
80. Schwab, F., et al. *Adult scoliosis: A health assessment analysis by SF-36. Spine*, 2003. **28**(6):602–6.
81. Walters, S.J., J.F. Munro, and J.E. Brazier. *Using the SF-36 with older adults: A cross-sectional community-based survey. Age Ageing*, 2001. **30**(4):337–43.
82. McHorney, C.A., et al. *The MOS 36–item Short-Form Health Survey (SF-36): III. Tests of data quality, scaling assumptions, and reliability across diverse patient groups. Med Care*, 1994. **32**(1):40–66.
83. Hays, R.D., C.D. Sherbourne, and R.M. Mazel. *The RAND 36–Item Health Survey 1.0. Health Econ*, 1993. **2**(3):217–27.
84. RAND. *Medical Outcomes Study (MOS): 36–Item Short Form Health Survey (SF-36)*. 2005. http://www.rand.org/health/surveys/sf36.htm/.
85. Jenkinson, C., A. Coulter, and L. Wright. *Short form 36 (SF36) health survey questionnaire: Normative data for adults of working age. BMJ*, 1993. **306**(6890):1437–40.

86. Brazier, J.E., et al. *Validating the SF-36 health survey questionnaire: New outcome measure for primary care. BMJ*, 1992. **305**(6846):160–4.
87. Ruta, D.A., et al. *SF 36 health survey questionnaire: I. Reliability in two patient based studies. Qual Health Care*, 1994. **3**(4):180–5.
88. Ware, J., Jr., M. Kosinski, and S.D. Keller. *A 12–item short-form health survey: Construction of scales and preliminary tests of reliability and validity. Med Care*, 1996. **34**(3):220–33.
89. Nelson, E.C., et al. *Dartmouth COOP functional health assessment charts: Brief measures for clinical practice*. In *More About the COOP Charts*. 2005. Hanover, NH: Dartmouth COOP Project, Dartmouth Medical School.
90. Nelson, E.C., and D.M. Berwick. *The measurement of health status in clinical practice. Med Care*, 1989. **27**(3 suppl):S77–90.
91. Nelson, E.C., et al. *The functional status of patients. How can it be measured in physicians' offices? Med Care*, 1990. **28**(12):1111–26.
92. Gilson, B.S., et al. *The Sickness Impact Profile. Development of an outcome measure of health care. Am J Public Health*, 1975. **65**(12):1304–10.
93. Stratford, P., et al. *Sensitivity of Sickness Impact Profile items to measure change over time in a low-back pain patient group. Spine*, 1993. **18**(13):1723–7.
94. Wahlgren, D.R., et al. *One-year follow-up of first onset low back pain. Pain*, 1997. **73**(2):213–21.
95. Beaton, D.E., C. Bombardier, and S.A. Hogg-Johnson. *Measuring health in injured workers: A cross-sectional comparison of five generic health status instruments in workers with musculoskeletal injuries. Am J Ind Med*, 1996. **29**(6):618–31.
96. Follick, M.J., T.W. Smith, and D.K. Ahern. *The Sickness Impact Profile: A global measure of disability in chronic low back pain. Pain*, 1985. **21**(1):67–76.
97. Deyo, R.A., and A.K. Diehl. *Measuring physical and psychosocial function in patients with low-back pain. Spine*, 1983. **8**(6):635–42.
98. Veterans Health Administration. *VHA Pain Outcomes Toolkit*. 2003. Washington, DC: Department of Veterans Affairs.
99. Sauer, P.M., et al. *Lumbar range of motion: Reliability and validity of the inclinometer technique in the clinical measurement of trunk flexibility. Spine*, 1996. 21(11):1332–8.
100. Hunt, D.G., et al. *Reliability of the lumbar flexion, lumbar extension, and passive straight leg raise test in normal populations embedded within a complete physical examination. Spine*, 2001. **26**(24):2714–8.
101. Mayer, T.G., et al. *Spinal range of motion. Accuracy and sources of error with inclinometric measurement. Spine*, 1997. **22**(17):1976–84.
102. Ensink, F.B., et al. *Lumbar range of motion: Influence of time of day and individual factors on measurements. Spine*, 1996. **21**(11):1339–43.
103. Chen, J., et al. *Meta-analysis of normative cervical motion. Spine*, 1999. **24**(15):1571–8.
104. Nattrass, C.L., et al. *Lumbar spine range of motion as a measure of physical and functional impairment: An investigation of validity. Clin Rehabil*, 1999. **13**(3):211–8.
105. Fischer, A.A. *Pressure algometry over normal muscles. Standard values, validity and reproducibility of pressure threshold. Pain*, 1987. **30**(1):115–26.
106. Goddard, G., H. Karibe, and C. McNeill, *Reproducibility of visual analog scale (VAS) pain scores to mechanical pressure. Cranio*, 2004. **22**(3):250–6.

107. Antonaci, F., et al. *Pain threshold in humans. A study with the pressure algometer.* Funct Neurol, 1992. **7**(4):283–8.
108. Reeves, J.L., B. Jaeger, and S.B. Graff-Radford. *Reliability of the pressure algometer as a measure of myofascial trigger point sensitivity.* Pain, 1986. **24**(3):313–21.
109. Bovim, G. *Cervicogenic headache, migraine, and tension-type headache. Pressure-pain threshold measurements.* Pain, 1992. **51**(2):169–73.
110. Delaney, G.A., and A.C. McKee. *Inter- and intra-rater reliability of the pressure threshold meter in measurement of myofascial trigger point sensitivity.* Am J Phys Med Rehabil, 1993. **72**(3):136–9.
111. Deyo, R.A., et al. *Outcome measures for low back pain research. A proposal for standardized use.* Spine, 1998. **23**(18):2003–13.

CHAPTER ELEVEN

Putting It All together

Thus far this book has introduced the evidence-based chiropractic (EBC) model and how the steps of EBC can be used to solve problems encountered in clinical practice. Information was also presented on how to find evidence in the health care literature, the types of research designs that are commonly used to investigate chiropractic topics, and how to appraise evidence after it has been located. This chapter presents some hypothetical examples of situations in which the use of EBC would be helpful in everyday practice. Although the five steps of EBC were originally developed for use in solving clinical questions that arise during patient encounters, the same principles can enable practitioners to find answers to many commonplace questions. For example, EBC can facilitate decision making about which continuing education seminars to attend, which educational materials to purchase (e.g., books, tapes, journal subscriptions), and even which equipment to purchase. Once mastered, practitioners can use EBC to assist with nearly all decisions that relate to clinical practice.

Practical Clinical Scenarios

Patient Encounters

It is Monday morning, and a practitioner is confronted with a 23-year-old female patient complaining of neck pain and a throbbing headache. The headache occurs several times per week and extends from behind the right eye to the occiput. The neck pain is constant, varying in intensity from 2 to 9 on the 11–point Numeric Rating Scale (NRS). The headaches typically last three to four hours and are not preceded by an aura. If the patient lies down in a darkened room at the onset of the headache, the pain only becomes a 4 on the 11–point NRS; if not, it may progress to an 8 or 9 with associated nausea and vomiting. On examination, there are several trigger points in the upper cervical musculature that exhibit grade 2 tenderness. Cervical range of motion is restricted and painful on extension and lateral bending to both sides. The Characteristic Pain Intensity score is 6, and the Headache Disability Inventory score is 55 (moderate).

The patient has been under the care of a neurologist for several years, but obtains little relief from prescribed medication. Consequently, she now wants to try chiropractic. How should one proceed with this patient? Does migraine headache respond to chiropractic care (i.e., is the care evidence-based)? Are there adjunctive therapies that may be beneficial? Does this patient actually have migraine, or is it in reality a cervicogenic headache? With these questions in mind, this would be an excellent opportunity to apply the five steps of EBC to a clinical problem.

The first step is to generate an appropriate foreground question. However, some background information on migraine may be helpful in this case, which can quickly be obtained from the online edition of *The Merck Manual*.[1] Merck defines migraine as "headache that lasts 4 to 72 hours, is throbbing, is moderate to severe in intensity, is unilateral, becomes worse with exertion, and is associated with nausea, vomiting, or sensitivity to light, sound, or smell." Three to four of these criteria must be present to make the diagnosis. There are no specific tests that are of use in diagnosing migraine. Merck also reports that the condition's onset is often between the ages of 10 to 40, it is more common in women, and there is often a family history of migraine. The cause of migraine has not been identified, although there are associated changes in the arterial blood flow of the brain and scalp. Migraine can be triggered by several factors, including estrogen cycles in females, changing barometric pressure, insomnia, and hunger. The headache is preceded by an aura in 10% to 20% of migraine cases. Medical treatment includes a variety of medications that are intended to prevent, abort, or relieve the headache symptoms; although rebound headache may occur with the use of analgesics. Merck does not include any information about cervicogenic headaches.

From this information, the following clinical question can be composed: *Is spinal manipulation and/or adjunctive physiotherapy effective at reducing pain in a young adult female headache patient?* A second part to this clinical question is called for to ascertain the best diagnostic tests to accurately diagnose the headache: *What are the appropriate diagnostic tests to differentiate migraine from cervicogenic headache?* These questions can be broken down into their PICO components as follows.

Patient or Problem: A young adult female headache patient.
Intervention: Manipulation and/or adjunctive physiotherapy, and appropriate diagnostic tests.
Comparison: Tests that can differentiate migraine from cervicogenic headache.
Outcome: Reducing pain, and accurate diagnosis.

At this point, search terms can be selected that are derived from these clinical questions.

Selecting search terms from a clinical question merely involves choosing several key words that convey the general idea of the topic. In this case, the terms *migraine* and *cervicogenic headache* are chosen. Other search terms could also be utilized (e.g., *manipulation* or *diagnosis*), depending on the search strategy. The next step is to determine if corresponding MeSH terms are available. When searching for **migraine** using the MeSH database, which can be accessed from the PubMed home page, we find that the MeSH term **migraine without aura** is most appropriate. This is based on the descriptions provided by MeSH, which indicate that headaches not preceded or accompanied by an aura are considered to be common migraines, as opposed to the MeSH term **classic migraine**, which is used when an aura is present.

There are no MeSH terms that directly correspond with *cervicogenic headache*, but the database suggests an alternate term, **generalized headache**. However, this search term is too broad and will most likely produce too many citations to be manageable. A text word search using the [tw] field tag after **cervicogenic headache** will be used instead. Thus, the PubMed search terms that are typed into the query box are as follows: **migraine without aura [MeSH] AND cervicogenic headache [tw]**. If desired, the specific clinical study categories "therapy" and "diagnosis" can be searched separately by clicking the Clinical Queries link from the PubMed home page.

The search retrieves three citations, with one by Antonaci and associates[2] being particularly applicable to this situation. This article reports that cervicogenic headache is very similar to common migraine, but is associated with symptoms and signs that link it to the neck. The fact that this patient has associated neck pain, tender trigger points, and reduced range of motion suggests that the patient's headache is of cervical origin rather than a common migraine. The article does not discuss treatment options, so another search of PubMed is called for. This time, a text word search will be performed using **cervicogenic headache**, but without the MeSH term **migraine without aura**. It would be preferable if a meta-analysis could be located; therefore, the PubMed Limits tab is selected, and Meta-Analysis is chosen from the Publication Types drop-down menu. Two articles are retrieved, with one of them pertaining to manipulation for tension and migraine headaches[3] and the other to electrotherapy for neck disorders.[4] The first article is positive, pointing to an effect with manipulation that is comparable to commonly used prescription medications and better than massage. On the other hand, the article on electrotherapy does not point to effectiveness, with evidence either lacking, limited, or having conflicting results. Just to be certain that there are no other meta-analyses available on this topic, another search is carried out using the same search terms on the MANTIS database. Using the same search terms with the High Clinical Relevancy option checked, 21 citations are retrieved, which comprise case reports, clinical trials, and review articles. One of the retrieved articles[5] is a systematic review that is at odds with the positive review mentioned previously. However, a letter to the editor by Vernon[6] pointed out numerous errors and omissions in this review, which leads to a decision to choose the former. Another study retrieved from MANTIS indicates that there is a dose-response relationship with chiropractic care for the treatment of cervicogenic headache, with larger doses (9 to 12 chiropractic treatments) being more beneficial than lower doses.[7]

The next step in the EBC process is to read and critique the articles that were retrieved during the literature search. The systematic review by Bronfort and colleagues,[7] *"Efficacy of Spinal Manipulation for Chronic Headache: A Systematic Review,"* is critiqued using the *checklist for the appraisal of review articles* found in Appendix 4. It appears that the study's methodology was sound, that a thorough search was carried out, and that the incorporated articles were accurately appraised and synthesized in an unbiased manner.

In the fourth step of EBC, the information gained from the selected articles is applied to the management of the patient's condition, along with the practitioner's clinical expertise and the patient's values. Based on the reviewed evidence and past experience with other headache patients, a series of chiropractic adjustments is recommended to the patient, but without the use of electrotherapy. The recommended visit frequency is three times per week, based on the study by Haas and associates[7] that reported better outcomes when larger doses of chiropractic treatment were utilized. The initial outcome measures are to be readministered at two and four weeks to monitor the patient's progress.

At this point the patient has a "values" issue and is hesitant to accept cervical manipulation because her neurologist told her that she might develop a stroke as a result. However, when informed that the chances of this occurring are 1 per 1,000,000 cervical manipulations or less and that these types of strokes have been reported following just about any activity that involves neck movement, she accepts the treatment recommendations.

The final EBC step in this case is to review the first four steps to see if anything could have been done differently to improve the process. In this case, the PubMed search may have been too limited, since a total of only five citations were retrieved from two searches. On the other hand, the MANTIS search, which is a much smaller database, produced 21 citations. Another issue that may be problematic in future patient encounters was the statement that the incidence of stroke following cervical manipulation was 1 per 1,000,000 or less. This statement was obtained from a practice management company brochure, but the accuracy of the statement was not verified. Since the issue regularly crops up in chiropractic practice, a separate literature search will be performed on the topic.

The PubMed search strategy this time will be as follows: **chiropractic manipulation AND (stroke OR dissection) AND incidence**. This search produces 12 citations, most of which are case reports or review articles. Some incidence estimates are provided, with the reported rate of vertebral artery dissection following cervical manipulation ranging from 1 in 400,000 to 1 in 5,846,381 cervical manipulation.[8,9] Therefore, the 1 in 1,000,000 estimate that was obtained from the practice management brochure is probably as close as can be ascertained, given the data available at this time.

Some additional information about manipulation and stroke that will be helpful in the future is derived from the articles that were discovered in the literature search. Based on a retrospective review of 64 medical legal cases, Haldeman and coworkers[10] reported that strokes following manipulation were not related to any particular manipulative technique that was used. Indeed, strokes were noted following rotation, extension, lateral flexion, neutral position, and even nonforce manipulations. The authors suggested that these types of strokes following manipulation were random and unpredictable and could be associated with virtually any neck movement. The authors went on to report that patients frequently seek chiropractic treatment for head or neck pain or both, but these symptoms are many times indistinguishable from those of cervical arterial dissection.[11] Therefore, practitioners should be especially attentive to patients with a sudden onset of acute and unusual head or neck pain that may actually be related to a dissection in progress. When these patients manifest signs or symptoms of brain ischemia (i.e., dizziness, diplopia, ataxia, Horner's syndrome, nystagmus), the best defense for chiropractors is to avoid cervical manipulation.[12,13] A patient with a sudden onset of acute and unusual head or neck pain or both is also dizzy may be managed with other nonmanipulative chiropractic procedures until the symptoms that could possibly be related to ischemia have subsided. On the other hand, patients with "hard" signs of brain involvement should immediately be referred for a neurological evaluation.

Selection of Postgraduate Education

The clinical scenario just described is an example of the most common application of the steps involved in evidence-based practice (EBP) and the primary reason that the method was developed. Another use has to do with choosing postgraduate training that is most likely to be of benefit. There are literally hundreds of seminars, conferences, and meetings to choose from. Some of them are very high quality, while some are poor quality and should be avoided.

When selecting postgraduate education, there are some other factors to consider in addition to the steps of EBP. One thing that is helpful is to make sure that the program is affiliated with a trustworthy sponsoring organization (e.g., a chiropractic college or association). These types of organizations generally have some basic criteria that must be met before sponsorship of educational programs is permitted. Such affiliation is not a guarantee that the instructional material of a particular seminar or conference is valid and worthwhile, but at least the worst offenders are usually eliminated.

The instructor or instructors should be well trained, with legitimate credentials and specialties in the topic being discussed. Beware of inflated or falsified credentials (e.g., Diplomate of the National Board of Chiropractic Examiners, mail-order degrees). The qualifications of all speakers should be provided in promotional materials or should at least be made available upon request. Lecture notes are not typically accessible prior to educational meetings, but once obtained, they should be critiqued using strategies similar to those used to evaluate journal articles. Brochures, web pages, and other forms of advertisement are usually available beforehand and should also be evaluated. Explanations of seemingly outlandish and unsupported claims can sometimes be obtained directly from the instructor.

A hypothetical example of how to make a decision on whether to participate in a postgraduate education event is as follows. A chiropractor is trying to decide whether to enroll in a technique seminar in response to an advertisement that was received in the mail. The first step is to determine if the seminar is sponsored by a reputable organization. In this case, a chiropractic college is listed as a co-sponsor, which contributes to its credibility. The second step is to ascertain whether the speaker's qualifications are legitimate. Indeed, the speaker has a chiropractic degree with diplomate status from a recognized and credible specialty organization.

The seminar brochure mentions that the speaker, who is also the developer of the technique, has conducted research on this topic for a number of years. It would be advantageous to review some of this research in advance; consequently, a literature search is conducted to retrieve articles that may shed some light on the technique. An author-specific PubMed search is carried out using the speaker's last name and first initial; however, no citations are found. To be thorough, similar searches are carried out using the MANTIS and Index to Chiropractic Literature databases. Two articles are retrieved from this search, one that appeared in *The American Chiropractor* and another in *Dynamic Chiropractic* (neither of these publications is peer-reviewed). Interestingly, both of these articles dealt with practice management issues and contained no research-related information that would give credibility to the technique under investigation.

The technique deals with the correction of scoliosis and involves the use of various weights of sandbags that are applied to "hyperaugmented" muscles along the prone patients' spinal column. (Keep in mind this is a hypothetical example!) The seminar brochure states that the technique has been 90% successful at reversing scoliosis in adolescents and adults under age 40. However, as was previously mentioned, no scientific articles can be found that were authored by the developer. Another literature search is carried out on several databases using the term **hyperaugmented muscles**, which is also unfruitful. It should be mentioned at this point that the use of nonstandard terminology is a red flag for untrustworthy information.

After performing these searches, the information that was gathered can now be used to help make a decision about whether to attend the seminar. Essentially, the investigation was unproductive, with no evidence being found that would support the statements that were made in the brochure. Accordingly, we can be quite confident that the technique developer's "research" has never been published. Likewise, one of the foundational terms used in the brochure, "hyperaugmented muscles," has not been reported in the literature.

There could be several possible explanations for these discrepancies. It is possible that the research was actually performed but was never published, either because it was never submitted or because it was of such poor quality that it was not accepted by a journal. Nonetheless, the findings of research do not actually become research until subjected to, and successfully passing, the scrutiny of the scientific community via peer review.[14] There may be another explanation for the lack of publications in this case. It is possible that no research was actually done—at least, what would be considered as legitimate research within the health care community. This may have been an innocent oversight, in that that the person did not truly realize what constitutes valid research. It has been my experience that some practitioners think that devising and then trying out innovative procedures on their patients can be considered research.

Should the chiropractor attend the hypothetical seminar that was just described, or choose another seminar that was more evidence-based? Ultimately, the decision about whether to attend a given seminar is up to the consumer. In reality, there is very little evidence that points to one chiropractic technique being more effective than any others, but there should at least be a solid anatomic and physiological basis for the therapeutic and diagnostic procedures that are involved. In this example case, however, one should seriously consider whether precious time should be invested in a seminar led by someone shown to be untrustworthy.

Practical Clinical Scenarios

Evidence-based methods can also be used to evaluate technique seminars after their attendance by appraising the material that was presented. Green and associates[15] suggest several criteria to evaluate chiropractic techniques:

1. Is there a reasonable anatomic and physiological basis for the procedures involved?
2. Is research available on the treatment and/or diagnostic methods?
3. Is literature available that covers indications and contraindications to the procedure?
4. Is a reliable test available to measure clinical change?
5. Is the procedure's response reproducible?
6. Is the procedure cost-effective?

The authors also mentioned that better-quality learning experiences should be interactive, with adequate time allotted for questions and answers. These sessions can be used to ask the instructor pertinent questions so that the seminar evaluation process can begin immediately.

Equipment Purchases

Decisions about purchasing diagnostic and treatment equipment are often complex, due to the multitude of choices available and the sometimes misleading claims made by manufacturers in their marketing. Choosing the wrong equipment can be wasteful monetarily and, most importantly, useless or even potentially harmful to patients. Diagnostic equipment should be valid and reliable, and therapeutic equipment should be backed by evidence that supports its safety and effectiveness. If patients were aware that they had received care from a doctor who used a device with doubtful validity they might feel cheated, especially if the device was the only decision-making tool utilized or a high fee was charged.

Verifying the validity and reliability of diagnostic equipment when contemplating equipment purchases essentially involves searching the literature to find appropriate studies that have tested the equipment. Often the specific brand name will not be the subject of a study, but the underlying theory has been tested. Also, a different version of a previously validated instrument may not require additional testing. For example, if a company developed a new type of dual inclinometer that is lighter and more portable than previous models, yet the fundamental mechanism is virtually the same as previous models that have been validated, the new version can be considered valid based on the earlier research.

Unfortunately, the literature is not always in agreement about the validity and reliability of a particular piece of equipment. For instance, the Scoliometer has been the topic of investigation for several validation studies that have produced conflicting conclusions.[16–18] Cote and colleagues[17] reported that the interexaminer measurement error of the Scoliometer was high, which limits its use as an instrument to measure clinical outcomes. These authors concluded that the Adam's forward bending test was more sensitive than the Scoliometer and that the Adam's test was the best noninvasive clinical test to evaluate scoliosis. Consequently, due to its poor validity, the Scoliometer is not appropriate for independent use as a diagnostic or patient management tool. On the other hand, it has been shown to be suitable for screening purposes.[18] A lesson that can be learned from this discussion is that it may be necessary to read several articles and related comments on a given topic in order to ascertain the worth of a diagnostic device. Furthermore, relying on the findings of one study, or just a minority of studies, on a topic may be misleading. This applies not only to validity and reliability studies, but also to any type of research. As was mentioned in Chapter 1, systematic reviews, when available, are the preferred source of information because they consider and amalgamate the diversity of opinions that are often present in the literature.

Another instrument that is even more controversial among chiropractors is used to measure side-to-side paraspinal temperature differences by means of a thermocouple device. Temperature variation is represented by a side-specific shift of a needle on the thermocouple's meter. When this occurs over a spinal segment, it is thought by some to represent neurophysiologic dysfunction caused by vertebral subluxation. Although these instruments are used by many chiropractors, their validity has been questioned. Furthermore, there is very little information available on this topic.[19] Following is an example of how to use EBC to make an informed decision about purchasing one of these devices.

The first step is to create a question that will give direction to the EBC process and facilitate the choice of search terms. The question in this case is somewhat different from the clinical foreground questions that were discussed in Chapter 1, because the validity of diagnostic equipment is involved rather than a patient or problem. Accordingly, the question is as follows: *Is the assessment of paraspinal temperature via thermocouple devices to detect spinal dysfunction valid and reliable?*

Searching for relevant literature is complicated in this case because different names are used to represent paraspinal temperature evaluation. The following search terms are selected for use on the PubMed and ICL databases: **thermocouple, nervoscope,** and **neurocalometer**. When searching PubMed, the term **thermocouple** is too broad, with nearly 800 citations being retrieved. However, when combined with **spine** using the AND operator, only 11 are produced. Two of these articles appear to be applicable to this investigation. Another PubMed search for **neurocalometer** retrieves only one article that discusses the instrument from a historical perspective. Searching ICL for **thermocouple** returns one article, **neurocalometer** three, and **nervoscope** zero. The article that resulted from the first of these three searches may be relevant, but the other three are also historical.

The three possibly suitable articles[20–22] that were retrieved during the search must now be evaluated to determine if they contain suitable information to help make a decision about the potential purchase. As is often the case, several more citations are discovered in the reference sections of the articles being reviewed. The most recent of these articles provides a brief review of the literature, reporting that the reliability of thermocouple devices was supported by a study done by Plaugher.[19] Of the retrieved articles, this is the only one that tested the paraspinal thermocouple instrument's reliability. Thus, its methodology should be carefully critiqued using the *checklist for the appraisal of diagnostic accuracy articles*, which can be found in Appendix 7.

Briefly, this study compared the findings of Nervoscope (a handheld paraspinal thermocouple instrument) scans of the cervical-thoracic, mid-thoracic, and lower lumbar regions for intraexaminer and interexaminer reliability. Data from the lumbar spine was not analyzable and weak interexaminer reliability was reported in the cervical-thoracic region. However, the authors indicated that there was good interexaminer agreement in the mid-thoracic spine (T4–8). In making this determination, the examiners were considered to be in agreement when both recorded a positive finding anywhere within the five vertebrae of the mid-thoracic region. However, since most chiropractors are interested in applying spinal adjustments to specific levels, it is questionable as to how applicable these findings are to the clinical setting. A review article published one year later commented on this study, indicating that there were many unresolved questions about these devices.[23]

After making use of the validity and reliability checklist, several deficiencies were found in this article. First, the study sample was made up of healthy chiropractic students who were selected out of convenience. If at all possible, patients in validity and reliability studies should be selected from a clearly identified population, and the spectrum of disease severity should be representative of what is typically seen in clinical practice. Second, no demographic data was presented to assess the makeup of the sample. Third, a potential problem exists because one of the funding sources was the Gonstead Clinical Studies Society, which encourages the use of these devices as part of the Gonstead technique. No gold standard was utilized, primarily because this was a reliability study.

Armed with this knowledge, a practitioner should now be able to make an educated decision about whether to purchase one of these devices. In this case, there is very little evidence available, and what is available does not effectively support the validity or reliability of paraspinal thermocouple devices. Accordingly, it would be more logical for a practitioner to choose other established methods of evaluation. On the other hand, the use of this instrument is integral to an adjustive technique system that is utilized, at least to some extent, by more than 50% of chiropractors in the United States.[24] Realizing the limitations of this instrument, a practitioner could reasonably opt to use a thermocouple device as an aid to spinal analysis, but it should be used alongside other valid tests. Those who do not use an adjustive technique that calls for this instrument would be prudent not to purchase one.

What If Evidence Is Lacking for Your Topic?

Many times little or no empirical evidence exists to assist with evidence-based decision making. In reality, it is not really appropriate to say that no evidence exists regarding a particular clinical problem, since there will always at least be an unsystematic observation or generalization from a physiological study that is available.[25] On the other hand, this type of evidence is extremely weak. In these cases, guidance may sometimes be obtained from a consensus viewpoint found in a practice guideline. This is not always possible, however, since guidelines are not available on every topic, and, when found, sometimes have inconsistencies. Other methods are required in these situations to help guide patient care decisions.

A number of different "ways of knowing" can be used when gathering evidence and attempting to make clinical decisions based on the knowledge acquired from that evidence. The ways of knowing have been categorized into six strategies ordered according to the amount of research available to support each level.[15] The strategies are intuition, tradition, authority, trial and error (experience), logical reasoning, and the scientific method. Intuition, although listed first and thus possessing the lowest research support, will be covered last.

Tradition is operational when a practitioner considers a matter to be true because of what was learned in the past. Sometimes practitioners have a great deal of confidence in tradition, usually in relation to the status of the knowledge source (e.g., the teacher). Tradition then is related to *authority*, which has the potential to be a reliable way of knowing, but the soundness of this knowledge hinges on the dependability of the teacher and whether the information he or she presents is valid.[26] Furthermore, the dependability of knowledge gained by tradition decreases as new information becomes available.

Knowledge gained through *experience* can be quite valuable, but is especially unsystematic because it is acquired by way of trial and error. Consequently, there is a strong tendency for clinicians who use this way of knowing to disregard or reinterpret information that challenges their past beliefs. When using this method to make clinical decisions, one should never conclude that the best answer has been found until it has been corroborated by more reliable means.[27]

Logical reasoning is commonly used in clinical practice by way of consistent and rational thought processes. Logical reasoning merges personal experiences, intellectual faculties, and formal systems of thought to answer everyday questions. Two distinct types of reasoning are utilized in this process: deductive (drawing conclusions that are based on general premises) and inductive (drawing conclusions based on specific observations). Conclusions that are based on logical reasoning in clinical practice are prone to error and should be verified through research evidence in order to be generalized.

The *scientific method* is the preferred approach to acquiring knowledge for use in the clinical setting. The scientific method assumes that nature is orderly, consistent, and predictable; therefore, events in nature are not accidental. Causes can then be discovered by identifying a research question, collecting related data, analyzing the data, and interpreting the findings. This form of inquiry must be carried out in a controlled environment where extraneous factors are minimized.

Intuition is a way of knowing that is derived from sudden insights that come about without conscious reasoning and are generally metaphysical.[15] Using intuition, practitioners assess whether a matter is correct based on the clarity of the enlightenment as well as the associated emotional experience. The developers of evidence-based medicine downplayed intuition and unsystematic clinical experience in the decision-making process.[28] However, a study reported that many primary care physicians consider research evidence and clinical intuition to be compatible.[29] These physicians thought that experience/intuition was a better form of evidence in some cases, particularly when the available evidence is conflicting or when patient preferences are at odds with what is presented in the evidence. The results of this study support the concept that clinicians regard intuition in the clinical setting to be as important as research evidence.

Greenhalgh[30] pointed out that intuition is not necessarily unscientific; it is in fact an integral part of hypothesis generation. She also reported that intuition is not easily accessed by novice practitioners, but that those who are experienced should be capable of creating and following clinical hunches in collaboration with the use of formal sources of evidence. Furthermore, practitioners can improve the efficiency of their intuition through the analysis of prior intuitive judgments, which can be accomplished by writing and talking with colleagues regarding past experiences. She also suggested that the status of intuition as an element of clinical decision making should be elevated.

The lack of evidence is a problem that affects all of the health care disciplines, not just chiropractic. Dieppe and Szebenyi[31] stated in an editorial in the *Journal of Rheumatology*: "A common misuse of EBM, for example, is the assumption that a lack of evidence for the efficacy of a particular treatment equates with its lacking efficacy; a potentially huge problem in rheumatology, where the treatments used frequently lack evidence of either efficacy or effectiveness." The rheumatology profession, like many others, is actively involved in conducting clinical trials and establishing practice guidelines that will assist practitioners with patient care.[32]

Actually, there is a good deal of support for many of the interventions commonly used by chiropractors. Wenban[33] carried out a study in a single chiropractic practice that was designed to find out what proportion of administered care was based on evidence from good-quality randomized controlled trials. After reviewing the case notes of 180 consecutive patients seen by a single chiropractor over the course of five working days, the author reported that 68.3% of patients received primary interventions for chief complaints that were supported by good-quality evidence. These findings were then contrasted with reports from other health care disciplines, which ranged from 11% for pediatric general surgery to 64.8% for internal medicine. A limitation of this study, which has been a problem with nearly every study that has considered this issue, is that in everyday practice, patients rarely present with an isolated, one-dimensional problem. Patients were considered in relation to only one primary complaint in this study, which artificially reduces the intricacies of clinical decision making.

Hunink[34] pointed out that there may be negative consequences associated with EBP if practitioners are required to blindly conform to the hierarchy of evidence by denying potentially beneficial treatments to patients simply because no randomized controlled trials or systematic reviews have been carried out on the topic. In these cases, practitioners should not withhold treatment, but should consider the best evidence that is available (i.e., observational studies) and then make the best decision possible. In fact, it would be wrong to deny treatment in such cases if there was no convincing evidence pointing to other therapies as being clearly superior. As stated by Shaughnessy and coworkers,[35] "From original research to clinical experience, each source of medical information is valuable; the trick is to learn which source is best for the specific information being sought."

Practitioners may sometimes choose to utilize diagnostic tests that lack validity or reliability, or both, for a variety of reasons. For instance, the tool may be a necessary part of a technique system, it may be illustrative to the patient (e.g., colorful computer printouts), or the practitioner may believe that some valuable information is actually derived from its use. In such cases, one should definitely incorporate other validated measures in conjunction with the unproven tests to ensure proper case management. Furthermore, patients should not be charged for invalid tests, and the practitioner should realize that insurance companies will often deny reimbursement for these services.

No matter how hard clinicians try, there will surely be aspects of clinical practice that are not supported by legitimate evidence. In these situations it is helpful to keep in mind some perceptive advice from Sackett and associates:[36]

> Although we promise to do our best for them, we do not guarantee them better health. (In fact, clinicians who do provide such guarantees are often labeled quacks and charlatans.) We diagnose and treat these symptomatic

patients as best we can, realizing that standard therapies for their conditions may never have been validated and may not even work, and that even the validated ones will not work for everyone. Their symptoms and their call for help force us to act, often on the basis of incomplete evidence, about the value of what we are about to do.

Improving the EBC Process

The material presented in this book will be of little benefit to readers unless the concepts are actually utilized in day-to-day practice. For a practitioner to become successful at using EBC, some preparations must be made. Most important, a commitment must be made to implement the procedures into a schedule that is doubtless already quite busy. The steps of EBC will likely be cumbersome and time consuming in the beginning, but will become dramatically less intrusive with continued practice. Also, having the right tools makes the practice of EBC much easier and can even have important effects on the quality of care that is rendered.[37] Minimally, at least one computer that is connected to the Internet should be readily accessible by the practitioner. Separate computers in each treatment room are not required, although that would be ideal. Once the computers are in place, the addresses to some of the websites mentioned in Chapters 2 and 3 should be placed in the web browser's Favorites menu. Quite a few of these resources are free; however, some of the better ones require paid subscriptions.

Bear in mind that it will probably not be possible to search the literature, obtain and read the retrieved articles, critique them, and then apply the evidence to the clinical situation while the patient is waiting in the treatment room. This process may take hours to do properly, especially when new to EBC. However, secondary sources of information, such as *eMedicine.com* or *uptodate.com*, can quickly provide the information necessary to solve many clinical problems. Moreover, these secondary sources utilize evidence-based methods to gather information on various clinical topics that is usually more reliable than what an individual practitioner can produce.

The Cochrane Database is another good secondary source of clinical information. The headache patient example presented earlier in this chapter could have aptly started off with a search of this database. Indeed, there is a *Cochrane Review* available on this topic, which reports that manipulation is safe and effective for the treatment of cervicogenic and posttraumatic headaches.[38] As was mentioned in Chapter 2, however, one should be cautious when using some medical sources in EBC, since information specific to chiropractic issues may be lacking and, if present, may at times be biased against chiropractic methods.

Several factors should be considered when contemplating which of the biomedical databases to use in practice. PubMed is free and, because of its enormity and powerful search capabilities, will be particularly useful in EBC. However, since PubMed does not include many chiropractic-specific citations, other databases are needed in order to carry out a complete search. The Index to Chiropractic Literature (ICL) is also free, but it does not include abstracts or links to sites where full-text articles may be obtained. MANTIS and CINAHL, on the other hand, do include abstracts, but both charge a fee. Recall that a journal abstract presents a synopsis of the associated article, which can be very helpful for assessing whether the article's complete text should be read.

Having subscriptions to relevant journals is another important aspect of EBC that should be carefully considered. One prime consideration is the fact that multiple journal subscriptions can be quite costly. For instance, a subscription to the *Journal of Manipulative and Physiological Therapeutics (JMPT)* is currently $124 USD per year. Another consideration is that it would be difficult to find the time to read all of the articles included in more than just a few journals. With these factors in mind, it is highly recommended that all chiropractors subscribe to JMPT, not only as a source of information but also to support the advancement of science in the chiropractic profession. Another highly recommended journal subscription is to *Chiropractic and Osteopathy*, which fortunately is free. Both of these journals will e-mail their table of contents from current issues as they are released at no cost. To register for this service, simply go to the journals' websites (see Chapter 2).

When reading literature, it is important to not get bogged down reading too many articles unnecessarily. Preferably, only highly relevant articles that are of the best quality should be read. Flaherty[39] developed a system that can be used to quickly decide whether to read a study by examining the abstract using the PP-ICONS approach (Table 11.1).

The key to becoming a successful evidence-based practitioner is to establish the habit of looking for evidence when needed and not being afraid to do it in front of patients. In fact, they appreciate the extra effort.

Beware of the trap that a few senior practitioners from all professions have a tendency to fall in to; that of placing "less importance on the need for anything as

TABLE 11.1 PP-ICONS approach to quickly deciding whether to read the entire article

Problem: Do I see this problem in my practice?

Patient population: Is the study population similar to my patient population?

Intervention: What intervention was used and can it realistically be used in my practice?

Comparison: What was the intervention compared to and was it a reasonable comparison?

Outcomes: Would the outcomes matter to my patients? (patien- oriented evidence that matters—POEMS).

Number: How many patients were in the study? Were the numbers sufficient?

Statistics: How does the study present its findings? Were the correct statistical tests used? Were the results statistically and clinically significant?

---

mundane as evidence."[40] It seems these practitioners consider that experience supersedes any amount of evidence that may be available and have steadfast confidence in their clinical experience. Unfortunately, as one repeatedly makes the same mistakes over the course of many years, confidence may indeed increase, but in light of current best evidence, patient care may suffer.

In addition to an undue reliance on experience by some practitioners, without regard for implementing EBP methods, there are four other reasons (excuses) why practitioners do not participate.[41] Especially within the context of busy practices, a lack of time is probably the most common excuse for disregarding EBP. A second often-used excuse is that practitioners do not have access to the required information because they do not subscribe to journals or do not have access to online resources. A third excuse, which is in effect a criticism of EBP, is the limited relevance of research to clinical practice.[42] Finally, some practitioners lack the skills that are needed to critically appraise evidence. None of these reasons is insurmountable, however, and with a strong commitment and follow-through, any health care practitioner can become proficient at EBP.

Evidence-based methods can also be used as a means to lifelong learning. In fact, the act of participating in the process of collecting evidence, appraising it, and then applying the results to solve specific clinical problems brings about better learning effects than didactic presentations.[43] This type of inquiry is highly relevant and is especially meaningful to the evidence-based practitioner. Thus, learning while doing not only improves EBC skills but also adds significantly to the practitioner's knowledge base. The results of a survey of medical practitioners about which educational methods they thought contributed most to their current practice performances indicated that practice-based independent learning was superior to formal continuing education, as well as to prior university education.[44]

To effectively integrate EBC into routine practice, it must be consistently utilized within that environment.[45] This style of practice will not only result in increased knowledge, but will also improve EBC skills, giving rise to increasing efficiency as time progresses. Keep in mind, however, that the steps of EBC are somewhat cumbersome in the beginning, which can lead to discouragement and the ultimate rejection of evidence-based methods. Therefore, if you are new to EBC, do not become disheartened if the process at first seems inefficient. Expect to spend progressively less time and generate more dependable information with continued use.

Some useful tips on implementing evidence-based methods into a busy practice can be extracted from an article that was originally intended for clinical teaching faculty.[46] For one thing, it is helpful to prepare ahead of time for certain problems and decisions that are commonly encountered in clinical practice. Certain questions can be anticipated and evidence-based answers can be discovered in advance so they are ready for use when needed. Otherwise, the practitioner runs the risk of having to rush to find answers after the fact or, worse yet, not having any available time at all. Another suggestion from the article is to obtain access to evidence resources in advance of when they will be needed. One final tip is to collect, and keep close at hand, concise summaries of the evidence on various topics, rather than trying to store the entire text of each article. This tip can appreciably speed up the process of finding and grasping the meaning of articles.

At some point, one should conduct a self-appraisal to determine the extent that one's practice is truly evidence-based. Indeed, the fifth step of traditional EBP is to evaluate one's performance. To assist with this process, Greenhalgh[47] listed six questions that practitioners can ask to assess the extent to which their own clinical circumstances measure up. In fact, one can ask the following questions with regard to any given clinical encounter:

1. Have I identified and prioritized the clinical, psychological, social, and other problems, taking into account the patient's perspective?

2. Have I performed a sufficiently competent and complete examination to establish the likelihood of competing diagnoses?
3. Have I considered additional problems and risk factors?
4. Where necessary, have I sought relevant evidence from systematic reviews, guidelines, clinical trials, and other sources?
5. Have I assessed and taken into account the completeness, quality, and strength of the evidence, and its relevance to this patient?
6. Have I presented the pros and cons of the different options to the patient in a way he or she can understand, and incorporated the patient's preferences into the final recommendations?

When possible, systematic, reproducible, and unbiased information derived from the health care literature should be used to answer questions about patient care. Although this method of practice de-emphasizes the reliance on pathophysiological rationale, intuition, or random clinical experience as **sufficient grounds** for clinical decision making, it does **not** devalue the importance of these factors in clinical practice. Yoder[48] said it quite well while referring to the practice of evidence-based nursing: "We must all be examining our practice daily; we must challenge tradition and determine whether our practice is based on scientific evidence, expert knowledge, and patient preferences."

When starting to implement evidence-based methods in an already existing practice, it may be necessary to do some catching up and find evidence for many of the clinical procedures that are already in use, especially if it has been a number of years since one has graduated from college. To accomplish this task most efficiently, one should focus on the most common and important conditions that are encountered in practice. The best information regarding each of these conditions should be systematically located by spending a set amount of time each day until the task is accomplished. Secondary resources (for example, the *Cochrane Database of Systematic Reviews*), are usually the best place to start. For instance, many chiropractors treat patients with lumbar disc herniations, yet it may have been years since they were updated on the current best practices for managing this condition.

As evidence on various clinical topics is collected, the practitioner should write a summary for each condition that can be used in the future when apposite patients present for care. A useful tool for recording this type of information is the *Critically Appraised Topic* (CAT),[49] which is essentially a short summary (i.e., one page or less) of the results of an EBP activity. Shannon[50] reported that CATs are able to serve several purposes: (1) reinforcing the link between clinical questions and available evidence, (2) serving as a resource to answer clinical questions, (3) providing a way to explore the literature on a given topic, and (4) keeping a record of clinical questions and answers.

For brave souls who would like to get more involved in the area of EBC and write an article for publication in a chiropractic or medical journal, supplementary information will be needed in addition to what was presented in this book. Although this book's contents should be very helpful in such an endeavor, it was not intended for, nor is it complete, for this purpose. Please refer to an article by Gleberzon and Killinger[51] entitled *"The Journal Article Cookbook,"* which straightforwardly provides practical instruction in this area. Two other resources that will help with scientific writing are also recommended: one is a brief, yet informative article by Perneger and Hudelson[52] and the other is a book by Huth.[53] Writing journal articles is not easy and is time-consuming; on the other hand, it can be very rewarding. The writing process can make one very familiar with the topic, and having publications in a curriculum vitae will significantly enhance one's professional image.

References

1. Beers, M.H. and R. Berkow. Migraine. In: *The Merck Manual of Diagnosis and Therapy*, 17th ed. 2005. Whitehouse Station, NJ: Merck. http://www.merck.com/mrkshared/mmanual/home.jsp.
2. Antonaci, F., et al. Cervicogenic headache: Evaluation of the original diagnostic criteria. Cephalalgia, 2001. **21**(5):573–83.
3. Bronfort, G., et al. *Efficacy of spinal manipulation for chronic headache: A systematic review. J Manipulative Physiol Ther*, 2001. **24**(7):457–66.
4. Kroeling, P., A. Gross, and P.E. Houghton. *Electrotherapy for neck disorders. Cochrane Database Syst Rev*, 2005. Issue 2, Article No. CD004251.
5. Astin, J., and E. Ernst. *The effectiveness of spinal manipulation for the treatment of headache disorders: A systematic review of randomized clinical trials. Cephalalgia*, 2002. **22**(8):617–23.
6. Vernon, H. *The effectiveness of spinal manipulation for the treatment of headache disorders: A systematic review of randomized clinical trials. Cephalalgia*, 2003. **23**(6): 479–80.
7. Haas, M., et al. *Dose response for chiropractic care of chronic cervicogenic headache and associated neck pain: A randomized pilot study. J Manipulative Physiol Ther*, 2004. **27**(9):547–53.
8. Haldeman, S., et al. *Clinical perceptions of the risk of vertebral artery dissection after cervical manipulation: The effect of referral bias. Spine J*, 2002. **2**(5):334–42.

9. Hurwitz, E.L., et al. *Manipulation and mobilization of the cervical spine. A systematic review of the literature. Spine*, 1996. **21**(15):1746–59; discussion 1759–60.
10. Haldeman, S., F.J. Kohlbeck, and M. McGregor. *Stroke, cerebral artery dissection, and cervical spine manipulation therapy. J Neurol*, 2002. **249**(8):1098–104.
11. Haneline, M.T., A.C. Croft, and B.M. Frishberg. *Association of internal carotid artery dissection and chiropractic manipulation. Neurologist*, 2003. **9**(1):35–44.
12. Thiel, H., and G. Rix. *Is it time to stop functional pre-manipulation testing of the cervical spine? Manual Therapy*, 2005. **10**(2):154–8.
13. Haneline, M., and G. Lewkovich. *Identification of internal carotid artery dissection in chiropractic practice. J Can Chiropr Assoc*, 2004. **48**(3):206–10.
14. Keating, J.C., Jr. *Toward a Philosophy of the Science of Chiropractic: A Primer for Clinicians*. 1992. Stockton, Calif: Stockton Foundation for Chiropractic Research, 314.
15. Green, B.N., C.D. Johnson, and A. Adams. *Caveat emptor! Evaluate and maximize your technique seminar experience. Topics in Clinical Chiropractic*, 1998. **5**(2):19–26.
16. Korovessis, P.G. *Scoliometer is useful instrument with high reliability and repeatability. Spine*, 1999. **24**(3):307–8.
17. Cote, P., et al. *A study of the diagnostic accuracy and reliability of the Scoliometer and Adam's forward bend test. Spine*, 1998. **23**(7):796–802; discussion 803.
18. Amendt, L.E., et al. *Validity and reliability testing of the Scoliometer. Phys Ther*, 1990. **70**(2):108–17.
19. Plaugher, G. *Skin temperature assessment for neuromusculoskeletal abnormalities of the spinal column. J Manipulative Physiol Ther*, 1992. **15**(6):365–81.
20. Owens, E.F., Jr., et al. *Paraspinal skin temperature patterns: An interexaminer and intraexaminer reliability study. J Manipulative Physiol Ther*, 2004. **27**(3):155–9.
21. Hart, J., and E.F. Owens, Jr. *Stability of paraspinal thermal patterns during acclimation. J Manipulative Physiol Ther*, 2004. **27**(2):109–17.
22. Schram, S.B., R.S. Hosek, and E.S. Owens, Jr. *Computerized paraspinal skin surface temperature scanning: A technical report. J Manipulative Physiol Ther*, 1982. **5**(3):117–21.
23. Boline, P.D., et al. *Interexaminer reliability of eight evaluative dimensions of lumbar segmental abnormality: Part II. J Manipulative Physiol Ther*, 1993. **16**(6):363–74.
24. Christensen, M. and M. Kollasch. *Job Analysis of Chiropractic*. 2005, Greeley, Colo: National Board of Chiropractic Examiners.
25. Guyatt, G.H., et al. *Users' guides to the medical literature: XXV. Evidence-based medicine: Principles for applying the Users' Guides to patient care. Evidence-Based Medicine Working Group. JAMA*, 2000. **284**(10):1290–6.
26. Playle, J. *The nature of research. J Community Nursing*, 2000. **14**(1):14–20.
27. Portney, L.G., and M.P. Watkins. *Foundations of Clinical Research: Applications to Practice*. 2nd ed. 2000. Upper Saddle River, NJ: Prentice Hall.
28. Evidence-Based Medicine Working Group. *Evidence-based medicine. A new approach to teaching the practice of medicine. JAMA*, 1992. **268**(17):2420–5.
29. Tracy, C.S., G. Dantas, and R. Upshur. *Evidence-based medicine in primary care: Qualitative study of family physicians*. BMC Family Practice, 2003. **4**(1):6.
30. Greenhalgh, T. *Intuition and evidence—uneasy bedfellows? Br J Gen Pract*, 2002. **52**(478):395–400.
31. Dieppe, P. and B. Szebenyi. *Evidence based rheumatology. J Rheumatol*, 2000. **27**(1):4–7.

32. Krishnan, L.L., and M.E. Suarez-Almazor. *Evidence-based rheumatology practice. Curr Opin Rheumatol*, 2005. **17**(2):117–23.
33. Wenban, A.B. *Is chiropractic evidence based? A pilot study. J Manipulative Physiol Ther*, 2003. **26**(1):47.
34. Hunink, M.G.M., *Does evidence based medicine do more good than harm? BMJ*, 2004. **329**(7473):1051.
35. Shaughnessy, A.F., D.C. Slawson, and J.H. Bennett. *Becoming an information master: A guidebook to the medical information jungle. J Fam Pract*, 1994. **39**(5):489–99.
36. Sackett, D.L., et al. *Clinical Epidemiology: A Basic Science for Clinical Medicine*. 2nd ed. Boston: Little, Brown & Company, 1991. 441.
37. Evidence-Based Care Resource Group. *Evidence-based care: 1. Setting priorities: How important is the problem? CMAJ*, 1994. **150**(8):1249–54.
38. Bronfort, G., et al. *Efficacy of spinal manipulation and mobilization for low back pain and neck pain: A systematic review and best evidence synthesis. The Spine Journal*, 2004. **4**(3):335–56.
39. Flaherty, R.J. *A simple method for evaluating the clinical literature. Fam Pract Manag*, 2004. **11**(5):47–52.
40. Isaacs, D. and D. Fitzgerald. *Seven alternatives to evidence-based medicine. Oncologist*, 2001. **6**(4):390–1.
41. Nieuwboer, A. *How self-evident is evidence-based practice in physiotherapy? Physiother Res Int*, 2004. **9**(2):iii–
42. McKenna, H.P., S. Ashton, and S. Keeney. *Barriers to evidence-based practice in primary care. J Adv Nurs*, 2004. **45**(2):178–89.
43. Evidence-Based Care Resource Group. *Evidence-based care: 5. Lifelong learning: How can we learn to be more effective? CMAJ*, 1994. **150**(12):1971–3.
44. Renschler, H.E., and U. Fuchs. *Lifelong learning of physicians: Contributions of different educational phases to practice performance. Acad Med*, 1993. **68**(2 suppl):S57–9.
45. Evidence-Based Care Resource Group. *Evidence-based care: 3. Measuring performance: How are we managing this problem? CMAJ*, 1994. **150**(10):1575–9.
46. Richardson, W.S. *Teaching evidence-based practice on foot. ACP J Club*, 2005. **143**(2):A10–2.
47. Greenhalgh, T. *"Is my practice evidence-based?" BMJ*, 1996. **313**(7063):957–8.
48. Yoder, L.H. *Evidence-based practice: The time is now! Medsurg Nurs*, 2005. **14**(2):91–2.
49. Strauss, S.E. *Evidence-Based Medicine: How to Practice and Teach EBM*. 3rd ed. 2005. Edinburgh and New York: Elsevier/Churchill Livingstone.
50. Shannon, S. *Critically appraised topics (CATs). Can Assoc Radiol J*, 2001. **52**(5):286–7.
51. Gleberzon, B. and L. Killinger. *The journal article cookbook. J Manipulative Physiol Ther*, 2004. **27**(7):481–92.
52. Perneger, T.V., and P.M. Hudelson. *Writing a research article: Advice to beginners. Int J Qual Health Care*, 2004. **16**(3):191–2.
53. Huth, E.J. *Writing and Publishing in Medicine*. 3rd ed. 1999. Baltimore: Williams & Wilkins.

APPENDIX ONE

Health Information Website Evaluation Checklist

Website Title _____

Sponsor _____ URL _____

Apparent conflicts of interest

Does the website allow advertising?	❑ Yes ❑ No
■ If yes, does the owner/sponsor market (a) specific product(s)?	❑ Yes ❑ No
• If yes, is the owner/sponsor the inventor/creator of the product?	❑ Yes ❑ No
○ If yes, be very wary of any health information that may be provided and cross-check with other, more reliable sources.	

Credibility

If an individual, does the author list his or her qualifications?	❑ Yes ❑ No
Does the author of the website have a relevant doctoral degree?	❑ Yes ❑ No
■ If no, does the author of the website have any relevant degree?	❑ Yes ❑ No
• If no, is there any other validation of the author's credibility?	❑ Yes ❑ No
○ If no, be very wary of any health information that may be provided and cross-check with other, more reliable sources.	
If an organization is involved, does it appear to be legitimate?	❑ Yes ❑ No
■ Does the organization have an adequate number of members?	❑ Yes ❑ No
■ Is the organization national or statewide?	❑ Yes ❑ No

References

Is a list of references in support of the website's opinions provided? ❑ Yes ❑ No
- If yes, are they relevant to the health topic being covered? ❑ Yes ❑ No
- Are the references from reliable sources? ❑ Yes ❑ No
- If no, is any other valid evidence presented that supports the opinions that are presented? ❑ Yes ❑ No
  - If no, be very wary of any health information that may be provided and cross-check with other, more reliable sources.

Content

Does the website cover the health issue(s) adequately?	❑ Yes ❑ No
Does the website have a professional appearance?	❑ Yes ❑ No
Is the grammar acceptable?	❑ Yes ❑ No
Is the information accurate?	❑ Yes ❑ No
Is the information presented in a consistent manner?	❑ Yes ❑ No
Is the website free of contradictions?	❑ Yes ❑ No
Are readers advised to contact a health professional with questions?	❑ Yes ❑ No
Is the information current?	❑ Yes ❑ No

Applicability

Does the website provide relevant health information?	❑ Yes ❑ No
Is the information relevant to the target population?	❑ Yes ❑ No
Does the website provide important information?	❑ Yes ❑ No

Overall impression regarding the trustworthiness of this website

❑ **Good**—Accept almost all of the material that is presented.

❑ **Fair**—Accept some material, but exclude: _____

_____

❑ **Poor**—Do not accept *any* of the material.

APPENDIX TWO

General Checklist for the Appraisal of Journal Articles

Title _____

Author _____ Journal _____

Vol. ____ Issue _____ Date _____

(Leave items blank that do not apply.)

The purpose of the study was conveyed plainly and rationally.	❏ Yes ❏ Partly ❏ No
A suitable literature review was presented that adequately covered the topic.	❏ Yes ❏ Partly ❏ No
The research design was clearly described.	❏ Yes ❏ Partly ❏ No
The research design was in concordance with the study question.	❏ Yes ❏ Partly ❏ No
The research design was adequately implemented.	❏ Yes ❏ Partly ❏ No
The target population was identified.	❏ Yes ❏ Partly ❏ No
A determination of the needed sample size was carried out.	❏ Yes ❏ Partly ❏ No
The sample size was adequate.	❏ Yes ❏ Partly ❏ No

Subjects were randomly assigned to groups.	❑ Yes ❑ Partly ❑ No
Groups were equivalent.	❑ Yes ❑ Partly ❑ No
Data collection methods were adequately described and were appropriate.	❑ Yes ❑ Partly ❑ No
Demographic characteristics of the groups were presented.	❑ Yes ❑ Partly ❑ No
The data were reported with sufficient detail.	❑ Yes ❑ Partly ❑ No
Statistical tests were described and were appropriate for the type of data involved.	❑ Yes ❑ Partly ❑ No
The discussion corresponded to and was supported by the data.	❑ Yes ❑ Partly ❑ No
Discussion statements were reasonable and logical.	❑ Yes ❑ Partly ❑ No
Conclusions were in agreement with the study's predetermined purpose.	❑ Yes ❑ Partly ❑ No
Study limitations were listed.	❑ Yes ❑ Partly ❑ No
References were accurate and appropriately used.	❑ Yes ❑ Partly ❑ No
References were from respected evidence sources.	❑ Yes ❑ Partly ❑ No
Was there any evidence of a 'fishing expedition'?	❑ Yes ❑ No

Overall impression about the trustworthiness of this article:

❑ **Good**—Accept all or most of the article's findings.

❑ **Fair**—Cautiously accept *some* of its findings.

❑ **Poor**—Do not accept *any* of its findings.

Key points to consider: _____

_____

If acceptable, how will I apply the results to my patient/practice? _____

_____

_____

APPENDIX THREE

Checklist for the Appraisal of Therapy Articles

Title _____

Author _____ Journal _____

Vol. ____ Issue _____ Date _____

(Leave items blank that do not apply.)

The topic of the article is relevant to the clinical question.	❏ Yes ❏ Partly ❏ No
An adequate literature review was conducted.	❏ Yes ❏ Partly ❏ No
A clear and focused study question is presented.	❏ Yes ❏ Partly ❏ No
Methods are described in enough detail so that the study could be duplicated.	❏ Yes ❏ Partly ❏ No
The patient selection criteria are provided.	❏ Yes ❏ Partly ❏ No
The inclusion/exclusion criteria are appropriate.	❏ Yes ❏ Partly ❏ No
Patients were randomized to treatment or control groups.	❏ Yes ❏ Partly ❏ No
Randomization was successful (groups are equivalent).	❏ Yes ❏ Partly ❏ No
Patients were blinded regarding group assignment.	❏ Yes ❏ Partly ❏ No
Study personnel were blinded regarding group assignment.	❏ Yes ❏ Partly ❏ No

All patients were accounted for at the end of the study.	❏ Yes ❏ Partly ❏ No
Patients were analyzed in the groups to which they were randomized (intention-to-treat).	❏ Yes ❏ Partly ❏ No
An estimate of the required sample size was calculated.	❏ Yes ❏ Partly ❏ No
The sample size was large enough to find a treatment effect if one was present.	❏ Yes ❏ Partly ❏ No
The groups were treated equally, except for the intervention.	❏ Yes ❏ Partly ❏ No
Appropriate statistical tests were utilized.	❏ Yes ❏ Partly ❏ No
The results of the study are statistically and clinically significant.	❏ Yes ❏ Partly ❏ No
Patient follow-up was adequate.	❏ Yes ❏ Partly ❏ No
Study limitations are reported and are reasonable.	❏ Yes ❏ Partly ❏ No
The conclusions are appropriate.	❏ Yes ❏ Partly ❏ No
Suggestions for future research are offered.	❏ Yes ❏ Partly ❏ No

Overall impression about the trustworthiness of this article.

❏ **Good**—Accept all or most of the article's findings.

❏ **Fair**—Cautiously accept *some* of its findings.

❏ **Poor**—Do not accept *any* of its findings.

Key points to consider: _____

_____

If acceptable, how will I apply the results to my patient/practice? _____

_____

_____

APPENDIX FOUR

Checklist for the Appraisal of Literature Review Articles

Title _____

Author _____ Journal _____

Vol. ____ Issue _____ Date _____

(Leave items blank that do not apply.)

The topic covered by the review is of interest.	❏ Yes ❏ Partly ❏ No
The introduction provides a compelling need for the review.	❏ Yes ❏ Partly ❏ No
A clear study question is presented.	❏ Yes ❏ Partly ❏ No
The study question is focused on a specific clinical issue.	❏ Yes ❏ Partly ❏ No
Methods are described in enough detail so that the study could be duplicated.	❏ Yes ❏ Partly ❏ No
The inclusion/exclusion criteria used to select articles are provided.	❏ Yes ❏ Partly ❏ No
The inclusion/exclusion criteria are appropriate.	❏ Yes ❏ Partly ❏ No
Query terms specified for the literature search are appropriate.	❏ Yes ❏ Partly ❏ No

The number and choice of databases utilized in the literature search are sufficient.	❏ Yes ❏ Partly ❏ No
The validity of the studies included in the review was assessed.	❏ Yes ❏ Partly ❏ No
Studies were appraised in a dependable manner.	❏ Yes ❏ Partly ❏ No
The included studies are randomized trials.	❏ Yes ❏ Partly ❏ No
The results of the studies are similar (homogeneity).	❏ Yes ❏ Partly ❏ No
Sources of heterogeneity are addressed.	❏ Yes ❏ Partly ❏ No
The synthesis logically flows from the results of the included studies.	❏ Yes ❏ Partly ❏ No
An estimate of treatment effect is provided.	❏ Yes ❏ Partly ❏ No
Statements made in the Discussion section are reasonable and logical.	❏ Yes ❏ Partly ❏ No
Study limitations are listed.	❏ Yes ❏ Partly ❏ No
References are accurate and appropriately used.	❏ Yes ❏ Partly ❏ No
References are from respected evidence sources.	❏ Yes ❏ Partly ❏ No
Suggestions for future research are offered.	❏ Yes ❏ Partly ❏ No

Overall impression about the trustworthiness of this article:

❏ **Good**—Accept all or most of the article's findings.

❏ **Fair**—Cautiously accept *some* of its findings.

❏ **Poor**—Do not accept *any* of its findings.

Key points to consider: _____

_____

If acceptable, how will I apply the results to my patient/practice? _____

_____

_____

APPENDIX FIVE

Checklist for the Appraisal of Case Reports

Title _____

Author _____ Journal _____

Vol. ___ Issue _____ Date _____

(Leave items blank that do not apply.)

The abstract presents an accurate description of the case and its implications.	❑ Yes ❑ Partly ❑ No
The case covers a new or unique feature of patient management.	❑ Yes ❑ Partly ❑ No
The reason for reporting the case is made clear.	❑ Yes ❑ Partly ❑ No
The impact of the health problem on society is stated.	❑ Yes ❑ Partly ❑ No
An adequate literature review was conducted.	❑ Yes ❑ Partly ❑ No
The references support the rationale for reporting the case.	❑ Yes ❑ Partly ❑ No
The patient is described adequately (chief complaint, history, etc.).	❑ Yes ❑ Partly ❑ No
The management of the case is effectively described.	❑ Yes ❑ Partly ❑ No
Valid and reliable outcome measures are utilized.	❑ Yes ❑ Partly ❑ No

The outcome measures are suitable for the given clinical circumstances.	❑ Yes ❑ Partly ❑ No
The results of diagnostic tests are presented adequately.	❑ Yes ❑ Partly ❑ No
Normal values of less common diagnostic tests are provided.	❑ Yes ❑ Partly ❑ No
An accurate diagnosis is provided.	❑ Yes ❑ Partly ❑ No
Convincing evidence in support of the diagnosis is presented.	❑ Yes ❑ Partly ❑ No
The case is compared with previously reported cases and studies.	❑ Yes ❑ Partly ❑ No
Study limitations are reported and are reasonable.	❑ Yes ❑ Partly ❑ No
Alternate explanations are considered and successfully refuted.	❑ Yes ❑ Partly ❑ No
Suggestions for future research are proposed.	❑ Yes ❑ Partly ❑ No
Implications for current clinical practice are pointed out.	❑ Yes ❑ Partly ❑ No
Enough evidence is presented to support the author's conclusions.	❑ Yes ❑ Partly ❑ No
The author communicates the importance of this case to the profession.	❑ Yes ❑ Partly ❑ No
The conclusions are appropriate.	❑ Yes ❑ Partly ❑ No

Overall impression about the quality of this case report:

❑ **Good** ❑ **Fair** ❑ **Poor**

Key points to consider: _____

_____

If acceptable, how will I apply the results to my patient/practice? _____

_____

APPENDIX SIX

Checklist for the Appraisal of Epidemiologic Articles

Title _____

Author _____ Journal _____

Vol. ____ Issue _____ Date _____
(Leave items blank that do not apply.)

The study's main objective was conveyed plainly and rationally.	❑ Yes ❑ Partly ❑ No
The study population was clearly identified.	❑ Yes ❑ Partly ❑ No
Case/cohort selection criteria were described and were adequate.	❑ Yes ❑ Partly ❑ No
Exposures were adequately described.	❑ Yes ❑ Partly ❑ No
Outcomes were adequately described.	❑ Yes ❑ Partly ❑ No
Cases/cohorts were representative of the population (i.e., low risk of selection bias).	❑ Yes ❑ Partly ❑ No
Non-exposed cohorts or controls were drawn from the defined study population.	❑ Yes ❑ Partly ❑ No
Controls were shown not to have a history of the condition under investigation.	❑ Yes ❑ Partly ❑ No

Cohorts were shown not to have the outcome of interest at the beginning of the study. ❑ Yes ❑ Partly ❑ No

Groups were matched or confounders were adjusted for in the analysis. ❑ Yes ❑ Partly ❑ No

The study design was appropriate. ❑ Yes ❑ Partly ❑ No

There was an independent blind assessment of outcomes. ❑ Yes ❑ Partly ❑ No

Follow-up of cohorts was long enough for the outcomes to occur. ❑ Yes ❑ Partly ❑ No

The study was completed by an acceptable number of subjects. ❑ Yes ❑ Partly ❑ No

Demographic characteristics of the groups were presented. ❑ Yes ❑ Partly ❑ No

The data were reported with sufficient detail. ❑ Yes ❑ Partly ❑ No

The discussion corresponded to and was supported by the data. ❑ Yes ❑ Partly ❑ No

Discussion statements were reasonable and logical. ❑ Yes ❑ Partly ❑ No

Conclusions were in agreement with the study's predetermined purpose. ❑ Yes ❑ Partly ❑ No

Study limitations were listed. ❑ Yes ❑ Partly ❑ No

References were acceptable. ❑ Yes ❑ Partly ❑ No

Overall impression about the trustworthiness of this article:

❑ **Good**—Accept all or most of the article's findings.

❑ **Fair**—Cautiously accept *some* of its findings.

❑ **Poor**—Do not accept *any* of its findings.

Key points to consider: _____

_____

If acceptable, how will I apply the results to my patient/practice? _____

SEVEN

APPENDIX

Checklist for the Appraisal of Diagnostic Accuracy Articles

Title _____

Author _____ Journal _____

Vol. ___ Issue ___ Date _____

(Leave items blank that do not apply.)

A reasonable question that can be answered by the study design is proposed.	❏ Yes ❏ Partly ❏ No
The methods for performing the test are described enough to permit replication.	❏ Yes ❏ Partly ❏ No
The test was compared with a suitable reference standard (gold standard).	❏ Yes ❏ Partly ❏ No
Comparison with the reference standard was blinded.	❏ Yes ❏ Partly ❏ No
The decision to perform the reference standard was independent of new test results.	❏ Yes ❏ Partly ❏ No
The setting where the data were collected is described adequately.	❏ Yes ❏ Partly ❏ No
Inclusion/exclusion criteria are presented and are reasonable.	❏ Yes ❏ Partly ❏ No

The spectrum of disease severity within the population
is described.   ❏ Yes ❏ Partly ❏ No

The sample size was adequate.   ❏ Yes ❏ Partly ❏ No

The demographic characteristics of the sample are
presented.   ❏ Yes ❏ Partly ❏ No

Participants in the study are similar to patients in your
practice.   ❏ Yes ❏ Partly ❏ No

The sample includes subjects with and without the
condition.   ❏ Yes ❏ Partly ❏ No

All subjects received both the new test and the reference
standard test.   ❏ Yes ❏ Partly ❏ No

The results of the test will facilitate the management of
your patient(s).   ❏ Yes ❏ Partly ❏ No

Calculations:

Condition
per gold standard

	Present	Absent	
Positive			___ $a+b$
	a	b	
	c	d	
Negative			___ $c+d$
	___ $a+c$	___ $b+d$	___ $a+b+c+d$

Test Result (Positive / Negative)

Sensitivity _____ $a/(a+c)$
Specificity _____ $d/(b+d)$
Positive predictive value _____ $a/(a+b)$
Negative predictive value _____ $d/(c+d)$
Likelihood ratio (+) _____ Sensitivity/(1 − Specificity)
Likelihood ratio (−) _____ (1 − Sensitivity)/Specificity

Checklist for the Appraisal of Diagnostic Accuracy Articles

Overall impression about the trustworthiness of this article:

❑ **Good**—Accept all or most of the article's findings.

❑ **Fair**—Cautiously accept *some* of its findings.

❑ **Poor**—Do not accept *any* of its findings.

Key points to consider: _____

_____

_____

If acceptable, how will I apply the results to my patient/practice? _____

_____

_____

APPENDIX

EIGHT

Characteristic Pain Intensity (CPI)

Patient _____ Date _____

Pain Scale

On the lines below, make straight vertical (up-and-down) marks to indicate how your neck pain feels RIGHT NOW, on AVERAGE, and when it is AT ITS WORST. If you do *not* have any pain, circle "NO PAIN."

How bad is your pain RIGHT NOW?

NO PAIN |————————————————————————| * WORST YOU HAVE EVER FELT

millimeters _____

How bad is your TYPICAL or AVERAGE pain?

NO PAIN |————————————————————————| * WORST YOU HAVE EVER FELT

millimeters _____

Appendix 8

How bad is your pain when it is AT ITS WORST?

NO PAIN |—————————————————|* WORST YOU HAVE EVER FELT

millimeters _____

Please circle what percentage of the time you notice neck pain:

0%   10%   20%   30%   40%   50%   60%   70%   80%   90%   100%

CPI = _____

$$CPI = \frac{\text{Pain right now} + \text{Worst pain} + \text{Average pain}}{3}$$

*Not shown at exact length, 100 mm.

NINE

APPENDIX

Short-Form McGill Pain Questionnaire and Pain Diagram

Date: _____

Name: _____

Check the column to indicate the level of your pain for each word, or leave blank if it does not apply to you.

	Mild	Moderate	Severe
1. Throbbing	___	___	___
2. Shooting	___	___	___
3. Stabbing	___	___	___
4. Sharp	___	___	___
5. Cramping	___	___	___
6. Gnawing	___	___	___
7. Hot-burning	___	___	___
8. Aching	___	___	___
9. Heavy	___	___	___
10. Tender	___	___	___
11. Splitting	___	___	___
12. Tiring-Exhausting	___	___	___
13. Sickening	___	___	___
14. Fearful	___	___	___
15. Cruel-Punishing	___	___	___

Mark or comment on the above figure where you have your pain or problems.

Appendix 9

Mark or comment on the above figure where you have your pain or problems.

Indicate on this line how bad your pain is—at the left end of line means no pain at all, at right end means worst pain possible.

No _____ *Worst Pain
Pain   Possible

   S /33   A   /12   VAS /10

Source: © R. Melzack, 1984, 1987. Reprinted with permission.
*Not shown at exact length, 100 mm.

TEN

APPENDIX

Revised Oswestry Low Back Disability Index

Patient name: _____ Date: _____

Please Read: This questionnaire is designed to enable us to understand how much your low back pain has affected your ability to manage your everyday activities. Please answer each Section by marking (☑) the ONE BOX that most applies to you. We realize that you may feel that more than one statement may relate to you, but PLEASE JUST MARK THE ONE BOX WHICH MOST CLOSELY DESCRIBES YOUR PROBLEM. Thank You.

Section 1—Pain Intensity

- ❑ The pain comes and goes and is very mild.
- ❑ The pain is mild and does not vary much.
- ❑ The pain comes and goes and is moderate.
- ❑ The pain is moderate and does not vary much.
- ❑ The pain comes and goes and is severe.
- ❑ The pain is severe and does not vary much.

Section 2—Personal Care [washing, dressing, etc.]

- ❑ I do not have to change my way of washing or dressing in order to avoid pain.
- ❑ I do not normally change my way of washing or dressing even though it causes some pain.

- ❑ Washing and dressing increases the pain but I manage not to change my way of doing it.
- ❑ Washing and dressing increases the pain and I find it necessary to change my way of doing it.
- ❑ Because of the pain I am unable to do some washing and dressing without help.
- ❑ Because of the pain I am unable to do any washing and dressing without help.

Section 3—Lifting

- ❑ I can lift heavy weights without extra pain.
- ❑ I can lift heavy weights, but it causes extra pain.
- ❑ Pain prevents me from lifting heavy weights off the floor.
- ❑ Pain prevents me from lifting heavy weights off the floor, but I can manage if they are conveniently positioned, for example, on a table.
- ❑ Pain prevents me from lifting heavy weights, but I can manage light to medium weights if they are conveniently positioned.
- ❑ I can only lift very light weights at the most.

Section 4—Walking

- ❑ I have no pain walking.
- ❑ I have some pain with walking but it does not increase with distance.
- ❑ I cannot walk more than 1 mile without increasing pain.
- ❑ I cannot walk more than 1/2 mile without increasing pain.
- ❑ I cannot walk more than 1/4 mile without increasing pain.
- ❑ I cannot walk at all without increasing pain.

Section 5—Sitting

- ❑ I can sit in any chair as long as I like.
- ❑ I can only sit in my favorite chair as long as I like.
- ❑ Pain prevents me from sitting for more than one hour.
- ❑ Pain prevents me from sitting for more than 1/2 hour.
- ❑ Pain prevents me from sitting for more than 10 minutes.
- ❑ Pain prevents me from sitting at all.

Section 6—Standing

- ❑ I can stand as long as I want without pain.
- ❑ I have some pain on standing but it does not increase with time.
- ❑ I cannot stand for longer than 1 hour without increasing pain.
- ❑ I cannot stand for longer than 1/2 hour without increasing pain.
- ❑ I cannot stand for longer than 10 minutes without increasing pain.
- ❑ I avoid standing because it increases the pain immediately.

Section 7—Sleeping

- ❑ I get no pain in bed.
- ❑ I get pain in bed but it does not prevent me from sleeping well.
- ❑ Because of pain my normal night's sleep is reduced by less than 1/4.
- ❑ Because of pain my normal night's sleep is reduced by less than 1/2.
- ❑ Because of pain my normal night's sleep is reduced by less than 3/4.
- ❑ Pain prevents me from sleeping at all.

Section 8—Social Life

- ❑ My social life is normal and gives me no pain.
- ❑ My social life is normal but increases the degree of pain.
- ❑ Pain has no significant effect on my social life apart from limiting my more energetic interests, e.g., dancing, etc.
- ❑ Pain has restricted my social life and I do not go out as often.
- ❑ Pain has restricted my social life to my home.
- ❑ I have no social life because of pain.

Section 9—Traveling

- ❑ I get no pain while traveling.
- ❑ I get some pain from traveling, but none of my usual forms of travel make it any worse.
- ❑ I get extra pain while traveling, but it does not compel me to seek alternative forms of travel.
- ❑ I get extra pain while traveling, which compels me to seek alternative forms of travel.

- ❑ Pain restricts all forms of travel.
- ❑ Pain prevents all forms of travel except that done lying down.

Section 10—Changing Degree of Pain

- ❑ My pain is rapidly getting better.
- ❑ My pain fluctuates but overall it is definitely getting better.
- ❑ My pain seems to be getting better but improvement is slow at present.
- ❑ My pain is neither getting better nor worse.
- ❑ My pain is gradually worsening.
- ❑ My pain is rapidly worsening.

$$\text{ODI score (\%)} = \frac{[\underline{\quad}] \text{ (total scored)}}{\underline{\hspace{3cm}}} \times 100 = \underline{\quad} \%$$

Source: From Hudson-Cook, N., K. Tormes-Nicholson, and A. Breen. A revised Oswestry disability questionnaire. In: *Back Pain: New Approaches to Rehabilitation and Education*, M.O. Roland and J.R. Jenner, eds. 1989. Manchester, United Kingdom: Manchester University Press, 187–204. Used with permission.

APPENDIX ELEVEN

The Roland-Morris Low Back Pain and Disability Questionnaire

Patient name: _____ Date: _____

Instructions

When your back hurts, you may find it difficult to do some of the things you normally do. This list contains some sentences that people have used to describe themselves when they have back pain. When you read them, you may find that some stand out because they describe you *today*. As you read the list, think of yourself *today*. When you read a sentence that describes you today, check (☑) the box to the left of it. If the sentence does not describe you, then leave the box blank and go on to the next one. Remember, only check the sentences that you are sure describe you today.

- ☐ 1. I stay at home most of the time because of my back.
- ☐ 2. I change position frequently to try to get my back comfortable.
- ☐ 3. I walk more slowly than usual because of my back.
- ☐ 4. Because of my back, I am not doing any jobs that I usually do around the house.
- ☐ 5. Because of my back, I use a handrail to get upstairs.
- ☐ 6. Because of my back, I lie down to rest more often.

- ❐ 7. Because of my back, I have to hold on to something to get out of an easy chair.
- ❐ 8. Because of my back, I try to get other people to do things for me.
- ❐ 9. I get dressed more slowly than usual because of my back.
- ❐ 10. I only stand up for short periods of time because of my back.
- ❐ 11. Because of my back, I try not to bend or kneel down.
- ❐ 12. I find it difficult to get out of a chair because of my back.
- ❐ 13. My back is painful almost all of the time.
- ❐ 14. I find it difficult to turn over in bed because of my back.
- ❐ 15. My appetite is not very good because of my back.
- ❐ 16. I have trouble putting on my socks (or stockings) because of the pain in my back.
- ❐ 17. I can only walk short distances because of my back pain.
- ❐ 18. I sleep less well because of my back.
- ❐ 19. Because of my back pain, I get dressed with the help of someone else.
- ❐ 20. I sit down for most of the day because of my back.
- ❐ 21. I avoid heavy jobs around the house because of my back.
- ❐ 22. Because of back pain, I am more irritable and bad tempered with people than usual.
- ❐ 23. Because of my back, I go upstairs more slowly than usual.
- ❐ 24. I stay in bed most of the time because of my back.

Source: Reprinted with permission from Roland, M., and R. Morris. A study of the natural history of back pain. Part I: Development of a reliable and sensitive measure of disability in low-back pain. *Spine*, 1983. **8**(2):141–4.

TWELVE

APPENDIX

Neck Disability Index

Patient name: _____ Date: _____

This questionnaire has been designed to give the doctor information as to how your neck has affected your ability to manage everyday life. Please answer every section and mark (☑) in each section only the ONE box which applies to you. We realize you may consider that two of the statements in any one section may relate to you, but please just mark the one box which most closely describes your problem.

Section 1—Pain Intensity

- ❏ I have no pain at the moment.
- ❏ The pain is mild at the moment.
- ❏ The pain comes and goes and is moderate.
- ❏ The pain is moderate and does not vary much.
- ❏ The pain is severe but comes and goes.
- ❏ The pain is severe and does not vary much.

Section 2—Personal Care (washing, dressing, etc.)

- ❏ I can look after myself without causing extra pain.
- ❏ I can look after myself normally but it causes extra pain.
- ❏ It is painful to look after myself and I am slow and careful.
- ❏ I need some help, but manage most of my personal care.
- ❏ I need help every day in most aspects of self-care.
- ❏ I do not get dressed, I wash with difficulty and stay in bed.

Section 3—Lifting

- ❏ I can lift heavy weights without extra pain.
- ❏ I can lift heavy weights, but it causes extra pain.
- ❏ Pain prevents me from lifting heavy weights off the floor, but I can manage if they are conveniently positioned, e.g. on the table.
- ❏ Pain prevents me from lofting heavy weights, but I can manage light to medium weights if they are conveniently positioned.
- ❏ I can lift very light weights.
- ❏ I cannot lift or carry anything at all.

Section 4—Reading

- ❏ I can read as much as I want to with no extra pain in my neck.
- ❏ I can read as much as I want with slight pain in my neck.
- ❏ I can read as much as I want with moderate pain in my neck.
- ❏ I cannot read as much as I want because of moderate pain in my neck.
- ❏ I cannot read as much as I want because of severe pain in my neck.
- ❏ I cannot read at all.

Section 5—Headache

- ❏ I have no headaches at all.
- ❏ I have slight headaches which come infrequently.
- ❏ I have moderate headaches which come infrequently.
- ❏ I have moderate headaches which come frequently.
- ❏ I have severe headaches which come frequently.
- ❏ I have headaches almost all the time .

Section 6—Concentration

- ❏ I can concentrate fully when I want to with no difficulty.
- ❏ I can concentrate fully when I want to with slight difficulty.
- ❏ I have a fair degree of difficulty in concentrating when I want to.
- ❏ I have a lot of difficulty in concentrating when I want to.
- ❏ I have a great deal of difficulty in concentrating when I want to.
- ❏ I cannot concentrate at all.

Section 7—Work

- ❏ I can do as much work as I want to.
- ❏ I can only do my usual work, but no more.
- ❏ I can do most of my usual work, but no more.
- ❏ I cannot do my usual work.
- ❏ I can hardly do any work at all.
- ❏ I cannot do any work at all.

Section 8—Driving

- ❏ I can drive my car without neck pain.
- ❏ I can drive my car as long as I want with slight pain in my neck.
- ❏ I can drive my car as long as I want with moderate pain in my neck.
- ❏ I cannot drive my car as long as I want because of moderate pain in my neck.
- ❏ I can hardly drive my car at all because of severe pain in my neck.
- ❏ I cannot drive my car at all.

Section 9—Sleeping

- ❏ I have no trouble sleeping.
- ❏ My sleep is slightly disturbed (less than 1 hour sleepless).
- ❏ My sleep is mildly disturbed (1–2 hours sleepless).
- ❏ My sleep is moderately disturbed (2–3 hours sleepless).
- ❏ My sleep is greatly disturbed (3–5 hours sleepless).
- ❏ My sleep is completely disturbed (5–7 hours sleepless).

Section 10—Recreation

- ❏ I am able to engage in all recreational activities with no pain in my neck at all.
- ❏ I am able to engage in all recreational activities with some pain in my neck.
- ❏ I am able to engage in most, but not all recreational activities because of pain in my neck.
- ❏ I am able to engage in a few of my usual recreational activities because of pain in my neck.

❑ I can hardly do any recreational activities because of pain in my neck.
❑ I cannot do any recreational activities at all.

Source: From Vernon, J., and S. Mior. The Neck Disability Index: A study of reliability and validity. *J Manipulative Physiol Ther*, 1991. **14**(7):409–15. Used with permission from the National University of Health Services.

THIRTEEN

APPENDIX

Whiplash Disability Questionnaire

Patient name: _____ Date: _____

This questionnaire has been designed to provide information on the impact that your whiplash injury and symptoms have upon your lifestyle. Please circle a number in each section to indicate how you have been affected by the whiplash injury and symptoms. If one or more questions are not relevant to you, please leave that section blank.

1. How much **pain** do you have today?

        0   1   2   3   4   5   6   7   8   9   10

    No pain   Worst pain imaginable

2. How much do your whiplash symptoms interfere with your **personal care** (washing, dressing, etc.)?

        0   1   2   3   4   5   6   7   8   9   10

    Not at all   Unable to perform

3. How much do your whiplash symptoms interfere with your **work home/study duties**?

   0   1   2   3   4   5   6   7   8   9   10

   Not at all   Unable to perform

4. How much have your whiplash symptoms interfered with **driving or using public transport**?

   0   1   2   3   4   5   6   7   8   9   10

   Not at all   Unable to travel in car/ use public transport

5. How much do your whiplash symptoms interfere with **sleep**?

   0   1   2   3   4   5   6   7   8   9   10

   Not at all   Cannot sleep

6. How **tired/fatigued** do you feel as a result of your whiplash injury/symptoms?

   0   1   2   3   4   5   6   7   8   9   10

   Not at all   Extreme tiredness/ fatigue all the time

7. How much do your whiplash symptoms interfere with **social activity**?

   0   1   2   3   4   5   6   7   8   9   10

   Not at all   Unable to socialize

8. How much do your whiplash symptoms interfere with **sporting activity**?

    0   1   2   3   4   5   6   7   8   9   10

    Not at all   Unable to
                                                        participate

9. How much do your whiplash symptoms interfere with **non-sporting leisure activity**?

    0   1   2   3   4   5   6   7   8   9   10

    Not at all   Unable to
                                                        participate

10. How much **sadness/depression** do you experience as a result of your whiplash injury/symptoms?

    0   1   2   3   4   5   6   7   8   9   10

    None   Extreme
                                                        sadness/
                                                        depression

11. How much **anger** do you experience as a result of your whiplash injury/symptoms?

    0   1   2   3   4   5   6   7   8   9   10

    None   Extreme anger

12. How much **anxiety** do you experience as a result of your whiplash injury/symptoms?

    0   1   2   3   4   5   6   7   8   9   10

    None   Extreme
                                                        anxiety

13. How much difficulty do you have **concentrating** as a result of your whiplash injury/symptoms?

| 0 | 1 | 2 | 3 | 4 | 5 | 6 | 7 | 8 | 9 | 10 |

No difficulty   Unable to concentrate

Source: Reprinted with permission from Pinfold, M., et al. Validity and internal consistency of a whiplash-specific disability measure. *Spine*, 2004. **29**(3):263–8.

APPENDIX FOURTEEN

Headache Disability Inventory

Patient name: _____ Date: _____

INSTRUCTIONS: Please mark (☑) the correct response:

I have a headache: ❏ 1 per month ❏ More than 1 but less than 4 per month ❏ More than 1 per week

My headache is: ❏ Mild ❏ Moderate ❏ Severe

The purpose of the scale is to identify difficulties that you may be experiencing because of your headache. Please answer "**YES**", "**SOMETIMES**", or "**NO**" to each item. Answer each question as it pertains to your headache only.

	YES	SOMETIMES	NO
E1. Because of my headaches I feel handicapped.	❏	❏	❏
F2. Because of my headaches I feel restricted in performing my routine daily activities.	❏	❏	❏
E3. No one understands the effect my headaches have on my life.	❏	❏	❏
F4. I restrict my recreational activities (e.g., sports, hobbies) because of my headaches.	❏	❏	❏
E5. My headaches make me angry.	❏	❏	❏

	YES	SOMETIMES	NO
E6. Sometimes I feel that I am going to lose control because of my headaches.	❏	❏	❏
F7. Because of my headaches I am less likely to socialize.	❏	❏	❏
E8. My spouse (significant other), or family and friends have no idea what I am going through because of my headaches.	❏	❏	❏
E9. My headaches are so bad that I feel that I am going to go insane.	❏	❏	❏
E10. My outlook on the world is affected by my headaches.	❏	❏	❏
E11. I am afraid to go outside when I feel that a headache is starting.	❏	❏	❏
E12. I feel desperate because of my headaches.	❏	❏	❏
F13. I am concerned that I am paying penalties at work or at home because of my headaches.	❏	❏	❏
E14. My headaches place stress on my relationships with family or friends.	❏	❏	❏
F15. I avoid being around people when I have a headache.	❏	❏	❏
F16. I believe my headaches are making it difficult for me to achieve my goals in life.	❏	❏	❏
F17. I am unable to think clearly because of my headaches.	❏	❏	❏

	YES	SOMETIMES	NO
F18. I get tense (e.g., muscle tension) because of my headaches.	❐	❐	❐
F19. I do not enjoy social gatherings because of my headaches.	❐	❐	❐
E20. I feel irritable because of my headaches.	❐	❐	❐
F21. I avoid traveling because of my headaches.	❐	❐	❐
E22. My headaches make me feel confused.	❐	❐	❐
E23. My headaches make me feel frustrated.	❐	❐	❐
F24. I find it difficult to read because of my headaches.	❐	❐	❐
F25. I find it difficult to focus my attention away from my headaches and on other things.	❐	❐	❐

Source: Reprinted with permission from Jacobson, G.P., et al. The Henry Ford Hospital Headache Disability Inventory (HDI). *Neurology*, 1994. **44**(5):837–42.

FIFTEEN

APPENDIX

Migraine Disability Assessment Score (MIDAS)

Patient name: _____ Date: _____

MIDAS Questionnaire

INSTRUCTIONS: Please answer the following questions about ALL the headaches you have had over the last 3 months. Write your answer in the box next to each question. Write zero if you did not do the activity in the last 3 months. (Please refer to the calendar below, if necessary.)

1. On how many days in the last 3 months did you miss work or school because of your headaches ☐ ☐ days

2. How many days in the last 3 months was your productivity at work or school reduced by half or more because of your headaches? (*Do not include days you counted in question 7 where you missed work or school*). ☐ ☐ days

3. On how many days in the last 3 months did you not do household work because of your headaches? ☐ ☐ days

4. How many days in the last 3 months was your productivity in household work reduced by half or more because of your headaches? (*Do not include days you counted in question 3 where you did not do household work*). ☐ ☐ days

5. On how many days in the last 3 months did you
    miss family, social, or leisure activities because
    of your headaches? ☐ ☐ days

A. On how many days in the last 3 months did you have
    any headache? (If a headache lasted more than one day,
    count each day). ☐ ☐ days

B. On a scale of 0–10, on average, how painful were these headaches?

Source: Reprinted with permission from W.F. Stewart.
(Note: Current year's calendar may be placed here.)

APPENDIX SIXTEEN

RAND 36-Item Health Survey Instrument (Version 1.0)

Patient name: _____ Date: _____

1. In general, would you say your health is:

(Circle One Number)

Excellent	1
Very good	2
Good	3
Fair	4
Poor	5

2. **Compared to one year ago**, how would your rate your health in general **now**?

(Circle One Number)

Much better now than one year ago	1
Somewhat better now than one year ago	2
About the same	3
Somewhat worse now than one year ago	4
Much worse now than one year ago	5

Appendix 16

The following items are about activities you might do during a typical day. Does **your health now limit you** in these activities? If so, how much?

(Circle One Number on Each Line)

	Yes, Limited a Lot	Yes, Limited a Little	No, Not Limited at all
3. **Vigorous activities**, such as running, lifting heavy objects, participating in strenuous sports	1	2	3
4. **Moderate activities**, such as moving a table, pushing a vacuum cleaner, bowling, or playing golf	1	2	3
5. Lifting or carrying groceries	1	2	3
6. Climbing **several** flights of stairs	1	2	3
7. Climbing **one** flight of stairs	1	2	3
8. Bending, kneeling, or stooping	1	2	3
9. Walking **more than a mile**	1	2	3
10. Walking **several blocks**	1	2	3
11. Walking **one block**	1	2	3
12. Bathing or dressing yourself	1	2	3

During the **past 4 weeks**, have you had any of the following problems with your work or other regular daily activities **as a result of your physical health**?

(Circle One Number on Each Line)

	Yes	No
13. Cut down the amount of time you spent on work or other activities	1	2
14. **Accomplished less** than you would like	1	2
15. Were limited in the **kind** of work or other activities	1	2
16. Had **difficulty** performing the work or other activities (for example, it took extra effort)	1	2

During the **past 4 weeks**, have you had any of the following problems with your work or other regular daily activities **as a result of any emotional problems** (such as feeling depressed or anxious)?

(Circle One Number on Each Line)

	Yes	No
17. Cut down the **amount of time** you spent on work or other activities	1	2
18. **Accomplished less** than you would like	1	2
19. Didn't do work or other activities as **carefully** as usual	1	2

20. During the **past 4 weeks**, to what extent has your physical health or emotional problems interfered with your normal social activities with family, friends, neighbors, or groups?

(Circle One Number)

Not at all	1
Slightly	2
Moderately	3
Quite a bit	4
Extremely	5

21. How much **bodily** pain have you had during the **past 4 weeks**?

(Circle One Number)

None	1
Very mild	2
Mild	3
Moderate	4
Severe	5
Very severe	6

22. During the **past 4 weeks**, how much did **pain** interfere with your normal work (including both work outside the home and housework)?

(Circle One Number)

Not at all	1
A little bit	2
Moderately	3
Quite a bit	4
Extremely	5

RAND 36-Item Health Survey Instrument (Version 1.0)

These questions are about how you feel and how things have been with you **during the past 4 weeks**. For each question, please give the one answer that comes closest to the way you have been feeling.

How much of the time during the **past 4 weeks** . . .

(Circle One Number on Each Line)

	All of the Time	Most of the Time	A Good Bit of the Time	Some of the Time	A Little of the Time	None of the Time
23. Did you feel full of pep?	1	2	3	4	5	6
24. Have you been a very nervous person?	1	2	3	4	5	6
25. Have you felt so down in the dumps that nothing could cheer you up?	1	2	3	4	5	6
26. Have you felt calm and peaceful?	1	2	3	4	5	6
27. Did you have a lot of energy?	1	2	3	4	5	6
28. Have you felt downhearted and blue?	1	2	3	4	5	6
29. Did you feel worn out?	1	2	3	4	5	6
30. Have you been a happy person?	1	2	3	4	5	6
31. Did you feel tired?	1	2	3	4	5	6

Appendix 16

32. During the **past 4 weeks**, how much of the time has your **physical health or emotional problems** interfered with your social activities (like visiting with friends, relatives, etc.)?

(Circle One Number)

All of the time	1
Most of the time	2
Some of the time	3
A little of the time	4
None of the time	5

How TRUE or FALSE is *each* of the following statements for you?

(Circle One Number on Each Line)

	Definitely True	Mostly True	Don't Know	Mostly False	Definitely False
33. I seem to get sick a little easier than other people.	1	2	3	4	5
34. I am as healthy as anybody I know.	1	2	3	4	5
35. I expect my health to get worse.	1	2	3	4	5
36. My health is excellent.	1	2	3	4	5

Source: Developed at RAND as part of a Medical Outcomes Study.

GLOSSARY

Absolute risk reduction (ARR) The difference in the probability of disease between the treatment and control groups. AAR describes how much of the difference in the reduction of disease incidence between the groups can be attributed to this treatment. It can be calculated using data from a two-by-two contingency table as follows:

$$[a / (a + b)] - [c / (c + d)]$$

Abstract A concise summary of the contents of a journal article or research proposal that is located at the beginning of the text.

Accuracy The degree to which a test or measurement truly represents the correct value of an attribute that is being measured. Accuracy of a test is determined by comparing results from the new test with the results of a reference standard (gold standard) test.

Alpha level (α) The probability of error that a researcher is willing to accept for a given research project; typically 0.05. Also known as *significance level*.

Alternative hypothesis (H_1) The hypothesis that states the expected relationship in a study and is only accepted following rejection of the null hypothesis. Also known as the *research hypothesis*.

Analysis of covariance (ANCOVA) A statistical technique used to compare the means of two or more groups, while controlling for extraneous variables (covariates).

Glossary

Analysis of variance (ANOVA)   A statistical method of comparing the means of three or more groups. The use of ANOVA is preferable to the use of multiple *t*-tests because it reduces the probability of a type I error.

Assessment bias   See *bias*

Attributable risk (AR)   A measure of association that represents the probability of disease in the exposed group minus the probability of disease in the unexposed group. AR represents the excess risk that is accounted for by exposure to the factor under investigation. The formula used to calculate AR is the same as that of the absolute risk reduction (ARR).

Baseline measure   The initial measurement carried out in a study that is the basis to which subsequent measurements are compared.

Baseline phase   The initial phase of a single-subject time series design where at least three repeated measures of the outcomes of interest are taken prior to beginning any treatment.

Beta   The probability of making a type II error.

Between-groups variance   A measure of how much the group means in a study differ from each other. Also known as *treatment variance*.

Bias   In research, bias refers to systematic errors introduced into a study that are attributable to problems with selection, assignment of participants to groups, or problems with the measurements involved in the study. Errors related to biases are not due to chance. Types of bias are as follows:

Assessment bias   Outcomes are assessed in systematically different ways. Also known as *detection bias* or *measurement bias*.

Exclusion bias   Subjects are lost to follow-up in a study who may somehow be different from those that remain. Also known as *attrition bias*.

Experimenter bias   Researchers may conduct themselves in a manner that influences study participants in such a way that the results of the study are distorted. Also known as *researcher bias*.

Performance bias   Study participants are cared for differently, other than the intervention under investigation. Also known as *intervention bias*.

Sampling bias Study participants are selected in such a way that each person from the source population does not have an equal chance of being selected.

Blinding A tactic used in research whereby certain study procedures are not disclosed to the researchers or study participants. Blinding takes several different forms: *single blinding* (participants are not aware of group assignment), *double blinding* (neither the patients nor the researchers know whether the treatment or placebo is involved), and *triple blinding* (neither the subject, the person providing the treatment, nor the evaluator is aware of group assignment). Also known as *masking*.

Boolean operator Used in database searches to combine query terms in ways that can either narrow or broaden the search, depending on which Boolean operator is used. Operators include AND, OR, and NOT which should always be capitalized. Also known as *logical operator*.

Case report An observational study that discusses the clinical management of one or a few patients. Case reports provide little or no evidence because of their many limitations. Also known as a *case study*.

Case-control study A retrospective observational study that compares exposures in two groups of subjects; participants in one group have the disease or condition under investigation (the cases), whereas those in the other group are free from the disease (the controls).

Case series A form of research wherein a single group of patients is treated and outcomes are assessed. Case series represent a low level of evidence because no comparison group is involved.

Central tendency A type of descriptive statistics that provides a measure of the location of the middle of a set of data. Measures of central tendency include the mean, median, and mode.

Chance In biomedical research, chance refers to random variation of data caused by such things as biological variability and measurement error. Chance findings are distinguished from real effects using statistical tests that provide P values or confidence intervals.

Chi-square test (χ^2) A statistical test used with nominal and ordinal data to determine whether one set of proportions is different from another by comparing frequencies. There are two versions of the chi-square test: the *chi-square goodness of fit* (tests whether the observed frequencies are different from what would be expected by chance) and the *chi-square test of independence* (tests whether the proportions or frequencies for one category differ significantly from those of another category).

Clinical practice guidelines   Statements systematically developed by experts in a particular field that are designed to assist practitioners and patients in choosing appropriate health care for specific conditions.

Clinical significance   Clinical significance has to do with whether the effect size in a study is large enough to be deemed worthwhile by patients. If a study's results are trivial in terms of practical implications, they may not apply, or have limited application, to clinical practice. Also known as *practical significance*.

Clinical trial   A type of human research study that evaluates an intervention to evaluate its safety and efficacy. Clinical trials have been categorized into four phases as follows:

Phase 1   The first step in the process of testing a new treatment in humans, which is concerned with determining how the intervention works physiologically and with observing any side effects. Phase 1 trials usually involve small numbers of healthy subjects with no comparison group. Consequently, they may provide early, but very limited, evidence of effectiveness and safety.

Phase 2   Phase 2 trials are conducted to test the effectiveness of the intervention on a larger sample of subjects, although they may not be conducted as randomized controlled trials.

Phase 3   Large studies that are usually randomized controlled trials involving a bigger sample of subjects and a longer period of time. Accordingly, they are capable of gathering more detailed and reliable information on the effectiveness and safety of a treatment.

Phase 4   Trials that are carried out after the treatment is commonly in use to determine additional risks, benefits, and best uses.

Coefficient of determination (r^2)   The square of the correlation coefficient (r). The coefficient of determination represents the amount of variation in the y variable can be explained by the x variable. Because r is squared in the process of calculating the coefficient of determination, it can have only positive values, which range from 0.0 to 1.0.

Cohort study   An observational study that involves two groups of subjects being followed forward in time. One group is exposed to some known or suspected cause of disease while the other group is not exposed. The outcomes of the groups are compared at the study's conclusion in an attempt to identify causal factors. Cohort studies are typically prospective, although they can be done retrospectively by identifying two groups at some point in time past and then assessing the development of outcomes from that time onward.

Concealment of allocation   A method used by researchers in randomized controlled trials to make sure blinding has actually occurred. Concealment of group allocation is often achieved by means of sealed sequentially numbered opaque envelopes that contain information on study assignment. As a result, awareness of group assignment is hidden from those charged with the task of randomizing study participants.

Concurrent validity   A pragmatic method of evaluating a test that involves comparing the results of a new test with an established (gold standard) test, both given at the same point in time, to determine if there is an adequate degree of correlation.

Confidence interval (CI)   The range of values within which a population parameter is expected to lie within a specified probability, usually 95%. The upper and lower boundaries of a 95% confidence interval are the 95% confidence limits.

Confounding   Interference by an extraneous factor that has an influence on the relationship between the variables in an experiment. The study's conclusion may be related to a confounding variable instead of the variable under study.

Confounding variable   A type of extraneous variable that introduces systematic error into a study because it affects the levels of the independent variables differently.

Consistency   One of the criteria required to establish causation in epidemiological studies; studies on the topic that are carried out by other researchers using different populations get similar results.

Construct validity   The extent to which a test adequately measures a theoretical construct (e.g., pain, disability). In construct validity, the characteristic being investigated is not observed directly; instead, an abstraction of the characteristic is observed (e.g., pain scale, disability questionnaire), which corresponds to the construct being considered.

Content validity   The ability of a test to include or represent all of the content of a particular construct.

Contingency table   A two-dimensional table of data that compares attributes of one variable with another. Examples include assessing the presence or absence of a condition in relation to positive or negative test results, as depicted in the accompanying table; the presence or absence of a condition in relation to exposure versus nonexposure to a risk factor; and the presence or absence of a condition in relation to the administration of a treatment versus no treatment. Contingency tables are used to perform a number of different calculations involved in health care. Also known as *two-by-two contingency table*.

		Condition		
		Present	Absent	
Test	Positive	a	b	$a+b$
	Negative	c	d	$c+d$
		$a+c$	$b+d$	$a+b+c+d$

Continuous variable   A variable that can take on any value within a range of values.

Control group   The group of subjects in a clinical study who are similar to the experimental group, but do not receive the intervention.

Convergent validity   The degree of correlation that exists between a new test and another measure of the same or similar constructs.

Correlation   A mathematical relationship between two or more events, characteristics, or other variables.

Correlation coefficient (r)   A measure of association between two variables that provides the information about the strength and direction of any mathematical relationship that may exist. The value of r ranges from -1.00 to $+1.00$, with $+1.00$ representing a perfect positive correlation and -1.00 representing a perfect negative correlation. Also known as Pearson product-moment correlation coefficient.

Covariate   A variable that is correlated with another variable. Also, in analysis of covariance (ANCOVA), it is the variable that is controlled for, so that the influence of the covariate on the relationship between the independent and dependent variables is statistically minimized.

Criterion-related validity   The degree to which a test corresponds with an external criterion that is an independent measure of the characteristic being tested. A criterion is the standard by which a measure is judged; thus, if a test is valid, it should correlate well with or predict some relevant criterion.

Critical appraisal   The process of systematically evaluating the validity of research evidence and determining its relevance to certain patients or circumstances.

Critical value   A threshold value used in a hypothesis test to which the computed test statistic is compared to determine whether the null hypothesis should be rejected or retained at a specified level of significance.

Cronbach's coefficient alpha   A statistical test used to evaluate the internal consistency of items in a questionnaire to determine whether they measure the same construct or if they are superfluous. It represents the mean correlation between each of a set of items in a questionnaire. The maximum value for coefficient alpha is 1, although it can have a value that is less than zero when numerous negatively correlating items are included in a questionnaire. An instrument with a reliability coefficient value of 0.70 or greater is generally considered to be acceptable. Also known as *alpha*.

Crossover design   A study design that involves two or more interventions, in which participants first receive one treatment and then are crossed over to receive the other treatment.

Cross-sectional study   An observational study that assesses both the health status as well as the exposure levels of individuals within a population simultaneously at one point in time. Also known as *prevalence study*.

Cutoff score   A score that is established as a cutoff point, so that scores above a specified value are considered positive and scores below that value are considered negative.

Deductive reasoning   Reasoning that is based on laws, rules, or other widely accepted principles. Deductive reasoning is utilized in research to test known theories or ideas to determine whether they are true.

Degrees of freedom (df)   The number of observations or values in a distribution that are free to vary. Degrees of freedom are used in t-tests, analysis of variance, and chi-square tests, among others.

Dependent variable   The outcome in a study that follows, and is hypothesized to be caused by, the independent variable.

Descriptive statistics   Statistics that summarize various aspects of a collection of data from a sample or a population in such a way that the data is easier to read and comprehend. Commonly used descriptive statistics include mean, median, and standard deviation.

Descriptive study   A study that is capable of describing various characteristics of persons in a particular population.

Directional hypothesis   A hypothesis where the researcher would be interested in either an increase or a decrease in the dependent variable, but not both. Thus, the results of the study would be expected to go in only one direction.

Discrete variable   A variable that can only take on certain values within the range of the variable and cannot be expressed in intervals less than 1.

Discriminant validity   A type of validity wherein a new test is found to be weakly related to or unrelated to another measure that it should actually be different from. Also known as *divergent validity*.

Dose-response   One of the criteria required to establish causation in epidemiological studies; it is present when greater exposure to a risk factor results in a greater effect on health.

In general, it is the relationship between the amount of exposure to a substance (which can include a treatment) and the consequential changes in body function or health.

Effect   The amount of difference between the outcomes of two treatments in a clinical trial.

Effectiveness   The assessment of how treatments or interventions work under real-life conditions and in terms that matter to patients.

Efficacy   The assessment of how treatments or interventions work under ideal conditions, as one would find in a controlled experiment.

Empirical observation   The process of gathering information that is derived from direct experience or observation.

Epidemiology   A branch of science that investigates the frequency and distribution of diseases in a distinct population in an attempt to determine their causes, to discover ways to alleviate them, and to prevent their reoccurrences.

Evidence-based chiropractic (EBC)   Actively seeking support for and improvement of chiropractic clinical practices through the integration of the best available research evidence, combined with clinical expertise and patient values.

Exclusion bias   See *bias*.

Experimental design   A study design in which the researcher randomly assigns subjects to groups, manipulates the independent variables, and then compares outcomes between subjects who receive an intervention and those in a control or comparison group.

Experimenter bias   See *bias*.

Exposed group   A group of research subjects who are exposed to a suspected risk factor.

External validity   The extent to which the results of a given study can be applied to another patient population or to real-world patients. Also known as *generalizability*.

Extraneous variable   An uncontrolled factor that has an influence on the relationship between the variables under study in an experiment. Extraneous variables affect the outcome of an experiment, even though they are not the variables that are actually being studied. They produce error in an experiment and, as a result, are undesirable.

Face validity Whether the test "on face value" appears to have merit, which is determined by deciding if it appears to measure what it was intended to measure.

Generalizability See *external validity*.

Gold standard A test that is commonly considered to be the best available (i.e., the most specific and sensitive). Gold standard tests are compared with new tests to ascertain their validity.

Goodness-of-fit test See *chi-square test*.

Hawthorne effect A phenomenon in which a research subject's behavior or response to an intervention is affected (usually favorably) simply because the individual is aware of the fact that he or she is participating in a study. The Hawthorne effect can therefore bias the results of a study.

Histogram A graphic representation of a frequency distribution that is composed of a series of bars that correspond to classes or groups of data. The height of each bar corresponds to the number of values that are contained in each class or group.

Homogeneity A term that describes a condition in which elements or ingredients of a set are similar and of uniform quality throughout. Examples of homogeneity are: studies included in a systematic review that are comparable and groups in a clinical trial that have similar baseline characteristics.

Hypothesis An assumption that seems to explain certain observations and that is proposed to be substantiated by further investigation.

Incidence The probability of a person being diagnosed with a disease during a specific period of time. It represents the number of newly diagnosed cases of a disease during a specified time period, which is usually one year.

Independent variable An intervention, exposure, or other characteristic in a study that is often manipulated by the researcher and is hypothesized to influence the dependent variable.

Inductive reasoning Reasoning that draws on observation to create an idea or theory.

Inferential statistics   The testing of hypotheses with specified degrees of uncertainty and then using sample data to make generalizations to other populations.

Informed consent   One of the cornerstones of ethical research, which involves obtaining consent from research subjects after informing them about a study's inherent benefits and risks.

Institutional review board (IRB)   Committee that oversees ethical concerns about research that involves human subjects at a given institution. Also known as *human subjects review board* or *ethics review board*.

Intention-to-treat   A way of analyzing data in a clinical trial in which patients are analyzed in the groups to which they were originally assigned, regardless of whether they received the intervention or completed the study.

Interexaminer reliability   Results of a measure are consistent between different examiners who are evaluating the same information. Assessing interexaminer reliability involves two or more examiners testing the same subjects for the same characteristic using the same measure and then ascertaining the degree to which their findings agree. Also known as *interobserver reliability* or *interrater reliability*.

Intermediate outcome measure   An outcome measure (e.g., blood pressure or a laboratory test) that substitutes for a truly important clinical outcome, especially one that would be considered important to a patient (e.g., less pain). Intermediate outcome measures are often assumed to represent clinical outcomes, but many times they do not. Also known as a *surrogate end point*.

Internal consistency   The extent to which items in a questionnaire measure the same characteristic.

Internal validity   The capacity of an experiment to show that the independent variables actually caused the changes that were observed in the dependent variables.

Interval measurement   A level of measurement in which measurements must exhibit equal intervals that are ordered, although the interval scale does not have a true zero. The classic example is the Fahrenheit scale, where 0° does not correspond to an absence of heat; thus, it does not represent a measurement of true zero.

Intervention phase The phase of a single-subject time series design in which an intervention is provided. At least three repeated measures of the outcomes of interest are taken during the intervention phase.

Intraclass correlation coefficient (ICC) A reliability coefficient that is often used to assess interexaminer reliability. The ICC is an index of reliability that ranges from below 0.0 to +1.0, with 1.0 representing strong reliability and 0.0 representing weak reliability.

Intraexaminer reliability Results of a measure are consistent when repeated by the same examiner. Assessing intraexaminer reliability involves a single examiner testing the same group of subjects on two or more occasions and then determining the degree to which the examiner agrees with himself or herself. Also known as *intraobserver reliability* or *intrarater reliability*.

Kappa statistic (κ) A measure of agreement that is capable of quantifying the amount of true agreement that exists between two examiners because it considers the proportion of agreement that would be expected beyond chance. Kappa is an appropriate statistic to use with dichotomous or nominal data.

Least squares line See *regression line*.

Likelihood ratio (LR) The probability that the results of a diagnostic test would be expected in a patient with the condition of interest (sensitivity) compared with the expected results of the same test in a patient without the condition (specificity).

LR of a negative test (LR^-) A ratio of the probability of a negative test in a person with the condition compared with the probability of a negative test in a person without the condition. $LR^- = (1 - \text{Sensitivity})/\text{Specificity}$.

LR of a positive test (LR^+) A ratio of the probability of a positive test in a person with the condition compared with the probability of a positive test in a person without the condition. $LR^+ = \text{Sensitivity}/(1 - \text{Specificity})$.

Longitudinal study An epidemiological study that follows a group or groups of subjects forward in time in order to observe any changes that may occur.

Masking See *blinding*.

Matching A method of group assignment that pairs subjects based on one or more variables, such as gender, age, conditions, severity, and so on. Matching has the potential of reducing the effects of selection bias by making groups more similar.

Mean A measure of central tendency that is the most commonly used descriptive statistic. The mean is calculated by adding all values of a series of numbers together, and then dividing by the number of elements. Also known as the *average*.

Measurement bias See *bias*.

Measurement error The difference between a theoretical true score and what was actually observed. There will always be a certain amount of measurement error attributable to both random and systematic effects.

Median A measure of central tendency that describes the midpoint of a set of data, such that 50% of the scores will be above the median and 50% will be below.

Meta-analysis A systematic review that incorporates an additional step of combining the quantitative data from the included articles using specific methodological and statistical procedures. Also known as *quantitative systematic review*.

Mode A measure of central tendency that identifies the score that occurs most frequently.

Multiple regression A type of regression in which more than one variable is used to predict the outcome variable. The equation used in multiple regression is $Y = a + b_1 X_1 + b_2 X_2 + \ldots + b_k X_k$, where X_1 is the value of the first predictor variable, X_2 is the value of the second, and X_k would continue for as many predictor variables as are being analyzed.

Multivariate analysis Statistical analyses that involve three or more variables.

Nominal measurement A scale of measurement that involves data that are coded in the form of a number, name, or letter that is assigned to the categories or groups that are involved. Order does not matter when nominal scale items are involved. Examples include gender (e.g., male or female), job category (e.g., managerial, clerical, or blue-collar), and hair color (e.g., black, brunette, blonde, or red). Also known as *classificatory scale*.

Nondirectional hypothesis A research hypothesis in which the researcher is interested in knowing if the scores between groups are different, but makes no predictions whether either of the scores will be higher or lower than the other.

Nonparametric data Data that is not normally distributed (skewed) or results from nominal or ordinal measurement.

Normal curve A fitted line that defines an underlying normal distribution. Also known as a *bell-shaped curve*.

Normal distribution A distribution of data with the following properties: (1) It is symmetric about its mean; (2) the highest point of the overlying normal curve is at the mean; and (3) as one moves away from the mean in either direction, the height of the curve decreases, approaching, but never reaching, zero. In a *standardized* normal distribution, the area under the curve is 1 and the standard deviation is 1. Also known as *Gaussian distribution*.

Null hypothesis (H_0) The assumption that there is no difference between the groups being tested in a study. The research hypothesis is adopted only if the null hypothesis proves to be unlikely. Since the null hypothesis asserts that there is no difference between the means, the idea is to reject it on the grounds that it is very doubtful that it is true. In biomedical research, it typically must be at least 95% unlikely that the null hypothesis is true before it can be rejected.

Number needed to treat (NNT) The number of patients who would need to be treated in order to prevent one additional bad outcome. NNT is calculated using data from a two-by-two contingency table as follows:

$$\frac{1}{[a/(a+b)]-[c/(c+d)]} = \frac{1}{\text{Absolute risk reduction}}$$

Observational study A type of epidemiological study that does not involve manipulation of the independent variable by the researchers. Observational studies are used when harmful interventions are involved (e.g., smoking, risky behaviors, overeating) that would be unethical for researchers to ask people to perform. Observational studies are more susceptible to the influence of biases and confounding than are randomized controlled trials. There are three types of observational studies: cross-sectional, cohort, and case-control.

Odds ratio (OR) A ratio of the odds of developing the disease under investigation in the exposed group divided by the odds of developing the disease in the unexposed group that is calculated from data in case-control studies. The OR is an estimate of the odds of developing the disease given that a person was exposed to a risk factor. Using data from a two-by-two contingency table, a/c is the odds that a case was exposed, and b/d is the odds that a control was exposed. The OR can then be calculated using either of the following formulas:

$$\frac{a/c}{b/d}$$

For easier calculation, this formula can be simplified to:

$$\frac{ad}{bc}$$

ORs are used in case-control studies because it is not possible to determine probability, since the disease rates in the study population are not known. ORs are also reported in other types of studies, such as meta-analyses.

One-tailed test   A statistical test that is based on a directional hypothesis, wherein the critical values are only in one tail of the distribution.

Ordinal measurement   A measurement scale that involves rank-ordered categorical data (e.g., rating pain severity as mild, moderate, and severe).

Outcome measures   The tools used to assess patients' health status and to track their progress in order to evaluate the effectiveness of a given treatment.

***P* value**   The probability of obtaining a statistical test value as extreme as or more extreme than what would be observed by chance alone, if the null hypothesis was true. Thus, the *P* value is the probability of incorrectly rejecting a null hypothesis that was actually true.

Parallel-forms reliability   Two versions of a questionnaire or test that measure the same constructs are compared. Also known as *alternate-forms reliability.*

Parameter   A measured characteristic of a population.

Parametric data   Data that is assumed to be normally distributed.

Pearson product-moment correlation coefficient   See *correlation coefficient.*

Placebo   An inert substance or treatment that is used as a comparison to the active substance or treatment in a randomized controlled trial.

Point estimate   A sample statistic that is an estimate of the true parameter in a population.

Population   In research, the units from which a sample is drawn and to whom the data will be generalized. A population may comprise people, but can also consist of events or observations.

Posttest probability   The probability that patients have a particular condition after considering their pretest probability of disease and the likelihood ratio of the test that they received. A high pretest probability coupled with a high likelihood ratio will generate a very high posttest probability, whereas a low pretest probability and low likelihood ratio will produce a very low posttest probability.

Power (1 − β)   The probability of correctly rejecting a false H_0. The power of a test is influenced by the size of the sample, the amount of the difference between group means (the bigger the better in both cases), and the value of alpha. By convention, the power of a study should be 80% or higher.

Precision   A term that is analogous to *reliability*; it describes how close repeated measurements of the same trait are to each other.

Predictive validity   The extent to which a test can accurately predict some future event. Predictive validity is determined by measuring some characteristic on one occasion and then waiting to see if the projected outcome actually occurs at some time in the future.

Predictive value   The ability of a positive or negative diagnostic test to predict the probability of having or not having a condition.

> **Negative predictive value (NPV)**   The probability that a person with a negative test does not have the condition. In other words, the probability that a negative test will correctly predict that the condition is not present. NPV can be calculated from data in a two-by-two contingency table as follows: $d/(c + d)$.
>
> **Positive predictive value (PPV)**   The probability that a person with a positive test actually has the condition. In other words, the probability that a positive test will correctly predict that the condition is present. PPV can be calculated from data in a two-by-two contingency table as follows: $a/(a + b)$.

Pretest probability The probability that a patient has the condition under consideration that is estimated before the test is actually carried out. Pretest probability is typically derived from the clinician's experience, the prevalence of the condition being considered, and published literature. It may be modified up or down for a particular patient in the presence of risk factors. Also known as *pretest likelihood* or *pretest odds*.

Prevalence The proportion of persons in a given population that have a disease or attribute at a certain point in time. It represents the total number of cases of disease in that population, regardless of when patients were diagnosed with the condition.

Prospective research A type of research in which data is collected contemporaneously with the temporal progression of the study.

Publication bias The tendency of journals to publish articles that report on studies with statistically significant positive results, to the exclusion of "failed" studies.

Qualitative research Research that makes use of qualitative data (e.g., words from questionnaires or interviews) and is typically based on inductive reasoning. Qualitative research is subjective because it is based on people providing estimations about things such as how they feel or their ability to function.

Quantitative research Research that involves quantitative data (e.g., numbers that are derived from taking measurements on participants in a study) and is typically based on deductive reasoning. Quantitative research is objective because data are founded on reliable measurements.

Quasi-experimental design A study design in which subjects are assigned to groups, the independent variables are manipulated, and outcomes compared, which is similar to experimental design; however, random group assignment is not involved. Because there is no randomization, it is much more difficult to make claims about causality based on quasi-experimental evidence.

Random assignment A method used to assign research subjects to study groups that is based on chance. A variety of legitimate randomization methods are available, including random number tables, computer-generated numbers, and coin tosses. Also known as *randomization*.

Random error Statistical variations in a measurement that may occur in either direction. Random error is due to limitations in the precision of the measuring instrument that are related to the researcher's inability to reliably take the same measurement from test to test.

Random sample A group of research participants that was selected in such a way that each subject had an equal chance of being chosen.

Randomized controlled trial (RCT) A type of research design wherein a sample of patients is randomly divided into two groups: one that receives the genuine treatment and another that receives a placebo or sham treatment.

Ratio measurement A level of measurement in which there are equal intervals between scores and a true zero. The ratio scale is the most advanced level of measurement that can accommodate the most types of arithmetic operations.

Recall bias A type of bias in which study participants do not report retrospective events accurately, which can be unintentional (e.g., inadequate memory) or intentional (e.g., concealing information about some sensitive issue).

Regression analysis A method for estimating the relationship of a predictor variable to an outcome variable (criterion variable) through a process that uses the observations in a set of data to calculate the best fit of a line passing through the data. Regression produces a formula for the least squares line that enables one to make predictions about the direction and amount of movement of the variables. The regression formula is $Y = a + bX$, where a is the Y intercept, b is the slope of the line, and X is the value of the variable X.

Regression line A line through the data points in a scatterplot, which is generated such that the total of all the squared distances of each data point from the line is as small as possible. Also known as the *least squares line*.

Regression to the mean A phenomenon wherein extreme test values on the pretest have a tendency to move toward the group's mean on subsequent evaluations, apart from any intervention.

This effect can often be identified by using a comparison group that does not receive the intervention.

Relative risk (RR) A ratio that compares the risk of some health-related event between two groups that are included in a prospective study. More specifically, it is the probability of disease occurrence in the exposed group, divided by the probability of disease in the unexposed group. The formula for calculating RR using data from a two-by-two contingency table is as follows:

$$\frac{a/(a+b)}{c/(c+d)} = \frac{\text{Probability of disease in exposed group}}{\text{Probability of disease in unexposed group}}$$

Relative risk reduction (RRR)   The comparative reduction in rates of bad outcomes between the experimental and control groups. RRR is calculated using data in a two-by-two contingency table as follows:

$$\frac{[a/(a+b)]-[c/(c+d)]}{c/(c+d)} = \frac{\text{Absolute risk reduction}}{\text{Probability of disease in unexposed group}}$$

Reliability   A test's reliability refers to its ability to provide consistent results when repeated by the same examiner or when more than one examiner tests the same attribute on the same group of subjects.

Representative sample   A sample having features that are similar to those of the source population. Representative samples are the result of random selection.

Research hypothesis (H_1)   The research hypothesis states that there is a difference between groups in an experiment. The research hypothesis is not tested directly, however; instead, the null hypothesis is tested first, and then, depending on the outcome of this test, there is either support for or against the research hypothesis being true. Also known as the *alternative hypothesis*.

Researcher bias   See *bias*.

Responsiveness   The capacity of a diagnostic test to accurately represent change in a patient's condition.

Retrospective research   A type of research in which data was collected in the past (e.g., from medical records or patient questionnaires).

Risk   The likelihood that a person will experience a given event.

Risk factor   An exposure, inherited trait, or behavior that magnifies the likelihood that a person will develop a disease.

Sample A subset of a population that is selected for a given study. Samples may be selected randomly (e.g., a representative sample) or nonrandomly (e.g., a nonrepresentative sample).

Sampling bias See *bias*.

Sensitivity The ability of a test to correctly identify people who have the target disorder. Sensitivity can be calculated from data in a two-by-two contingency table as follows:

$$\frac{a}{a+c}$$

Significance level See *alpha level*.

Single-subject time series design A study that involves a single patient in which repeated measurements are taken while an intervention is systematically applied and withdrawn. The objective of this type of study is to compare measures of outcomes between phases of treatment and observational phases. Sometimes an alternate form of treatment is utilized rather than no treatment during the observational phase. Also known as *n-of-1 trial*.

Specificity The ability of a test to correctly identify people who do not have the target disorder. Specificity can be calculated from data in a two-by-two contingency table as follows:

$$\frac{d}{b+d}$$

Standard deviation (S) A measure of the dispersion of scores about the mean. Standard deviation is the square root of the variance.

Statistic A measured characteristic of a sample.

Statistical adjustment A statistical technique that can minimize differences between the study and comparison groups.

Statistical significance A term that indicates that a study's results are unlikely to be the result of chance at a specified probability level, leading to rejection of the null hypothesis and acceptance of the research hypothesis.

Surrogate end points See *intermediate outcome measure*.

Systematic error Inaccurate test results that consistently occur in the same direction and persist throughout the entire study. Systematic error is due to malfunction of the measuring device, such as an elongated tape measure that always produces measurements that are too long. It is not possible to detect this type of error statistically, because all of the data are shifted in the same direction.

Systematic review A type of review that utilizes very strict, well-defined methods of locating, appraising and synthesizing all of the research that is available on a given topic. Also known as *qualitative systematic review*.

***t*-test** A statistical test that is used to determine whether the means of two groups are statistically different from each other. Also known as *Student's t-test*.

Target population The population to which the results of a study are generalized.

Temporality One of the criteria required to establish causation in epidemiological studies, wherein an exposure must occur prior to the onset of a disease when attempting to determine whether exposure to a specific risk factor is a cause of a particular disease within a population. Also known as *temporal precedence*.

Test-retest reliability The reliability of a test that is administered to the same group of individuals on more than one occasion. There should be a high degree of correlation between repeated test scores in order to have acceptable test-retest reliability.

Two-tailed test A statistical test that is based on a nondirectional hypothesis, wherein the critical values could be in either tail of the distribution.

Type I error Erroneous rejection of a true null hypothesis. In this type of error, the researcher reports that there is a difference between the groups, but there is actually no difference.

Type II error Erroneous acceptance of a false null hypothesis. In this type of error, the researcher reports that there is no difference between the groups, but there actually is a difference.

Validity The degree to which a test or measuring device actually measures what it was intended to measure. Validity also applies to research design. A study is considered to be valid if its measures actually measure what they claim to and if there are no logical errors in drawing conclusions from the data.

Variable A characteristic that can be observed or manipulated and can take on different values. When referring to data from a population, these characteristics are known as *parameters*; when referring to data from samples, they are known as *statistics*.

Variance (S^2) A measure of the variability of a set of data that is equal to the square of the standard deviation.

Visual Analogue Scale (VAS) A 10-centimeter line with descriptive phrases at each end depicting the extremes of some characteristic that is being measured (e.g., pain).

Washout period A period of time without treatment that is allocated prior to switching treatments in a crossover study. The purpose of this no treatment interval is to allow the effects of the first treatment to disappear before starting the second treatment.

INDEX

Absolute risk reduction (ARR), 264, 421
Abstract
    of case report, 216, 237
    explanation of, 198, 421
AccessMedicine, 50
Accuracy, 421
ACP Journal Club, 50
Admission rate bias, 256
Agency for Health Care Policy and Research, 6
Agency for Healthcare Research and Quality (AHRQ), 27–29
Algometry, 340, 341
Alpha level
    explanation of, 115–118, 421
    in nondirectional test, 124
Alternative hypothesis, 114, 421
AMED database, 43, 68
American College of Occupational and Environmental Medicine (ACOEM), 15
Analysis of covariance (ANCOVA), 162–163, 421
Analysis of variance (ANOVA)
    calculations for, 128–130
    explanation of, 127–128, 421, 422
    one-way, 130
    use of, 130–131, 227
AND operator, 76–79
Appraisal
    of randomized controlled trials, 173–176
    of research studies, 172–173
Appraisal of Case Reports Checklist, 236, 383–384

Appraisal of Diagnostic Accuracy Articles Checklist, 387–389
Appraisal of Epidemiologic Articles Checklist, 385–386
Appraisal of Journal Articles General Checklist, 377–378
Appraisal of Literature Review Articles Checklist, 381–382
Appraisal of Therapy Articles General Checklist, 379–380
Arithmetic mean, 94
Assendelft, W.J.J., 190
Assessment bias, 422
Association of Chiropractic Colleges, 32
Asthma, manipulation for childhood, 14, 168
Attributable risk (AR), 262, 422
Automatic term mapping, 81

Background questions, 20–23
The Back Letter, 49
Baseline measure, 422
Baseline phase, 223, 422
Beck Depression Inventory (BDI), 326–327
Bell-shaped curve, 98
Belmont Report (1979), 170, 171
Berkson's bias, 256
Best fit, 139
Best practice, 13–15, 316
Beta error, 116, 118, 422
Between-groups variance, 128, 129, 422
Bias
    assessment, 422
    Berkson's, 256

Bias (*continued*)
 in case-control studies, 256
 in case series, 221, 222
 dropout rates and, 267
 exclusion, 422
 experimenter, 157, 422
 explanation of, 151–152, 422
 in group clinical trial designs, 156–158
 in narrative reviews, 182, 187
 observation, 221
 in peer-review process, 59
 performance, 422
 publication, 187, 437
 recall, 256, 270, 438
 sampling, 156, 423
 selection, 157, 182, 221
 in systematic reviews, 183–184, 187
 types of, 156–158
 work-up, 304
Binomial variables, 135
Biostatistics
 descriptive statistics and, 91–109
 inferential statistics and, 109–119
 overview of, 89–90
 populations and samples and, 90–91
 statistics tests and, 119–141
Blinding
 assessment of, 174–175
 double, 157
 explanation of, 8, 423
 importance of, 40, 44
 of treatment providers, 157–158
 triple, 157
 use of, 157
Blocking, 155
Block randomization, 155
Bonferroni method, 128
Boolean operators, 76–82, 423
British Medical Journal, 219
Bronfort, G., 10

CAMLINE, 69
CAM on PubMed, 68
Canadian Stroke Consortium (CSS), 251
Carry-over effects, 165
Case-control studies
 advantages and disadvantages of, 257
 bias in, 256
 categories of, 260
 cummulative incidence, 260
 design aspects of, 267
 example of, 257–259
 explanation of, 254, 423
 odds ratio and, 254–256
 prevalent, 260
Case reports
 appraisal tactics for, 236–239
 case series, 220–222
 evidence-based, 219–220
 explanation of, 211, 423
 limitations of, 214–216, 218–219
 overview of, 211–213
 retrospective, 212
 single-subject time series design, 223–236
 storied, 217–218
 structure of, 215–218, 236
 types of, 213–214
Case series
 bias in, 221, 222
 cohort studies and, 222
 explanation of, 211, 220–221, 423
 function of, 222
Case studies
 cohort studies vs., 222
 explanation of, 220, 224
 meta-analysis of, 222
Causal research, 148
Causation
 criteria for, 249
 in epidemiology, 246–252
Center for Evidence Based Medicine, 50
Center for Integrative Medicine (University of Maryland), 53
Central tendency
 explanation of, 97, 423
 measures of, 93–95
Centre for Evidence-Based Medicine (CEBM), University of Toronto, 265
Centre for Reviews and Dissemination, 50
Chance, 423
Characteristic Pain Intensity (CPI) Scale, 321, 391–392

Checklist for the Appraisal of Case Reports, 383–384
Checklist for the Appraisal of Diagnostic Accuracy Articles, 387–389
Checklist for the Appraisal of Epidemiologic Articles, 266, 385–386
Checklist for the Appraisal of Literature Review Articles, 352, 381–382
Checklist for the Appraisal of Therapy Articles, 173, 379–380
Chiropractic and Osteopathy, 42, 46, 365
Chiropractic care
 best practices in, 13–15
 clinical practice guidelines for, 313–317
 documentation in, 311–313
 function measures in, 327–341
 information explosion and, 12–13
 outcome measures used in, 317–319
 pain drawings and, 323–325
 pain questionnaires and, 325–326
 pain scales and, 319–323
 prejudice of medical authors against, 10
 psychometric measures and, 326–327
 reimbursement issues in, 15
Chiropractic History, 42, 46
Chiropractic interventions, experimental methods and, 167–169
Chiropractic Journal of Australia (CJA), 46
Chiropractic philosophy, 32–34
Chiropractic Research Review, 49
Chiropractic Resource Organization, 50, 52
The Chiropractic Report, 49
Chi-square distribution, 113
Chi-square tests
 explanation of, 131–132, 423–424
 goodness-of-fit, 131–132
 of independence, 131–135
 use of, 135
Clinical Chiropractic, 46
Clinical Evidence, 50
Clinical practice guidelines
 development of, 314–315
 documentation and, 311–313
 explanation of, 313–314, 424
 updates of, 315–316
 use of, 316–317

Clinical significance
 assessment of, 175–176
 explanation of, 119, 424
The Clinical Application of Outcomes Assessment (Yeomans), 317
Clinical trials, 424
Cochrane Database, 364, 368
The Cochrane Library, 51, 69
Coefficient of determination, 136–137, 424–425
Cohen's *d,* 192
Cohort studies
 advantages ad disadvantages of, 262
 case studies vs., 222
 design aspects of, 267–268
 determining risk in, 261–265
 explanation of, 222, 260–261, 425
 types of, 265
Comparison tests, 128
Concealed assignment, 155–156
Concealment of allocation, 425
Concurrent validity, 287, 290, 425
Conferences, 43–44
Confidence intervals (CIs)
 explanation of, 112–114, 425
 hypothesis testing and, 118
Confidence level, 118
Confounding, 159–160, 425
Confounding variable, 159, 257, 425
Consistency, 248, 425
Content validity, 286–287, 290, 426
Contingency tables
 explanation of, 426
 2 × 2, 132, 133, 255, 261, 263, 281–282
 use of, 135
Continuous data, 93
Continuous variables, 426
Control groups, 426
Controls, 254
Convenience sampling, 151
Convergent validity, 288–289, 426
COOP/WONCA, 337
Copenhagen Neck Functional disability Scale, 333
Correlation
 explanation of, 135–136, 427

Correlation (*continued*)
  graphic representations of, 137, 138
  measures of, 136–137
Correlation coefficient *(r)*
  explanation of, 136, 427
  intraclass, 284–285, 330
  Pearson product-moment, 136, 435
Covariate, 427
Cox, James M., 48
Criterion-related validity, 287, 290, 427
Critical appraisal, 427
Critically Appraised Topic (CAT), 368–369
Critical value, 427
Cronbach's coefficient alpha, 281, 336, 427
Crossover designs, 165–166, 427
Cross-sectional studies
  design aspects of, 268
  example of, 253–254
  explanation of, 252, 428
  function of, 252–253
Cross-tabulation table, 132
Cummulative incidence case-control studies, 260
Cumulative Index to Nursing and Allied Health Literature (CINAHL), 43, 68
Cumulative meta-analysis, 194–195
Cutoff score, 292, 428

Dartmouth Primary Care Cooperative Information Project (COOP), 336–338
Data
  continuous, 93
  discrete, 93
  explanation of, 89–90
  qualitative, 145
  quantitative, 145
  shape of, 97–109
Databases
  explanation of, 66–67
  list of, 68–69
  organization of, 66
  searches of, 70
Declaration of Helsinki (1964), 170
Deductive reasoning, 146, 428
Degrees of freedom *(df)*, 122, 428
Delphi method, 315

Dependent variables, 90, 428
Descriptive research, 148
Descriptive statistics
  explanation of, 91–93, 148, 428
  levels of measurement and, 91, 95–97
  measures of central tendency and, 91, 93–95
  shape of data and, 91, 97–109
  uses for, 91, 92
Descriptive studies, 250, 428
Directional hypothesis, 428
Discrete data, 93
Discrete variable, 428
Discriminant validity, 289, 290, 428
Disease-oriented evidence (DOE), 23
Dispersion, 91
DOCLINE, 70
Documentation, 311–313
Dose-response, 248, 428–429
Double blinding, 157
Dropout rates
  bias and, 267
  in crossover designs, 165–166
Drug trials, 8

EBC. *See* Evidence-based chiropractic (EBC)
EBM. *See* Evidence-based medicine (EBM)
EBP. *See* Evidence-based practice (EBP)
Education, postgraduate, 354–357
Effectiveness, 146, 429
Effects
  explanation of, 429
  treatment, 153, 154, 190–194
Effect size, meta-analysis and, 190–192
Efficacy, 429
Efficacy of Spinal Manipulation for Chronic Headache: A Systematic Review (Bronfort et al.), 352
eMedicine.com, 50, 364
Empirical observation, 429
Epidemiology
  appraisal tactics and, 265–271
  case-control studies and, 254–260
  causation in, 246–251
  cohort studies and, 260–265

cross-sectional studies and, 252–254
disease frequency and occurrence
  measurement and, 244–246
explanation of, 243–244, 429
measure selection and, 251–252
Equipment purchases, 352–360
Errors
  beta, 116, 118, 422
  random, 277, 438
  systematic, 159, 277–278, 441
  Type I, 116, 117, 441
  Type II, 116, 117, 441
Error variance, 278
Estimation approach, 119
Ethical issues
  in research, 169–171
  in SSTSDs, 233–234
Evidence
  comparison of levels of, 28–29
  guidelines for lack of, 360–364
  hierarchy of research, 24–27
  indexing and, 42–43
  overview of, 39
  peer review and, 40–42
  rating systems for, 27, 30–31
  where to find, 24
Evidence-based case report, 219–220
Evidence-based chiropractic (EBC)
  background of, 7–8
  chiropractic philosophy vs., 32–34
  clinical scenario in, 349–354
  essential components of, 11–12
  evidence-based practice vs., 7–10
  explanation of, 3–7, 19, 429
  function of, 9, 311
  methods to improve process of, 364–369
  steps involved in practice of, 18–23, 364
  when to use, 16–18
Evidence-based medicine (EBM)
  background of, 7–8
  explanation of, 3–4
Evidence-based practice (EBP)
  application of steps involved in, 349–354
  background of, 3–4, 8
  criticisms of, 5–7
  evidence-based chiropractic vs., 7–10

negative consequences associated with, 363
Evidence sources
  explanation of, 43–44
  journals as, 44–47
  newsletters as, 45, 48, 49
  red flags for untrustworthy, 58–59
  scholarly articles as, 55–58
  steps for appraising, 59–61
  websites as, 48–55
Exclusion bias, 422
Experimental designs
  explanation of, 148–149, 161, 429
  options for, 162–167
Experimental methods, 167–169
Experimenter bias, 157, 422
Explanatory research, 146–147
Exposed groups, 429
External validity, 161, 429
Extraneous variables, 159, 429–430

Face validity, 286, 290, 430
Factorial design, 164, 165
FCER Advance, 49
Field tags, 76, 79
Fisher's exact test, 135
Food and Nutrition Science Alliance, 59, 60
Foreground questions, 20–23
Forest plot, 190
Foundations of Clinical Research: Applications to Practice (Portney & Watkins), 227, 285
F-ratio, 128
Function measures
  explanation of, 327
  general health questionnaires, 335–339
  headache-specific questionnaires, 334–335
  low back-specific questionnaires, 328–332
  neck-specific questionnaires, 332–334
  physiologic, 339–341
Fundamentals of Biostatistics (Rosner), 89

Gaussian distribution. *See* Normal distribution

General Checklist for the Appraisal of
   Journal Articles, 172–173, 377–378
Generalizability, of research findings,
   161–162
Gold standard, 287, 293, 303, 430
Gossett, W. S., 120
Gray's Anatomy of the Human Body, 50
Greenhalgh, T., 367
Group clinical trial designs
   bias and, 156–158
   explanation of, 151–154
   extraneous and confounding variables
      and, 158–161
   generalizability of findings and, 161–162
   randomization and, 154–156
Guidelines for Chiropractic Quality
   Assurance and Practice Parameters
   (Mercy guidelines), 314–316
Guyatt, Gordon, 7–8, 119

Harrison's Online, 43
Hawthorne effect, 156, 430
Headache Disability Inventory (HDI), 334,
   409–411
Headache-specific questionnaires, 334–335
Health Information Website Evaluation
   Checklist, 373–375
Health insurance, 15
Health on the Net Foundation, 53, 54
Health-related quality of life (HRQL)
   measures, 318
Health-related quality of life questionnaires,
   318
HerbMed, 69
Heterogeneity
   explanation of, 188
   in meta-analysis, 189–190
   statistical, 189
High-Yield Biostatistics (Glaser), 89
Hill, A. B., 248, 249
Histograms
   explanation of, 93, 97–98, 430
   illustration of, 92, 99
Homogeneity, 188–189, 430
The Hom-Inform Database, 69
Hypotheses

   alternative, 114
   explanation of, 114, 430
   nondirectional, 124
   null, 114–115, 118
   research, 114
Hypothesis testing
   explanation of, 114–119
   use of, 106

Inception cohort studies, 265
Incidence
   estimates for, 146
   explanation of, 244, 246, 430
Independent variables, 90, 430
Indexing, 42–43
Index to Chiropractic Literature (ICL), 43,
   68, 365
Inductive reasoning, 146, 430
Inferential statistics
   confidence intervals and, 112–114
   explanation of, 109, 111–112, 431
   hypothesis testing and, 114–119
Informed consent
   explanation of, 171, 431
   for SSTSDs, 234
Institutional review boards (IRBs), 170
Intention-to-treat, 175, 431
Interexaminer reliability, 279, 280, 431
Intermediate outcome measure, 431
Internal consistency reliability, 281, 431
Internal validity
   explanation of, 158–159, 431
   threats to, 160–161
International Bibliographic Information on
   Dietary Supplements (IBIDS), 69
Internet. *See also* Websites
   checklist for evaluating information on,
      373–375
   evaluating information on, 52–55
   information explosion due to, 12–13
   as information source, 48, 52
Interval measurement
   explanation of, 96, 431
   mathematical operations to correspond
      with, 97
Intervention phase, 223, 432

Intraclass correlation coefficient (ICC), 284–285, 330, 432
Intraexaminer reliability, 279, 280, 432
Intuition, 362

Johnson, Debbie, 338
Journal articles
  anatomy of, 55–58
  literature searches for, 65–87. *See also* Literature searches
Journal of Manipularive and Psysiological Therapeutics (JMPT), 42, 47, 211, 216, 220, 365
Journal of the American Chiropractic Association (JACA) Online, 46
Journal of the Canadian Chiropractic Association (JCCA), 46
Journal of the Chiropractic Education (JCA), 47
Journal of the Chiropractic Humanities, 47
Journal of the Chiropractic Medicine, 47
Journal of the Clinical Chiropractic Pediatrics (JCCP), 47
Journal of Vertebral Subluxation Research (JVSR), 47
Journals
  indexing of, 42–43
  as information source, 43–45
  list of chiropractic, 46–47
  peer-reviewed, 40–42
The Journal Article Cookbook (Gleberzon & Killinger), 369
Junk science, 58

Kappa statistic
  calculation of, 283–284
  explanation of, 281–283, 432
Keating, J. C., Jr., 18
Kruskal-Wallis test, 130–131

Landon, Alfred, 156
Level of Evidence (Oxford Centre for Evidence-based Medicine), 27
Likelihood ratio (LR), 296–298, 432
Linear regression equation, 140
Literature reviews
  appraisal tactics for, 202–206, 237
  comparison of, 195–198
  explanation of, 179
  format of, 198–201
  meta-analysis, 180–181, 187–195
  narrative, 179–183, 198
  systematic, 179–187, 198
Literature searches. *See also* PubMed
  Boolean operators and, 76–82
  databases and, 66–70
  explanation of, 24
  filters and, 86
  medical subject headings and, 83–86
  methods for, 70–76, 86–87
  overview of, 65–66
  phrase searching and, 83
  truncation and wildcards and, 82–83
Loansome Doc, 70
Logical operators. *See* Boolean operators
Logical reasoning, 361
Longitudinal studies, 260, 265, 432
Low back pain, 10

Manipulation, for low back pain, 10
Mann-Whitney *U*-test, 122
MANTIS (Manual Alternative and Natural Therapy Index System)
  explanation of, 43, 67, 68
  searching on, 71–73, 76, 84, 352, 355
Margolis, R. B., 324
Masking. *See* Blinding
Matching, 432–433
McGill Pain Questionnaire (MPQ), 325–326
McMaster's University, 3, 8
Mean
  confidence interval of, 112–113
  explanation of, 93–94, 433
  regression to the, 160–161, 221, 438
  skewed data and, 100
  standard error of, 111
Measurement, levels of, 91, 95–97
Measurement error, 433
Measures of central tendency
  explanation of, 93–95
  levels of measurement and, 97
  nature of, 98, 100

Index

Measures of explained variance, 128
Median
 explanation of, 94, 433
 skewed data and, 100
MEDLINE
 explanation of, 42, 43
 literature review articles and, 202
 use of, 67, 70, 83
The Merck Manual of Diagnosis and Therapy (Merck & Company), 51, 350
Mercy guidelines, 15, 314–316
MeSH (medical subject heading) terms
 explanation of, 70, 72, 83
 method for finding, 83–86
Meta-analysis. *See also* Literature reviews
 benefits and drawbacks of, 196–197
 of case reports or case studies, 222
 cummulative, 194–195
 explanation of, 180, 187–188, 433
 homogeneity and heterogeneity in, 188–190
 techniques used in, 194
 treatment effects and, 190–194
Meta-regression, 194
Microsoft Excel, *t*-test using, 125, 126
Migraine Disability Assessment Score (MIDAS), 334–335, 413–414
Mode, 94, 433
Motion palpation, investigations of, 14
Motion Sensitivity Test (MST), 289
Multiple-baseline design, 229–231
Multiple regression, 140–141, 433
Multivariate analysis, 433

Narrative reviews. *See also* Literature reviews
 advantages and disadvantages of, 195–196, 198
 explanation of, 179–182
 publication bias and, 187
 systematic reviews vs., 183
National Center for Complementary and Alternative Medicine, 9
National Commission for the Protection of Human Subjects of Biomedical and Behavioral Research, 170

National Guideline Clearinghouse (NGC), 51
National Library of Medicine (NLM)
 journal indexing and, 42, 67, 83
 Loansome Doc, 70
Neck Disability Index (NDI), 318, 332–333, 401–404
Neck Pain and Disability Scale, 333
Neck-specific questionnaires, 332–334
Negative predictive value (NPV), 291, 292, 436
Nesting, 79
Newsletters
 as information source, 45, 48
 list of useful, 49
Nominal measurement
 explanation of, 95, 433
 mathematical operations to correspond with, 97
Nonconcurrent multiple-baseline design, 229
Nondirectional hypothesis, 124, 433–434
Nonexperimental designs, 167
Nonparametric data, 434
Normal curves
 explanation of, 98, 434
 properties of, 102
 standard deviation and, 108
Normal distribution
 explanation of, 98–99, 434
 properties of, 99, 100, 102
Northwick Park Neck Pain Questionnaire, 333
NOT operator, 76–79
Null hypothesis
 decisions regarding, 116, 117
 explanation of, 114–115, 118, 434
Number needed to treat (NNT), 264–265, 434
Numeric Rating Scale (NRS), 319–321
Nuremberg Code, 169–171

Observational research, 148
Observational studies, 250, 434
Observation bias, 221
Observed score variance, 278

Index

Odds ratio (OR)
  case-control studies and, 254–256, 258–259
  explanation of, 192, 434–435
  study assessment and, 269, 270
101-point numeric rating scale (NRS-101), 320
One-tailed tests, 435
One-way ANOVA, 130
Ordinal measurement
  explanation of, 95–96, 435
  mathematical operations to correspond with, 97
OR operator, 76, 78, 79
Oswestry Disability Index (ODI), 318, 328–330, 332
Outcome measures (OMs). *See also specific outcome measures*
  assessment of, 176
  in epidemiologic studies, 250–251
  evaluation of, 238
  explanation of, 435
  SSTSDs and, 223
  use of, 312, 317–319, 341
Outliers, 138–139
Oxford Centre for Evidence-based Medicine (CEBM), 27–29
Oxman, Andrew, 8

Pain
  emotional and psychological state and, 326–327
  measures of, 319–322
Pain drawings, 323–325
Pain questionnaires, 325–326
Pain scales, 319–322
Pain threshold meter, 340
Paired t-test
  explanation of, 127
  SSTSDs and, 227
Parallel-forms reliability, 280, 281, 435
Parameters, 90, 435
Parametric data, 435
Patient-oriented evidence that matters (POEMs), 23
Patients
  behavior modification based on study risk factors and, 271
  benefit of tests for, 304–305
  evidence-based practice and, 16
Patient-Specific Functional Scale, 333–334
Pearson product-moment correlation coefficient, 136, 435
Peer-review process
  bias in, 59
  explanation of, 40–41
  points considered in, 41
  safeguards in, 41–42, 44
Percentage, of population, 246
Performance bias, 422
Period prevalence, 245
Phase 1 trials, 424
Phase 2 trials, 424
Phase 3 trials, 424
Phase 4 trials, 424
Phrase searching, 83
Physical Therapy, 218
Physiologic measures, 339–341
Physiotherapy Evidence Database (PEDro), 67
Phytotherapies.org, 69
P-ICONS approach, 365, 366
PICO questions, 21–23
Placebo effect, 153–154, 167–168
Placebos
  in chiropractic trials, 8–9
  explanation of, 152–153, 435
Point estimate, 111, 436
Point prevalence, 245
Population
  assessment of selection of, 174, 266–267
  defining target, 150–151
  explanation of, 90, 150, 436
  making inferences about, 90–91
  percentage of, 246
Positive predictive value (PPV), 291, 292, 436
Postgraduate education, 354–357
Posttest-only randomized controlled trial, 164
Posttest probability, 297, 299, 436
Power, 118, 436

Index

Pragmatic research, 146, 147
Precision, 436
Predictive validity, 288, 290, 436
Predictive value, 436
Predictor variable. *See* Risk factors
Prefiltered information, 20–21
Pressure threshold, 341
Pressure tolerance, 341
Pretest-posttest randomized experimental design, 161
Pretest probability, 297, 299, 437
Prevalence
   estimates for, 146
   explanation of, 245, 246, 437
   period, 245
   point, 245
Prevalent case-control studies, 260
Primary sources, 20, 45
Probabilistic equivalence, 155
Prospective case reports, 212
Prospective research, 437
Prospective studies, 260
Pseudoscience, 58–59
Psychometric measures, 326–327
Publication bias, 187, 437
PubMed. *See also* Literature searches
   Boolean operators and, 76–82
   CAM on, 68
   explanation of, 43, 44, 68
   field tags for, 79–81
   limitations of, 365
   literature reviews on, 181
   literature searches on, 65, 66, 70–87
   MeSH terms and, 84–86
   phrase searching on, 83
   search filters and, 86
   truncation and wildcards and, 83
PubMed Central (PMC), 51
PubMed/MEDLINE, 43, 67
P values
   explanation of, 116, 435
   use of, 118

Qualitative data, 145
Qualitative research, 145, 146, 437
Quantitative data, 145
Quantitative research, 145–146, 437
Quasi-experimental design
   explanation of, 148–149, 437
   function of, 166
Questionnaires
   design of, 251
   general health, 335–339
   headache-specific, 334–335
   health-related quality of life, 318
   low back-specific, 328–332
   neck-specific, 332–334
   pain, 325–326
   test-retest reliability of, 280
Questions
   asking appropriate clinical, 20–23
   background vs. foreground, 20–23
QUOROM (Quality of Reporting of Meta-analysis) Statement, 196–197

RAND 36-Item Health Survey Instrument, 336–338, 415–420
Random assignment
   assessment of, 173
   explanation of, 148–149, 437
   selection bias and, 157
Random errors, 277, 438
Randomization
   assessment of, 174
   block, 155
   explanation of, 91, 148–149
   function of, 154–155, 162
   methods for accomplishing, 155–156
   SSTSDs and, 231–232
   stratified, 155
Randomized controlled trials (RCTs)
   appraisal of, 173–176
   bias in, 156–158
   design of, 152
   explanation of, 24–26, 145, 151–152, 438
   extraneous and confounding variables and, 158–161
   meta-analysis and, 193
   placebo and, 152–154, 168
   randomization and, 154–156
   systematic reviews and, 184
   use of, 166–167, 250

Index

Random samples, 151, 438
Range of motion (ROM) assessment, 339–340
Ratio measurement
 explanation of, 96, 438
 mathematical operations to correspond with, 97
RCTs. *See* Randomized controlled trials (RCTs)
Recall bias, 256, 270, 438
Recommended Clinical Protocols and Guidelines for the Practice of Chiropractic (International Chiropractor's Association), 314
Regression analysis, 139, 438
Regression line, 438
Regression to the mean, 160–161, 221, 438
Relational research, 148
Relative risk reduction (RRR), 264, 439
Relative risk (RR), 193, 262, 269, 438–439
Reliability
 appraisal tactics for, 301–306
 clinical disagreement and, 300–301
 in epidemiologic studies, 250
 estimation of, 278–281
 explanation of, 275–277, 289, 291, 439
 interexaminer, 279
 intraclass correlation coefficient and, 284–285
 intraexaminer, 279
 kappa statistic and, 281–284
 of measures, 160
 types of test, 280
Reliability coefficient, 279
Representative sample, 439
Research
 appraisal tactics for, 172–176
 design options for, 162–167
 ethics in, 169–171
 funding of, 176
Researcher bias, 157
Research hypothesis, 114, 439
Research methods
 descriptive, relational, and causal, 147–148
 experimental and quasi-experimental, 148–149, 167–169

populations and samples and, 150-151
 pragmatic and explanatory, 146–147
 quantitative and qualitative, 145–146
Responsiveness, 439
Retrospective case reports, 212
Retrospective research, 439
Revised Oswestry Low Back Disability Index, 395–398
Risk
 attributable, 262, 422
 cohort studies to determine, 261–265
 estimate of, 254–255
 explanation of, 245, 439
 relative, 193, 262, 269, 438–439
 type II error, 175
Risk factors, 243, 439
Roland-Morris Low Back Pain and Disability Questionnaire (RMQ), 329–332, 399–400
Roosevelt, Franklin D., 156

Sackett, David, 3, 8, 311, 316–317, 363–364
Samples
 assessment of, 175
 explanation of, 90–91, 440
Sampling bias, 156, 423
Sampling distribution, 111
Scatterplots, 137–138
Scheffé test, 128
Scholarly articles, anatomy of, 55–58
The Science of Chiropractic; It's Principles and Adjustments (Palmer & Palmer), 33
Scientific method, 361
Scoliometer, 358
Scottish Intercollegiate Guidelines Network (SIGN), 27–31
Searches. *See* Literature searches
Search filters, 86
Secondary sources, 20, 45
Selection bias
 in case series, 221
 explanation of, 157, 182
Self-education, 17
Sensitivity
 explanation of, 291, 440
 test validity and, 291–299, 306

Index

Sensitivity analysis, 194
SF-36 health survey, 318, 319
Sham treatments, 153, 167
Shannon, S., 369
Shekelle, Paul, 48
Short-Form McGill Pain Questionnaire and Pain Diagram, 393–394
Sickness Impact Profile (SIP), 318, 338–339
Simultaneous replication design, 231
Single-group cohort studies, 265
Single-subject time series design (SSTDs)
　design variations and, 224–225, 227–231
　ethical issues related to, 233–234
　explanation of, 211, 223–224, 440
　plotting of, 225–226
　statistical analysis of, 226–227
　tally-sheet for, 234–236
　use of, 228–229, 232–233
Skewed distributions
　explanation of, 98, 100
　positively and negatively, 101
Snow, John, 243–244
Specificity
　explanation of, 291, 440
　test validity and, 291–299, 306, 440
Split-half reliability, 280
SSTSDs. *See* Single-subject time series design (SSTDs)
Standard deviation
　calculation of, 104–106
　explanation of, 102–104, 111, 440
　illustrations of, 107, 108
　skewed data and, 100
Standard error of the difference, 122
Standard error (SE), 111–112
Standardization, 109
Standardized Finger-Nose Test (SFNT), 289
Standard mean difference, 191–192
Statistic
　explanation of, 440
　kappa, 281–284
Statistical adjustment, 440
Statistical heterogeneity, 189
Statistical significance
　assessment of, 175
　explanation of, 115, 440

Statistical tests
　analysis of variance, 127–131
　chi-square test, 131–135
　correlation and, 135–141
　overview of, 119–120
　t-test, 120–127
　used in EBC, 120
Statistics
　descriptive, 91–109
　explanation of, 90
　inferential, 109–119
Statistics (Witte & Witte), 89
Storied case reports, 217–218
Stratified analysis, 258
Stratified randomization, 155
Subgroup analysis, 193–194
Surrogate end points, 440
Survey methods, design of, 251
Symptom Checklist-90 - Revised (SCL-90-R), 327
Systematic errors, 159, 277, 441
Systematic reviews. *See also* Literature reviews
　advantages and disadvantages of, 196–198
　design of, 184–185
　explanation of, 179–184, 441
　narrative vs., 183
　process for writing, 185–186
　publication bias and, 187
　weighting of studies for, 186–187

Target population, 441
t-distribution, 113, 122
Temporality, 246–247, 441
Tenderness rating scales, 321–322
Test-retest reliability
　explanation of, 280, 441
　of pain drawings, 325
Textbooks, as information source, 43
36-item short form (SF-36), 335–336
Tradition, 361
t-ratio, 122
Treatment effects
　explanation of, 153, 154
　meta-analysis and, 190–194
　RCTs and, 224

TRIP Database, 51
Triple blinding, 157
True score variance, 278
Truncation, 82
t-score
  calculation of, 122–124
  explanation of, 122
t-table, 124, 125
t-test
  explanation of, 121–124, 441
  paired, 127, 227
  as reported in literature, 124–127
  steps involved in, 127
  use of, 120–121
Turkey HSD test, 130, 131
Turkey-Kramer test, 128
Tuskegee Syphilis Study, 169
Two-group pretest-posttest design, 163
Two-tailed tests, 441
2×2 contingency tables
  in case-control studies, 255
  in cohort studies, 261, 263
  explanation of, 132, 133, 255
  use of, 281–282
Type I error, 116, 117, 441
Type II error, 116, 117, 175, 441

Unfiltered information, 20
University of Maryland, Center for Integrative Medicine, 53
University of Toronto, Centre for Evidence-Based Medicine (CEBM), 265
uptodate.com, 51, 364

Validity
  appraisal tactics for, 301–306
  clinical disagreement and, 300–301
  concurrent, 287, 290, 425
  construct, 288, 290, 426
  content, 286–287, 290, 426
  convergent, 288–289, 426
  criterion-related, 287, 290, 427
  discriminant, 289, 290, 428
  explanation of, 158–161, 276, 285, 431, 441
  external, 161, 429
  face, 286, 290, 430
  internal, 158–161
  of literature reviews, 204
  methods for determining test, 285–291
  predictive, 288, 290, 436
  sensitivity and specificity and, 291–299
Variables
  confounding, 159, 257, 425
  dependent, 90
  explanation of, 90, 442
  extraneous, 159
  independent, 90
Variance
  calculation of, 103–105
  explanation of, 103, 442
  within-group and between-group, 128, 129
Verbal Rating Scale (VRS), 321, 322
Vertebral Subluxation in Chiropractic Practice (Council on Chiropractic Practice), 314
Visual Analogue Scale (VAS), 320–321, 329, 442

Washout period, 442
Websites. *See also* Internet
  chiropractic journal, 46–47
  evaluation checklist for, 373–375
  evaluation of, 52–55
  Health on the Net Foundation code of conduct for, 54
  as information source, 48, 52
  list of useful, 50–51
  newsletter, 49
The Week in Chiropractic, 49
Whiplash Disability Questionnaire (WDQ), 333, 405–408
Wilcoxon test, 122
Wildcards, 83
Withdrawal design, 225
Within-group variance, 128, 129
Work-up bias, 304
World Medical Association, 170

z-score, 106, 109
Z-tables, 109, 111